Chapter 8: Fish and Seafood........69

Chapter 9: Pork, Beef, and Lamb..87

THE DIABETIC COOKBOOK FOR BEGINNERS

500 Easy and Healthy Diabetic Diet Recipes for the Newly Diagnosed | 21-Day Meal Plan to Manage Type 2 Diabetes and Prediabetes

Tiara R. Barrett

21/11/22.   Maureen Sheehan Lonine

Hummus

Tahini   —   1 Tablespoon.
Olive Oil   —   4 Tablespoons

Squeesed Lemon.
Salt.   —   Pinch.
1 Tin of Chick Peas

TEFAL Pots + Pans
                Sainsbury

NESVITTS for
        Knives.

Guacamole

Avocado.
Ripe Choped Tomatoe.
Fresh Lemon Juice
Cracked black Pepper.
Corriander.
Sweet Chilli. Sauce

Table of Content

Introduction

I know, it's scary. When you irst get the news you have diabetes, it can hit you

like a Mack truck. Many of us suspect the diagnosis, but it doesn't take hold and become real until your doctor tells you, straight up: **you have diabetes.**

As I walked from the doctors clinic the day, I found out about my diabetes, I felt like someone had just gut-punched me. Yeah, I'd thought maybe I had it and I probably dealt with some of the symptoms, but until the 'episode' which caused me to consult my doctor came up, I just fleetingly played with the idea in my head. Maybe it was, and maybe it wasn't diabetes. For some reason it was easier to put the realization off until tomorrow. I'll deal with it later.

Well, 'later' finally happened, and when I got home, I just sat on my couch, looking out the window with my springer spaniel at my side. She knew I was upset.

Was 'upset' the real word for it? I was swirling with all kinds of emotions: despair, regret, confusion, fear, loss. And did I mention fear?

What was I going to do? Take the medicine, sure. But I was even unsure about that. My diabetes is type 2, so there were some options my doctor had suggested.

My diet needed to be regimented (I hate that, why can't I just eat what I want to eat and be healthy?) and I needed to exercise more (so what else is new? I've had this hanging over my head ever since I was very young).

Diabetes runs in my family. I shouldn't have been surprised about the diagnosis at all. But it always seemed like it was at arms length, like it would never be my problem, always theirs, they were the 'sick' ones.

Surprise. It was mine now, and I needed to own up to it.

I wallowed in my own desperation for a couple of weeks. When it got to the point of my friends dropping over to see if I was okay (I never answered the door, just texted them later with an excuse of being out or in the shower), I figured I should at least come clean and be honest. One of my voice messages rang loud and clear.

"Jo, I know you're scared. I know you're avoiding the subject, and I know you also know you can't avoid it. I talked to your aunt, and she said you'd had an appointment with her doctor who specializes in diabetes. Not hard to come to a conclusion. Please, can we have an afternoon together? I want to tell you how I deal with my problems and what you can do to live with it, no matter how severe it is or how scared you are. PLEASE call me!"

Olivia had diabetes? I never knew, and we'd been friends since college. She was more active than I, but not to the point of being a gym addict, at least not that I saw. And her diet seems decent. Healthy, but she had goodies (probably not as much as I did) and normal food, too. Maybe she could show me a way out of this hole I'd dug myself into.

So, shortly thereafter, Olivia and I met for tea at a nice little sidewalk cafe, and we spent the next two hours discussing the ways she restructured her life to work with her ailment. That's what she called it, and it seemed a lot better, if only for my own comfort, than calling it a disease.

First of all, she gave me some figures, which made me think twice. A lot of people have type 2 diabetes and it isn't necessarily my fault that I do. Americans are subjected to non-stop advertising which lures us into horrible habits of eating food loaded with preservatives, sugar, and other horrible non-nutrients which make people develop pre-diabetes. It strikes the young and the old and, in recent years, more children, teens, and young people than ever before in medical history have been afflicted.

Mine is type 2 diabetes, which doesn't let natural pancreatic insulin enter cells to turn carbohydrate sugars into energy. Fat surrounding and inside the cells inhibit the insulins' job, causing bloodstream to contain higher levels of sugar and glucose than is healthy. If not treated, the high levels can not only cause weight gain, but destroy tissues which keep the heart healthy, the blood and brain, eyesight and more.

In other words, it knocks your body out of whack enough to make you feel lethargic, dizzy, ill, and short-of-breath.

As we spoke, I remembered my doctor telling me that because of my poor health history, he wanted to put me on insulin. It wouldn't be a strong dose, and we'd regulate it to make sure I wouldn't be taking more than I needed.

Poor health history? What did that mean? Olivia seemed to think it meant I ate poorly and didn't exercise. But she also said, with some adjustments, I could change my lifestyle to probably not need insulin at all.

I was up for that!

And what you are reading now is a compilation of the next 2 years of learning about type 2 diabetes, experimenting with a whole grain plant-based diet, eating healthy, and changing my lifestyle, including the dreaded exercising!

Today, I don't take insulin, and I've become a nutritionist by profession. I have been a nutritionist for 8 years now. And I feel great!

You must be ready to learn more about changing your lifestyle too, or you wouldn't be reading this book right now.

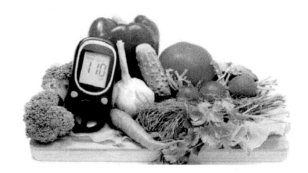

And I admire you for your courage. I know how hard it can be to feel like you need to change instead of wanting to change. You probably want to change too, which is what will get you past the little bumps you might experience along the way.

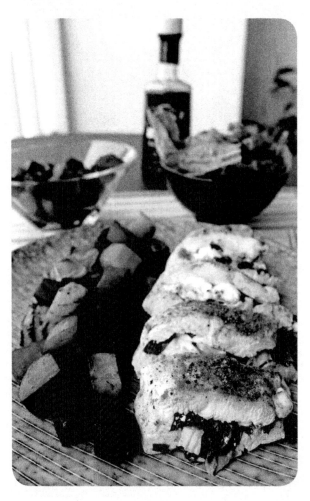

As you read through this handbook, you'll:

- understand thoroughly what diabetes is and why regulating it with your diet and exercise is the best way to manage it;

- see how the symptoms of diabetes are recognized and the difference between type 1 and type 2;

- discover how to overcome diabetes and regulate your blood sugars to healthy levels;

- learn how to arrange a delicious meal plate consisting of exactly what you need, nutritious ingredients, as well as portion-control;

- get over 500 recipes which will help you adjust to your new you;

- develop a 4 - week menu plan to help you shop for the recipe ingredients and pantry items you'll want on hand.

All the above will happen as you understand and start to control your panic and anxiety. And while it's natural to feel fearful and hesitant, your concerns can be laid to rest with a bit of education and a few changes to your lifestyle and nutrition.

Welcome to living with diabetes on your terms!

Chapter 1: Before Getting Started

The Basics of Diabetes

I'm sure you feel like a victim, especially if diabetes crept up on you from nowhere. It can seem like you are carrying a notorious villain within you, which you can't control and you want nothing to do with. And you are justified in feeling like this.

Also know, however, that this frame of mind is your choice, because you can live with diabetes and you can live a great life, without giving it a second thought. But you will have to change a few things and devote yourself to YOURSELF. Afterall, no one will benefit from your adjustments other than you, and what better way to control your ailment than to be the one calling the shots?

Diabetes is unlike almost any other disease known to man, because it is possible to manage. You'll want to have a few people in your corner to help you as you begin your journey though, such as your doctor, dietitian, nutritionist, diabetes educator, and pharmacist. Once you know the advantages of certain methods, how to avoid the pitfalls, and adapt to the changes which improve your health, there isn't any reason in the world why you can't live on your terms and be incredibly happy and healthy at the same time!

Managing your diabetes may need medications to get your insulin regulated. You may be able to wean off of these or you may need to have a dose included in your daily diet. Your blood sugar levels will determine this. By keeping your blood sugar level as close to your target as possible, you will be able to prevent or delay diabetes-related complications, which is the main reason all of us are scared when diagnosed. We've all heard about the horrors.

I'm not going to give you a talk about how easy this will be and how you can ignore the obvious; you really can't. But by simply checking your blood sugar levels and adjusting where you can (the key to this being the knowledge of what can be changed!), you'll soon see that diabetes doesn't have to be the monster you originally thought it to be.

Some people choose to do this and abstain from making necessary changes to improve their well-being and health. I get that. But you are different and you will soon know how you can tweak a few things here and there to feel better, look better, manage your ailment, and continue with life in a robust and adventurous style!

Whether you have type 1 diabetes (insulin-deficiency) or type 2 diabetes (insulin-resistance), diabetes is the result of too much sugar building up in your blood. If left unchecked, it will overwhelm your kidneys and spill into your urine. Because too much sugar in the bloodstream can break down tissue, diabetes can lead to blindness, kidney failure, stroke, and heart attacks.

High blood sugar can also damage your nerves, which creates the condition of neuropathy. This damage shows signs of numbness, tingling, and pain. Poor circulation can also develop, leaving a lack of feeling in the extremities, which eventually can lead to poor healing injuries and end up as amputations.

Diabetes has tripled in the last 30 years, with more than 20 million Americans diagnosed with either type 1 (5% to 10% cases) or type 2 (90% to 95% cases) diabetes[1].

I don't mean to scare you with these facts, but knowing them will help you veer from temptations down the road. They certainly did me. You need to understand, these small but necessary changes, if left unchecked, will lead to the fear you felt when you were first given the news of having diabetes. If you don't heed the warnings and change detrimental damage, you may just have justified the fear you originally felt.

The major reason your cells can't assimilate the sugars they need to create energy and regenerate cells and growth, is they have developed a gooey substance which resists insulin (type 2 diabetes). Do you have any idea of what this gooey substance is? It is FAT. Plain and simple.

The good news is that type 1 diabetes is regulated with insulin, which reconstructs the insulin to be used in the cells. Type 2 diabetes can be regulated with medications also, but the best and healthiest way is with an active lifestyle and nutritious diet. You are in control of both these things!

Develop Good Habits

Here are some good habits to develop for whatever level your diabetes is at:

- Drink more water and no sugary drinks;

- Eat more vegetables and make healthier food choices and find some new favorites;

- Devise an exercise program you really enjoy;

- Keep regular records of your daily blood sugar levels;

- Recognize the signs of high or low blood sugar, and then apply your knowledge to correct the irregularities;

- If necessary, take medication correctly and diligently;

- Keep a close watch on your feet, eyes, and skin to find possible symptoms before they develop;

- Store your diabetic supplies and food properly (both medications and meal ingredients) for optimum benefit;

- Manage stress and anxiety with exercise and suggested routines by your doctor.

Make sure you have a support team for any slip-ups you might find yourself making, especially in the beginning, while you are learning and developing new routines. And find a buddy you can call when you feel lost or stressed; this person will become your lifeline to not only health, but also to your sanity. As time passes, this person will also be one of your most trusted allies, a relationship you both will treasure.

Chapter 2: Designing Your Menu

What do you think you need to know in order to cook an appealing and great tasting meal?

- Fresh ingredients

- Careful preparation

- Experience with herb and spice combinations

- Presenting the meal in an appealing way

If you agree with these few basic things, you've been paying attention to your meals, haven't you? You know when a dish is good and when it isn't. Mostly, because you have had both the good and the bad.

And, you may be thinking you'll have to learn how to like eating healthily, because nothing you have ever liked was on a healthy menu. You probably thought of that as rabbit food.

Well, I'm here to tell you, though you may think eating healthily will be hard to plan, boring, tasteless, and include ingredients you hate, think again. If you use the ingredients and preparation methods as I suggest here, your menus will be more flavorful and interesting, take less time to prepare, and give you lots of room for customizing for a delicious and nutritious diet.

Before we dive into meal planning, it will serve you well to know the basics of food and why some food is tasty while others are not.

Nutrients and Diabetes

Foods are made up of 3 basic macronutrients: proteins, carbohydrates, and fats. If you look at a nutrition label on a packaged food item, you will not only see these ingredients listed along with their percentage of a daily recommended allowance, you'll also see a breakdown of these nutrients, which can contain fiber, sugar, saturated and trans fats, and sodium. You can also see the ingredients which have been used to make the product of whatever is inside the package from the highest to the lowest percentage.

It's these ingredients which have, no doubt, made diabetes one of the highest health risks in America (7th highest death rate, 30% increase in cases[1]). The wonderful thing about knowing the packaged ingredients however, is not for what is inside them (we're pretty sure most of it is processed and contains huge amounts of sugar), but for what is not found in them. And this is why you choose to put most of them back on the shelf after reading the label.

Rarely, will you see a list of two to five ingredients, which is pretty much what the recipes you'll be using in your new diet will have.

You'll also notice many, if not most, are ingredients you would never find in the produce section, meat section, or baking aisle.

Preservatives riddle processed products and because the manufacturers of these products need a long shelf life, most often these preservatives are linked to sugar or fructose syrups (what began as natural preservatives, long ago). Eating all these chemicals and processed ingredients has led to obesity and, yes, you guessed it, type 2 diabetes.

Enough of the bad - let's focus on the good stuff.

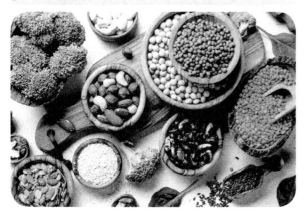

Proteins: meat, poultry, beans, nuts, eggs, seafood, soy products, and seeds, all share the identity of being a protein (peas and beans are also listed as vegetables). Proteins can be lean or have excessive amounts of fat, and must be managed accordingly when assessing their place in your daily menu. Proteins are made up of amino acids, and aid in building tissue, strengthening muscles, and aiding in the health of the blood.

Carbohydrates: made up of sugars and starches, carbohydrates' primary function is to provide energy to cells, including the brain, which is the only carbohydrate-dependent organ in the body. The Recommended Dietary Allowance (RDA) for carb intake is 130 grams per day for adults, though most adults consume between 220 and 330 grams as men and 180 to 230 grams as women. Carbs are found in starchy root vegetables, breads and grains, fruit, and rice.

Fat: There are four types of fat: saturated fat, which is solid at room temperature and consists of animal fat; unsaturated fat, which is liquid at room temperature and is plant-based and can further broken down into monounsaturated and polyunsaturated fat (olive oil, nuts and seeds).

Fiber is important to our digestive system, as well as our blood and organ health. Fiber keeps antioxidants from accumulating and 'scrubs' toxins and free-radicals from intestines and digestive organs.

Water is a natural lubricant for all systems in our body. Because we are made of 85% water, it is important to keep water intake high to maintain these levels, due its constant evaporation through sweat, toxin elimination (urine), and sodium excess.

As you become familiar with the function of each food you enjoy, you'll see how they affect your body systems and the general overall well-being of your body.

For example, if you aren't accustomed to eating 3 portions of leafy greens a day, when you begin to add this power food into your diet, you will notice clarity of vision (improved night vision), improved digestive tract health (less blotting, cramps, and constipation), and an improved sense of taste (sodium and sugar are cleansed from the tongue and inside the mouth).

Many whole foods and plant-based diet ingredients will awaken your dulled senses too, by not only tasting better, but smelling better and appreciating the combination of flavor mixes. It's like a veil being lifted from your taste buds, and almost every other system responding to your upgrades. If food is the fuel for your body, premium is the desired fuel!

Do I need to mention what improving your diet will do for your skin? Suppleness will return, wrinkles will fade, elasticity will improve, and a youthful 'glow' will radiate from every pore.

How Much Should I Eat?

When contemplating portions and combinations of the food groups you will base your diet plan on, try to focus on consuming between 2000 and 2800 calories a day. Ask your doctor what caloric intake you should be at, adjusting it to your exercise level, age, and how your diabetes is managed. There are a few factors which can play a part in coming up with the perfect figure.

Keep your meals well-rounded, with additions from proteins, carbs, and fat. Focusing on a whole grain plant-based diet will give you a few basics you can incorporate in every meal.

Suggested portions for each meal should roughly follow this outline:

- ½ plate of non-starchy vegetables - broccoli, green beans, asparagus, peppers, carrots, cucumbers, onions, and cauliflower.

- ¼ plate of healthy protein - seafood, eggs, edamame, low fat dairy and yogurt, chicken or turkey, tuna, beans, and soy products (tofu).

- ¼ plate carbs - berries, peas, lentils, whole grains (no sugar), oats, quinoa.

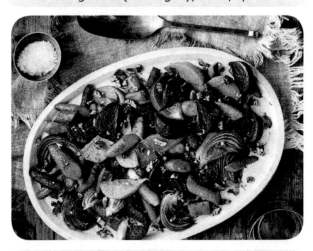

By keeping to this basic outline, you can put together a delicious meal with many varied and flavorful foods.

Also, by using the recipes in this book, you can substitute the ingredients while still keeping the basic cooking method to change a dish and your menu.

If, for example, you wanted to make a basic eggs, cheese, and potatoes dish, but didn't have any potatoes, you could easily substitute sweet potatoes, beets, squash (zucchini or butternut) for the potatoes and have a brand new dish. Don't be afraid to mix things up and move food groups around!

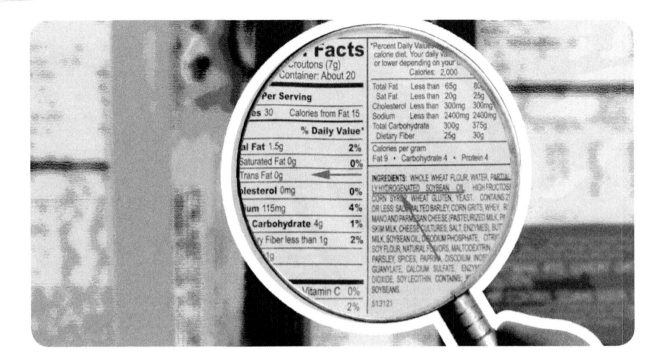

There are also some 'tricks' you can use to entice meal flavors and enhance your eating experience, while lessening your risk of diabetes.

- Eat your meals at the table, not in front of the TV (where temptations are most likely to be experienced!),

- Eat slowly and chew every bite. Take at least 20 minutes to eat your meal; this is how long it takes your stomach to feel full.

- Drink more water, which is great for your body and fills you up with zero calories.

- Adjust your own foods and dishes you like to a healthier version.

- Involve others when you cook, make it a 'party.'

- Shop for food on a full stomach so you won't be tempted by unhealthy foods.

- Read labels and educate yourself on the ingredients of all pre-packaged foods.

- Don't feel like you need to 'clean' your plate. Have baggies or plastic storage containers on hand to save leftovers in.

- Serve smaller portions.

- Plate your meals at the kitchen counter, not at the table.

Follow these suggestions and guidelines. By doing so, you will not only lower your blood sugar levels and improve your health, but you will create a life-long ability to regulate, manage, and control diabetes.

Chapter 3: Pantry and Craving Lists

Do you feel better now about planning your meals?

Are you confident you'll change the necessary things to design an enjoyable, healthy, and happy life, well-lived?

Creating a healthy and nutritious diet plan for yourself isn't rocket science, but sometimes it can seem daunting, especially when your stomach is growling and there's nothing in the kitchen to fix.

Here's a list of items to keep on hand as back-ups when the weekend sneaks up on you, or the unprepared work-week leaves you tired with the cupboard bare.

Pantry List:

Have a number of these items on hand at any given time. Use them as main ingredients or supplemental ingredients in a meal. Don't ever just rely on 'carrots' or 'blueberries.' Get creative and mix and match as you prepare a smoothie, an omelette, or an asian bowl. Also, make sure you have healthy 'snacks' to fall back on, such as nuts, seeds, berries, or olives. Apple

- Raspberries
- Loganberries
- Strawberries
- Blueberries
- Wild salmon
- Haddock
- Tuna
- Swordfish
- Mackerel

- Avocados
- Dark chocolate (75% plus)
- Red onions
- Carrots
- Greek yogurt
- Oats
- Cinnamon
- Turmeric

- Leafy greens
- Garlic
- Flaxseed
- Nuts
- Olive oil
- Coconut oil
- Bell peppers
- Black coffee
- Green juice

Cravings List:

The infamous 'craving' - oh how it can topple an otherwise well structured week. By knowing what you are in need of, physically, you can stay one step ahead of the game to out-play those binges.

Below are a few of the craving-based supplements our bodies need, yet it can be a hit and miss if a holiday plays into the mix or you've been too busy to pay close attention.

Keep a few of each food substitute at hand, so when you feel the urge to splurge, you're giving your body what it actually needs. By always having options for your 'munchies,' you will teach your body it will always receive exactly the nutritious food it is in need of, thereby satisfying the immediate craving as well as slowly suppressing the urges.

You Want	What You Need	What to Eat Instead
Chocolate	Magnesium	Raw cacao, nuts, seeds, veggies, fruits
Sugary Foods	Chromium Carbon Phosphorus Sulphur Tryptophan	Broccoli, grapes, cheese, chicken Fresh fruit (berries, apples) Chicken, fish, eggs, dairy, nuts, veggies Cranberries, cabbage, cauliflower Cheese, raisins, sweet potato, spinach
Bread, pasta & other carbs	Nitrogen	High protein foods, meat, fish, nuts, beans, chia seeds
Oily Foods	Calcium	Organic milk, cheese, leafy greens
Salty Foods	Chloride	Fatty fish, goat milk, radishes

* There you have it, all the basics you need to begin your adventure into becoming a diabetic 'foodie'. Not only are you prepared to revamp your diet, but you can do it with confidence, enthusiasm, and the assurance of creating many healthy habits in the kitchen.

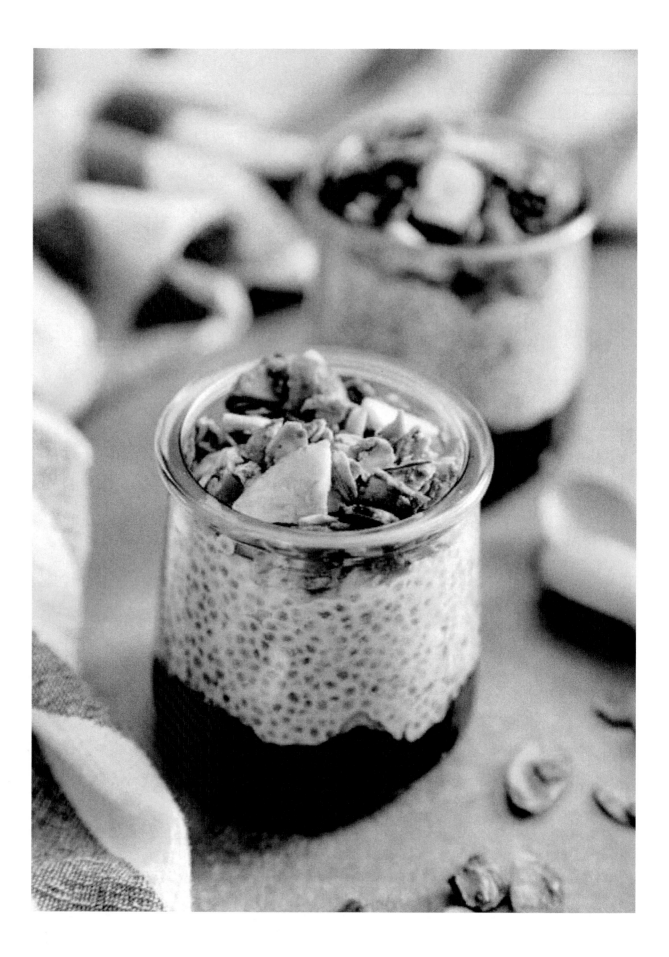

Chapter 4: Breakfast

Coconut and Berry Smoothie

Prep time: 5 minutes | Cook time: 0 minutes | Serves 2

½ cup mixed berries (blueberries, strawberries, blackberries)
1 tablespoon ground flaxseed
2 tablespoons unsweetened coconut flakes
½ cup unsweetened plain coconut milk
½ cup leafy greens (kale, spinach)
¼ cup unsweetened vanilla nonfat yogurt
½ cup ice

1. In a blender jar, combine the berries, flaxseed, coconut flakes, coconut milk, greens, yogurt, and ice.
2. Process until smooth. Serve.

Per Serving
calories: 182 | fat: 14.9g | protein: 5.9g
carbs: 8.1g | fiber: 4.1g | sugar: 2.9g
sodium: 25mg

Tropical Yogurt Kiwi Bowl

Prep time: 5 minutes | Cook time: 0 minutes | Serves 2

1½ cups plain low-fat Greek yogurt
2 kiwis, peeled and sliced
2 tablespoons shredded unsweetened coconut flakes
2 tablespoons halved walnuts
1 tablespoon chia seeds
2 teaspoons honey, divided (optional)

1. Divide the yogurt between two small bowls.
2. Top each serving of yogurt with half of the kiwi slices, coconut flakes, walnuts, chia seeds, and honey (if using).

Per Serving
calories: 261 | fat: 9.1g | protein: 21.1g
carbs: 23.1g | fiber: 6.1g | sugar: 14.1g
sodium: 84mg

Blueberry Muffins

Prep time: 10 minutes | Cook time: 25 minutes | Serves 18 muffins

2 cups whole-wheat pastry flour
1 cup almond flour
½ cup granulated sweetener
1 tablespoon baking powder
2 teaspoons freshly grated lemon zest
¾ teaspoon baking soda
¾ teaspoon ground nutmeg
Pinch sea salt
2 eggs
1 cup skim milk, at room temperature
¾ cup 2 percent plain Greek yogurt
½ cup melted coconut oil
1 tablespoon freshly squeezed lemon juice
1 teaspoon pure vanilla extract
1 cup fresh blueberries

1. Preheat the oven to 350ºF (180ºC).
2. Line 18 muffin cups with paper liners and set the tray aside.
3. In a large bowl, stir together the flour, almond flour, sweetener, baking powder, lemon zest, baking soda, nutmeg, and salt.
4. In a small bowl, whisk together the eggs, milk, yogurt, coconut oil, lemon juice, and vanilla.
5. Add the wet ingredients to the dry ingredients and stir until just combined.
6. Fold in the blueberries without crushing them.
7. Spoon the batter evenly into the muffin cups. Bake the muffins until a toothpick inserted in the middle comes out clean, about 25 minutes.
8. Cool the muffins completely and serve.
9. Store leftover muffins in a sealed container in the refrigerator for up to 3 days or in the freezer for up to 1 month.

Per Serving
calories: 166 | fat: 9.1g | protein: 3.9g
carbs: 18.1g | fiber: 2.1g | sugar: 6.9g
sodium: 75mg

Walnut and Oat Granola

Prep time: 10 minutes | Cook time: 30 minutes | Serves 16

4 cups rolled oats
1 cup walnut pieces
½ cup pepitas
¼ teaspoon salt
1 teaspoon ground cinnamon
1 teaspoon ground ginger
½ cup coconut oil, melted
½ cup unsweetened applesauce
1 teaspoon vanilla extract
½ cup dried cherries

1. Preheat the oven to 350ºF (180ºC). Line a baking sheet with parchment paper.
2. In a large bowl, toss the oats, walnuts, pepitas, salt, cinnamon, and ginger.
3. In a large measuring cup, combine the coconut oil, applesauce, and vanilla. Pour over the dry mixture and mix well.
4. Transfer the mixture to the prepared baking sheet. Cook for 30 minutes, stirring about halfway through. Remove from the oven and let the granola sit undisturbed until completely cool. Break the granola into pieces, and stir in the dried cherries.
5. Transfer to an airtight container, and store at room temperature for up to 2 weeks.

Per Serving
calories: 225 | fat: 14.9g | protein: 4.9g
carbs: 20.1g | fiber: 3.1g | sugar: 4.9g
sodium: 31mg

Ratatouille Egg Bake

Prep time: 20 minutes | Cook time: 50 minutes | Serves 4

2 teaspoons extra-virgin olive oil
½ sweet onion, finely chopped
2 teaspoons minced garlic
½ small eggplant, peeled and diced
1 green zucchini, diced
1 yellow zucchini, diced
1 red bell pepper, seeded and diced
3 tomatoes, seeded and chopped
1 tablespoon chopped fresh oregano
1 tablespoon chopped fresh basil
Pinch red pepper flakes
Sea salt and freshly ground black pepper, to taste
4 large eggs

1. Preheat the oven to 350ºF (180ºC).
2. Place a large ovenproof skillet over medium heat and add the olive oil.
3. Sauté the onion and garlic until softened and translucent, about 3 minutes. Stir in the eggplant and sauté for about 10 minutes, stirring occasionally. Stir in the zucchini and pepper and sauté for 5 minutes.
4. Reduce the heat to low and cover. Cook until the vegetables are soft, about 15 minutes.
5. Stir in the tomatoes, oregano, basil, and red pepper flakes, and cook 10 minutes more. Season the ratatouille with salt and pepper.
6. Use a spoon to create four wells in the mixture. Crack an egg into each well.
7. Place the skillet in the oven and bake until the eggs are firm, about 5 minutes.
8. Remove from the oven. Serve the eggs with a generous scoop of vegetables.

Per Serving
calories: 148 | fat: 7.9g | protein: 9.1g
carbs: 13.1g | fiber: 4.1g | sugar: 7.1g
sodium: 99mg

Quick Breakfast Yogurt Sundae

Prep time: 5 minutes | Cook time: 0 minutes | Serves 1

¾ cup plain Greek yogurt
¼ cup mixed berries (blueberries, strawberries, blackberries)
2 tablespoons
cashew, walnut, or almond pieces
1 tablespoon ground flaxseed
2 fresh mint leaves, shredded

1. Pour the yogurt into a tall parfait glass and scatter the top with the berries, cashew pieces, and flaxseed.
2. Sprinkle the mint leaves on top for garnish and serve chilled.

Per Serving
calories: 238 | fat: 11.2g | protein: 20.9g
carbs: 15.8g | fiber: 4.1g | sugar: 8.9g
sodium: 63mg

Cottage Pancakes

Prep time: 10 minutes | Cook time: 20 minutes | Serves 4

2 cups low-fat cottage cheese
4 egg whites
2 eggs
1 tablespoon pure
vanilla extract
1½ cups almond flour
Nonstick cooking spray

1. Place the cottage cheese, egg whites, eggs, and vanilla in a blender and pulse to combine.
2. Add the almond flour to the blender and blend until smooth.
3. Place a large nonstick skillet over medium heat and lightly coat it with cooking spray.
4. Spoon ¼ cup of batter per pancake, 4 at a time, into the skillet. Cook the pancakes until the bottoms are firm and golden, about 4 minutes.
5. Flip the pancakes over and cook the other side until they are cooked through, about 3 minutes.
6. Remove the pancakes to a plate and repeat with the remaining batter.
7. Serve with fresh fruit.

Per Serving
calories: 345 | fat: 22.1g | protein: 29.1g
carbs: 11.1g | fiber: 4.1g | sugar: 5.1g
sodium: 560mg

Crispy Pita with Canadian Bacon

Prep time: 5 minutes | Cook time: 15 minutes | Serves 2

1 (6-inch) whole-grain pita bread
3 teaspoons extra-virgin olive oil, divided
2 eggs
2 Canadian bacon slices
Juice of ½ lemon
1 cup microgreens
2 tablespoons crumbled goat cheese
Freshly ground black pepper, to taste

1. Heat a large skillet over medium heat. Cut the pita bread in half and brush each side of both halves with ¼ teaspoon of olive oil (using a total of 1 teaspoon oil). Cook for 2 to 3 minutes on each side, then remove from the skillet.
2. In the same skillet, heat 1 teaspoon of oil over medium heat. Crack the eggs into the skillet and cook until the eggs are set, 2 to 3 minutes. Remove from the skillet.
3. In the same skillet, cook the Canadian bacon for 3 to 5 minutes, flipping once.
4. In a large bowl, whisk together the remaining 1 teaspoon of oil and the lemon juice. Add the microgreens and toss to combine.
5. Top each pita half with half of the microgreens, 1 piece of bacon, 1 egg, and 1 tablespoon of goat cheese. Season with pepper and serve.

Per Serving
calories: 251 | fat: 13.9g | protein: 13.1g
carbs: 20.1g | fiber: 3.1g | sugar: 0.9g
sodium: 400mg

Coconut and Chia Pudding

Prep time: 5 minutes | Cook time: 0 minutes | Serves 2

7 ounces (198 g) light coconut milk
¼ cup chia seeds
3 to 4 drops liquid stevia
1 clementine
1 kiwi
Shredded coconut (unsweetened)

1. Start by taking a mixing bowl and adding in the light coconut milk. Add in the liquid stevia to sweeten the milk. Mix well.
2. Add the chia seeds to the milk and whisk until well-combined. Set aside.
3. Peel the clementine and carefully remove the skin from the wedges. Set aside.
4. Also, peel the kiwi and dice it into small pieces.
5. Take a glass jar and assemble the pudding. For this, place the fruits at the bottom of the jar; then add a dollop of chia pudding. Now spread the fruits and then add another layer of chia pudding.
6. Finish by garnishing with the remaining fruits and shredded coconut.

Per Serving
calories: 486 | fat: 40.5g | protein: 8.5g
carbs: 30.8g | fiber: 15.6g | sugar: 11.6g
sodium: 24mg

Spinach and Cheese Breakfast Tacos

Prep time: 5 minutes | Cook time: 10 minutes | Serves 4

Taco:

Avocado oil cooking spray
1 medium green bell pepper, chopped
8 large eggs
¼ cup sharp Cheddar cheese, shredded
4 (6-inch) whole-wheat tortillas

1 cup fresh spinach leaves
½ cup Pico de Gallo (see below)
Chopped scallions, for garnish (optional)
Avocado slices, for garnish (optional)

Pico De Gallo:

1 tomato, diced
½ large white onion, diced
½ jalapeño pepper, stemmed, seeded, and diced

2 tablespoons fresh cilantro, chopped
1 tablespoon freshly squeezed lime juice
⅛ teaspoon salt

Make the Tacos

1. Heat a skillet over medium-low heat until hot, then spray the skillet with cooking spray.
2. Add the chopped bell pepper and sauté for 4 minutes until tender, stirring occasionally.
3. Meanwhile, whisk together the eggs and shredded cheese in a medium bowl until well blended.
4. Slowly pour the egg mixture into the skillet with the bell pepper. Scramble for about 5 minutes until the eggs are soft and the cheese melts.
5. Remove the egg mixture from the pan to a platter and set aside.
6. Put the tortillas on a plate and microwave for 8 seconds until warm and pliable.
7. Top each tortilla evenly with ¼ cup of spinach leaves and scrambled eggs, followed by the Pico de Gallo.
8. Sprinkle the scallions and avocado slices on top for garnish before serving, if desired.

Make the Pico De Gallo

1. Mix together the tomato, onion, pepper, cilantro, lime juice, and salt in a bowl. Stir well with a fork to incorporate.

Per Serving

calories: 279 | fat: 15.3g | protein: 16.2g
carbs: 28.3g | fiber: 3.1g | sugar: 8.2g
sodium: 560mg

Easy and Creamy Grits

Prep time: 5 minutes | Cook time: 10 minutes | Serves 4

1 cup fat-free milk
2 cups water

1 cup stone-ground corn grits

1. Pour the milk and water into a saucepan over medium heat, then bring to a simmer until warmed through.
2. Add the corn grits and stir well. Reduce the heat to low and cook covered for 5 to 7 minutes, whisking continuously, or until the grits become tender.
3. Remove from the heat and serve warm.

Per Serving

calories: 168 | fat: 1.1g | protein: 6.2g
carbs: 33.8g | fiber: 1.1g | sugar: 2.8g
sodium: 33mg

Sausage and Pepper Burrito

Prep time: 10 minutes | Cook time: 15 minutes | Serves 4

8 ounces (227 g) bulk pork breakfast sausage
½ onion, chopped
1 green bell pepper, seeded and chopped
8 large eggs, beaten
4 (6-inch) low-carb

tortillas
1 cup shredded pepper Jack cheese
½ cup sour cream (optional, for serving)
½ cup prepared salsa (optional, for serving)

1. In a large nonstick skillet on medium-high heat, cook the sausage, crumbling it with a spoon, until browned, about 5 minutes. Add the onion and bell pepper. Cook, stirring, until the veggies are soft, about 3 minutes. Add the eggs and cook, stirring, until eggs are set, about 3 minutes more.
2. Spoon the egg mixture onto the 4 tortillas. Top each with the cheese and fold into a burrito shape.
3. Serve with sour cream and salsa, if desired.

Per Serving

calories: 487 | fat: 36.1g | protein: 31.8g
carbs: 13.1g | fiber: 7.9g | sugar: 5.1g
sodium: 811mg

Coconut Berry Smoothie

Prep time: 10 minutes | Cook time: 0 minutes | Serves 2

½ cup mixed berries (blueberries, strawberries, blackberries)
½ cup leafy greens (kale, spinach)
¼ cup unsweetened vanilla nonfat yogurt

½ cup unsweetened plain coconut milk
2 tablespoons unsweetened coconut flakes
1 tablespoon ground flaxseed
½ cup ice

1. Process the mixed berries, leafy greens, yogurt, coconut milk, coconut flakes, flaxseed, and ice in a blender until all ingredients are combined into a smooth mixture. Pour the mixture into two smoothie glasses.
2. Serve chilled or at room temperature.

Per Serving
calories: 183 | fat: 15.3g | protein: 6.2g
carbs: 8.2g | fiber: 4.1g | sugar: 3.2g
sodium: 26mg

Buckwheat Crêpes

Prep time: 20 minutes | Cook time: 20 minutes | Serves 5

1½ cups skim milk
3 eggs
1 teaspoon extra-virgin olive oil, plus more for the skillet
1 cup buckwheat flour

½ cup whole-wheat flour
½ cup 2 percent plain Greek yogurt
1 cup sliced strawberries
1 cup blueberries

1. In a large bowl, whisk together the milk, eggs, and 1 teaspoon of oil until well combined.
2. Into a medium bowl, sift together the buckwheat and whole-wheat flours. Add the dry ingredients to the wet ingredients and whisk until well combined and very smooth.
3. Allow the batter to rest for at least 2 hours before cooking.
4. Place a large skillet or crêpe pan over medium-high heat and lightly coat the bottom with oil.
5. Pour about ¼ cup of batter into the skillet. Swirl the pan until the batter completely coats the bottom.
6. Cook the crêpe for about 1 minute, then flip it over. Cook the other side of the crêpe for another minute, until lightly browned. Transfer the cooked crêpe to a plate and cover with a clean dish towel to keep warm.
7. Repeat until the batter is used up; you should have about 10 crêpes.
8. Spoon 1 tablespoon of yogurt onto each crêpe and place two crêpes on each plate.
9. Top with berries and serve.

Per Serving (2 Crêpes)
calories: 330 | fat: 6.9g | protein: 15.9g
carbs: 54.1g | fiber: 7.9g | sugar: 11.1g
sodium: 100mg

Apple and Pumpkin Waffles

Prep time: 10 minutes | Cook time: 20 minutes | Serves 6

2¼ cups whole-wheat pastry flour
2 tablespoons granulated sweetener
1 tablespoon baking powder
1 teaspoon ground cinnamon
1 teaspoon ground

nutmeg
4 eggs
1¼ cups pure pumpkin purée
1 apple, peeled, cored, and finely chopped
Melted coconut oil, for cooking

1. In a large bowl, stir together the flour, sweetener, baking powder, cinnamon, and nutmeg.
2. In a small bowl, whisk together the eggs and pumpkin.
3. Add the wet ingredients to the dry and whisk until smooth.
4. Stir the apple into the batter.
5. Cook the waffles according to the waffle maker manufacturer's directions, brushing your waffle iron with melted coconut oil, until all the batter is gone.
6. Serve immediately.

Per Serving
calories: 232 | fat: 4.1g | protein: 10.9g
carbs: 40.1g | fiber: 7.1g | sugar: 5.1g
sodium: 52mg

Swiss Chard Shakshuka

Prep time: 15 minutes | Cook time: 20 minutes | Serves 4

4 ounces (113 g) Swiss chard (about 4 large stems and leaves)
2 tablespoons extra-virgin olive oil
½ medium onion, chopped
½ teaspoon kosher salt
½ teaspoon freshly ground black pepper
½ tablespoon Italian seasoning
2 teaspoons minced garlic
1½ cups Marinara Sauce with Red Lentils or tomato-based pasta sauce
4 large eggs
1 tablespoon chopped fresh parsley
2 tablespoons freshly grated Parmesan cheese

1. Separate the stems from the leaves of the Swiss chard. Finely chop the stems; you'll need about ½ cup. Stack the leaves, slice into thin strips, then chop. Set aside.
2. Set the electric pressure cooker to the Sauté setting. When the pot is hot, pour in the olive oil.
3. Add the Swiss chard stems, onion, salt, pepper, and Italian seasoning to the pot, and sauté for 3 to 5 minutes or until the vegetables begin to soften.
4. Add the Swiss chard leaves and garlic, and sauté for 2 more minutes.
5. Hit Cancel. Add the pasta sauce and let the pot cool for 5 minutes.
6. Make 4 evenly spaced indentions in the sauce mixture. Carefully crack an egg into a custard cup, then pour it into one of the indentions. Repeat with the remaining eggs. (Note you can crack the eggs directly into the pot, but the whites will spread out more and the eggs won't look as nice.)
7. Close and lock the lid of the pressure cooker. Set the valve to sealing.
8. Select low pressure and set the timer for 0 minutes.
9. When the cooking is complete, hit Cancel and quick release the pressure.
10. Once the pin drops, unlock and remove the lid.
11. Sprinkle with parsley and Parmesan, and serve immediately.

Per Serving
calories: 183 | fat: 12.1g | protein: 8.1g
carbs: 11.1g | fiber: 2.9g | sugar: 5.9g
sodium: 850mg

Tacos with Pico De Gallo

Prep time: 5 minutes | Cook time: 10 minutes | Serves 4

For the Taco Filling:
Avocado oil cooking spray
1 medium green bell pepper, chopped
8 large eggs
¼ cup shredded sharp Cheddar cheese
4 (6-inch) whole-wheat tortillas
1 cup fresh spinach leaves
½ cup Pico de Gallo
Scallions, chopped, for garnish (optional)
Avocado slices, for garnish (optional)

For the Pico De Gallo:
1 tomato, diced
½ large white onion, diced
2 tablespoons chopped fresh cilantro
½ jalapeño pepper, stemmed, seeded, and diced
1 tablespoon freshly squeezed lime juice
⅛ teaspoon salt

To Make the Taco Filling
1. Heat a medium skillet over medium-low heat. When hot, coat the cooking surface with cooking spray and put the pepper in the skillet. Cook for 4 minutes.
2. Meanwhile, whisk the eggs in a medium bowl, then add the cheese and whisk to combine. Pour the eggs and cheese into the skillet with the green peppers and scramble until the eggs are fully cooked, about 5 minutes.
3. Microwave the tortillas very briefly, about 8 seconds.
4. For each serving, top a tortilla with one-quarter of the spinach, eggs, and pico de gallo. Garnish with scallions and avocado slices (if using).

To Make the Pico De Gallo
1. In a medium bowl, combine the tomato, onion, cilantro, pepper, lime juice, and salt. Mix well and serve.

Per Serving
calories: 277 | fat: 12.1g | protein: 16.1g
carbs: 28.1g | fiber: 2.9g | sugar: 8.1g
sodium: 563mg

Almond Berry Smoothie

Prep time: 5 minutes | Cook time: 0 minutes | Serves 4

2 cups frozen berries of choice
1 cup plain low-fat Greek yogurt
1 cup unsweetened vanilla almond milk
½ cup natural almond butter

1. In a blender, add the berries, almond milk, yogurt, and almond butter. Process until fully mixed and creamy. Pour into four smoothie glasses.
2. Serve chilled or at room temperature.

Per Serving
calories: 279 | fat: 18.2g | protein: 13.4g
carbs: 19.1g | fiber: 6.1g | sugar: 11.1g
sodium: 138mg

Blueberry and Banana Breakfast Cookies

Prep time: 10 minutes | Cook time: 15 minutes | Serves 4

4 tablespoons unsalted butter, at room temperature
2 medium bananas
4 large eggs, whisked
½ cup unsweetened applesauce
1 teaspoon vanilla extract
$^2/_3$ cup coconut flour
¼ teaspoon salt
1 cup fresh or frozen blueberries

1. Preheat the oven to 375ºC (190ºC). Line a baking sheet with parchment paper and set aside.
2. With the back of a fork, mash the butter and bananas in a large bowl until a uniform consistency is achieved.
3. Add the whisked eggs, applesauce, and vanilla extract. Stir to combine well. Add the coconut flour and salt and give the mixture a good stir, then fold in the blueberries.
4. Using a cookie scoop to drop about 2 tablespoons of the mixture onto the prepared baking sheet and flatten each into a rounded biscuit shape with the back of a spoon.

5. Bake in the preheated oven for about 12 minutes, or until the cookies are firm to the touch and lightly browned.
6. Remove from the oven and let the cookies cool for 5 minutes before serving.

Per Serving
calories: 307 | fat: 18.2g | protein: 8.1g
carbs: 28.1g | fiber: 7.3g | sugar: 15.3g
sodium: 220mg

Mushroom Frittata

Prep time: 10 minutes | Cook time: 15 minutes | Serves 4

8 large eggs
½ cup skim milk
¼ teaspoon ground nutmeg
Sea salt and freshly ground black pepper, to taste
2 teaspoons extra-virgin olive oil
2 cups sliced wild mushrooms (cremini, oyster, shiitake, portobello, etc.)
½ red onion, chopped
1 teaspoon minced garlic
½ cup goat cheese, crumbled

1. Preheat the broiler.
2. In a medium bowl, whisk together the eggs, milk, and nutmeg until well combined. Season the egg mixture lightly with salt and pepper and set it aside.
3. Place an ovenproof skillet over medium heat and add the oil, coating the bottom completely by tilting the pan.
4. Sauté the mushrooms, onion, and garlic until translucent, about 7 minutes.
5. Pour the egg mixture into the skillet and cook until the bottom of the frittata is set, lifting the edges of the cooked egg to allow the uncooked egg to seep under.
6. Place the skillet under the broiler until the top is set, about 1 minute.
7. Sprinkle the goat cheese on the frittata and broil until the cheese is melted, about 1 minute more.
8. Remove from the oven. Cut into 4 wedges to serve.

Per Serving
calories: 227 | fat: 15.1g | protein: 17.1g
carbs: 5.1g | fiber: 0.9g | sugar: 4.1g
sodium: 224mg

Portobello and Chicken Sausage Frittata

Prep time: 10 minutes | Cook time: 15 minutes | Serves 4

Avocado oil cooking spray
1 cup roughly chopped portobello mushrooms
1 medium green bell pepper, diced
1 medium red bell pepper, diced

8 large eggs
¾ cup half-and-half
¼ cup unsweetened almond milk
6 links maple-flavored chicken or turkey breakfast sausage, cut into ¼-inch pieces

1. Preheat the oven to 375ºF (190ºC).
2. Heat a large, oven-safe skillet over medium-low heat. When hot, coat the cooking surface with cooking spray.
3. Heat the mushrooms, green bell pepper, and red bell pepper in the skillet. Cook for 5 minutes.
4. Meanwhile, in a medium bowl, whisk the eggs, half-and-half, and almond milk.
5. Add the sausage to the skillet and cook for 2 minutes.
6. Pour the egg mixture into the skillet, then transfer the skillet from the stove to the oven, and bake for 15 minutes, or until the middle is firm and spongy.

Per Serving
calories: 281 | fat: 17.1g | protein: 20.9g
carbs: 10.1g | fiber: 2.1g | sugar: 7.1g
sodium: 445mg

Egg Salad Sandwiches

Prep time: 10 minutes | Cook time: 0 minutes | Serves 4

8 large hardboiled eggs
3 tablespoons plain low-fat Greek yogurt
1 tablespoon mustard
½ teaspoon freshly ground black pepper

1 teaspoon chopped fresh chives
4 slices 100% whole-wheat bread
2 cups fresh spinach, loosely packed

1. Peel the eggs and cut them in half.
2. In a large bowl, mash the eggs with a fork, leaving chunks.
3. Add the yogurt, mustard, pepper, and chives, and mix.
4. For each portion, layer 1 slice of bread with one-quarter of the egg salad and spinach.

Per Serving
calories: 278 | fat: 12.1g | protein: 20.1g
carbs: 23.1g | fiber: 2.9g | sugar: 3.1g
sodium: 365mg

Apple and Bran Muffins

Prep time: 10 minutes | Cook time: 20 minutes | Makes 18 muffins

2 cups whole-wheat flour
1 cup wheat bran
1/3 cup granulated sweetener
1 tablespoon baking powder
2 teaspoons ground cinnamon
½ teaspoon ground ginger
¼ teaspoon ground

nutmeg
Pinch sea salt
2 eggs
1½ cups skim milk, at room temperature
½ cup melted coconut oil
2 teaspoons pure vanilla extract
2 apples, peeled, cored, and diced

1. Preheat the oven to 350ºF (180ºC).
2. Line 18 muffin cups with paper liners and set the tray aside.
3. In a large bowl, stir together the flour, bran, sweetener, baking powder, cinnamon, ginger, nutmeg, and salt.
4. In a small bowl, whisk the eggs, milk, coconut oil, and vanilla until blended.
5. Add the wet ingredients to the dry ingredients, stirring until just blended.
6. Stir in the apples and spoon equal amounts of batter into each muffin cup.
7. Bake the muffins until a toothpick inserted in the center of a muffin comes out clean, about 20 minutes.
8. Cool the muffins completely and serve.
9. Store leftover muffins in a sealed container in the refrigerator for up to 3 days or in the freezer for up to 1 month.

Per Serving
calories: 142 | fat: 7.1g | protein: 4.1g
carbs: 19.1g | fiber: 3.1g | sugar: 6.1g
sodium: 21mg

Banana Crêpe Cakes

Prep time: 5 minutes | Cook time: 20 minutes | Serves 4

Avocado oil cooking spray
4 ounces (113 g) reduced-fat plain cream cheese, softened

2 medium bananas
4 large eggs
½ teaspoon vanilla extract
⅛ teaspoon salt

1. Heat a large skillet over low heat. Coat the cooking surface with cooking spray, and allow the pan to heat for another 2 to 3 minutes.
2. Meanwhile, in a medium bowl, mash the cream cheese and bananas together with a fork until combined. The bananas can be a little chunky.
3. Add the eggs, vanilla, and salt, and mix well.
4. For each cake, drop 2 tablespoons of the batter onto the warmed skillet and use the bottom of a large spoon or ladle to spread it thin. Let it cook for 7 to 9 minutes.
5. Flip the cake over and cook briefly, about 1 minute.

Per Serving
calories: 176 | fat: 9.1g | protein: 9.1g
carbs: 15.1g | fiber: 2.1g | sugar: 8.1g
sodium: 214mg

Shrimp with Scallion Grits

Prep time: 15 minutes | Cook time: 20 minutes | Serves 6 to 8

1½ cups fat-free milk
1½ cups water
2 bay leaves
1 cup stone-ground corn grits
¼ cup seafood broth
2 garlic cloves, minced
2 scallions, white and green parts, thinly

sliced
1 pound (454 g) medium shrimp, shelled and deveined
½ teaspoon dried dill
½ teaspoon smoked paprika
¼ teaspoon celery seeds

1. In a medium stockpot, combine the milk, water, and bay leaves and bring to a boil over high heat.

2. Gradually add the grits, stirring continuously.
3. Reduce the heat to low, cover, and cook for 5 to 7 minutes, stirring often, or until the grits are soft and tender. Remove from the heat and discard the bay leaves.
4. In a small cast iron skillet, bring the broth to a simmer over medium heat.
5. Add the garlic and scallions, and sauté for 3 to 5 minutes, or until softened.
6. Add the shrimp, dill, paprika, and celery seeds and cook for about 7 minutes, or until the shrimp is light pink but not overcooked.
7. Plate each dish with ¼ cup of grits, topped with shrimp.

Per Serving
calories: 198 | fat: 1.0g | protein: 20.1g
carbs: 24.9g | fiber: 1.0g | sugar: 3.1g
sodium: 204mg

Breakfast Cheddar Zucchini Casserole

Prep time: 10 minutes | Cook time: 35 minutes | Serves 12 to 15

Nonstick cooking spray
6 medium brown eggs
8 medium egg whites
1 green bell pepper, chopped
½ small yellow onion, chopped

1 zucchini, finely grated, with water pressed out
1 cup shredded reduced-fat Cheddar cheese
1 teaspoon paprika
½ teaspoon garlic powder

1. Preheat the oven to 350ºF (180ºC). Spray a large cast iron skillet with cooking spray.
2. In a medium bowl, whisk the eggs and egg whites together.
3. Add the bell pepper, onion, zucchini, cheese, paprika, and garlic powder, mix well, and pour into the prepared skillet.
4. Transfer the skillet to the oven, and bake for 35 minutes. Remove from the oven, and let rest for 5 minutes before serving with Broccoli Stalk Slaw.

Per Serving
calories: 79 | fat: 4.1g | protein: 8.1g
carbs: 2.1g | fiber: 1.1g | sugar: 1.2g
sodium: 133mg

Peanut Butter and Berry Oatmeal

Prep time: 5 minutes | Cook time: 5 minutes | Serves 2

1½ cups unsweetened vanilla almond milk
¾ cup rolled oats
1 tablespoon chia seeds
2 tablespoons natural

peanut butter
¼ cup fresh berries, divided (optional)
2 tablespoons walnut pieces, divided (optional)

1. Add the almond milk, oats, and chia seeds to a small saucepan and bring to a boil.
2. Cover and continue cooking, stirring often, or until the oats have absorbed the milk.
3. Add the peanut butter and keep stirring until the oats are thick and creamy.
4. Divide the oatmeal into two serving bowls. Serve topped with the berries and walnut pieces, if desired.

Per Serving
calories: 260 | fat: 13.9g | protein: 10.1g
carbs: 26.9g | fiber: 7.1g | sugar: 1.0g
sodium: 130mg

Coconut and Berry Oatmeal

Prep time: 10 minutes | Cook time: 35 minutes | Serves 6

2 cups rolled oats
¼ cup shredded unsweetened coconut
1 teaspoon baking powder
½ teaspoon ground cinnamon
¼ teaspoon sea salt
2 cups skim milk
¼ cup melted coconut oil, plus extra for greasing the

baking dish
1 egg
1 teaspoon pure vanilla extract
2 cups fresh blueberries
⅛ cup chopped pecans, for garnish
1 teaspoon chopped fresh mint leaves, for garnish

1. Preheat the oven to 350°F (180°C).
2. Lightly oil a baking dish and set it aside.
3. In a medium bowl, stir together the oats, coconut, baking powder, cinnamon, and salt.

4. In a small bowl, whisk together the milk, oil, egg, and vanilla until well blended.
5. Layer half the dry ingredients in the baking dish, top with half the berries, then spoon the remaining half of the dry ingredients and the rest of the berries on top.
6. Pour the wet ingredients evenly into the baking dish. Tap it lightly on the counter to disperse the wet ingredients throughout.
7. Bake the casserole, uncovered, until the oats are tender, about 35 minutes.
8. Serve immediately, topped with the pecans and mint.

Per Serving
calories: 296 | fat: 17.1g | protein: 10.2g
carbs: 26.9g | fiber: 4.1g | sugar: 10.9g
sodium: 154mg

Goat Cheese and Avocado Toast

Prep time: 10 minutes | Cook time: 5 minutes | Serves 2

2 slices whole-wheat bread, thinly sliced
½ avocado
2 tablespoons goat cheese, crumbled

Salt, to taste
2 slices of crumbled bacon, for topping (optional)

1. Toast the bread slices in a toaster for 2 to 3 minutes on each side until golden brown.
2. Using a large spoon, scoop the avocado flesh out of the skin and transfer to a medium bowl. Mash the flesh with a potato masher or the back of a fork until it has a spreadable consistency.
3. Spoon the mashed avocado onto the bread slices and evenly spread it all over.
4. Scatter with crumbled goat cheese and lightly season with salt.
5. Serve topped with crumbled bacon, if desired.

Per Serving
calories: 140 | fat: 6.2g | protein: 5.2g
carbs: 18.2g | fiber: 5.1g | sugar: 0g
sodium: 197mg

Tropical Fruity Steel Cut Oats

Prep time: 5 minutes | Cook time: 20 minutes | Serves 4

1 cup steel cut oats
1 cup unsweetened almond milk
2 cups coconut water or water
¾ cup frozen chopped peaches
¾ cup frozen mango

chunks
1 (2-inch) vanilla bean, scraped (seeds and pod)
Ground cinnamon
¼ cup chopped unsalted macadamia nuts

1. In the electric pressure cooker, combine the oats, almond milk, coconut water, peaches, mango chunks, and vanilla bean seeds and pod. Stir well.
2. Close and lock the lid of the pressure cooker. Set the valve to sealing.
3. Cook on high pressure for 5 minutes.
4. When the cooking is complete, allow the pressure to release naturally for 10 minutes, then quick release any remaining pressure. Hit Cancel.
5. Once the pin drops, unlock and remove the lid.
6. Discard the vanilla bean pod and stir well.
7. Spoon the oats into 4 bowls. Top each serving with a sprinkle of cinnamon and 1 tablespoon of the macadamia nuts.

Per Serving
calories: 126 | fat: 7.1g | protein: 1.9g
carbs: 14.2g | fiber: 2.9g | sugar: 8.1g
sodium: 166mg

Farro with Walnuts and Berries

Prep time: 8 minutes | Cook time: 15 minutes | Serves 6

1 cup farro, rinsed and drained
1 cup unsweetened almond milk
¼ teaspoon kosher salt
½ teaspoon pure vanilla extract
1 teaspoon ground cinnamon

1 tablespoon pure maple syrup
1½ cups fresh blueberries, raspberries, or strawberries (or a combination)
6 tablespoons chopped walnuts

1. In the electric pressure cooker, combine the farro, almond milk, 1 cup of water, salt, vanilla, cinnamon, and maple syrup.
2. Close and lock the lid. Set the valve to sealing.
3. Cook on high pressure for 10 minutes.
4. When the cooking is complete, allow the pressure to release naturally for 10 minutes, then quick release any remaining pressure. Hit Cancel.
5. Once the pin drops, unlock and remove the lid.
6. Stir the farro. Spoon into bowls and top each serving with ¼ cup of berries and 1 tablespoon of walnuts.

Per Serving
calories: 190 | fat: 4.9g | protein: 5.1g
carbs: 31.9g | fiber: 2.9g | sugar: 6.0g
sodium: 112mg

Cranberry Grits

Prep time: 10 minutes | Cook time: 15 minutes | Serves 5

¾ cup stone-ground grits or polenta (not instant)
½ cup unsweetened dried cranberries
Pinch kosher salt
1 tablespoon

unsalted butter or ghee (optional)
1 tablespoon half-and-half
¼ cup sliced almonds, toasted

1. In the electric pressure cooker, stir together the grits, cranberries, salt, and 3 cups of water.
2. Close and lock the lid. Set the valve to sealing.
3. Cook on high pressure for 10 minutes.
4. When the cooking is complete, hit Cancel and quick release the pressure.
5. Once the pin drops, unlock and remove the lid.
6. Add the butter (if using) and half-and-half. Stir until the mixture is creamy, adding more half-and-half if necessary.
7. Spoon into serving bowls and sprinkle with almonds.

Per Serving
calories: 219 | fat: 10.2g | protein: 4.9g
carbs: 32.1g | fiber: 4.1g | sugar: 6.9g
sodium: 30mg

Feta Brussels Sprouts and Scrambled Eggs

Prep time: 5 minutes | Cook time: 15 minutes | Serves 4

Avocado oil cooking spray
4 slices low-sodium turkey bacon
20 Brussels sprouts,
halved lengthwise
8 large eggs, whisked
¼ cup crumbled feta cheese, for garnish

1. Heat a large skillet over medium heat until hot. Coat the skillet with cooking spray.
2. Fry the bacon slices for about 8 minutes until evenly crisp, flipping occasionally.
3. With a slotted spoon, transfer the bacon to a paper towel-lined plate to drain and cool. Leave the bacon grease in the skillet.
4. Add the Brussels sprouts to the bacon grease in the skillet and cook as you stir for about 6 minutes until browned on both side.
5. Push the Brussels sprouts to one side of the skillet, add the whisked eggs and scramble for about 3 to 4 minutes until almost set.
6. Once the bacon is cooled, crumble into small pieces.
7. Divide the Brussels sprouts and scrambled eggs among four serving plates. Scatter the tops with crumbled bacon pieces and garnish with feta cheese before serving.

Per Serving
calories: 255 | fat: 15.3g | protein: 21.3g carbs: 10.2g | fiber: 4.2g | sugar: 4.2g sodium: 340mg

Breakfast Grain Porridge

Prep time: 5 minutes | Cook time: 35 minutes | Serves 8

1 cup teff
1 cup stone-ground corn grits
1 cup quinoa
¼ teaspoon whole cloves
1 tablespoon
sunflower seed oil
5 cups water
2 cups roughly chopped fresh fruit
2 cups unsalted crushed nuts

1. In an electric pressure cooker, combine the teff, grits, quinoa, and cloves.
2. Add the oil and water, mixing together with a fork.
3. Close and lock the lid, and set the pressure valve to sealing.
4. Select the Porridge setting, and cook for 20 minutes.
5. Once cooking is complete, allow the pressure to release naturally. Carefully remove the lid.
6. Serve each portion with ¼ cup fresh fruit and ¼ cup nuts of your choice.

Per Serving
calories: 418 | fat: 19.1g | protein: 13.2g carbs: 49.1g | fiber: 9.1g | sugar: 5.1g sodium: 6mg

Brussels Sprout with Fried Eggs

Prep time: 10 minutes | Cook time: 15 minutes | Serves 4

3 teaspoons extra-virgin olive oil, divided
1 pound (454 g) Brussels sprouts, sliced
2 garlic cloves, thinly sliced
¼ teaspoon salt
Juice of 1 lemon
4 eggs

1. Heat 1½ teaspoons of olive oil in a large skillet over medium heat.
2. Add the Brussels sprouts and sauté for 6 to 8 minutes until crispy and tender, stirring frequently.
3. Stir in the garlic and cook for about 1 minute until fragrant. Sprinkle with the salt and lemon juice.
4. Remove from the skillet to a plate and set aside.
5. Heat the remaining oil in the skillet over medium-high heat. Crack the eggs one at a time into the skillet and fry for about 3 minutes. Flip the eggs and continue cooking, or until the egg whites are set and the yolks are cooked to your liking.
6. Serve the fried eggs over the crispy Brussels sprouts.

Per Serving
calories: 157 | fat: 8.9g | protein: 10.1g carbs: 11.8g | fiber: 4.1g | sugar: 4.0g sodium: 233mg

Cheesy Spinach, Artichoke, and Egg Casserole

Prep time: 10 minutes | Cook time: 35 minutes | Serves 8

1 (10-ounce / 284-g) package frozen spinach, thawed and drained
1 (14-ounce / 397-g) can artichoke hearts, drained
¼ cup finely chopped red bell pepper
8 eggs, lightly beaten
¼ cup unsweetened plain almond milk
2 garlic cloves, minced
½ teaspoon salt
½ teaspoon freshly ground black pepper
½ cup crumbled goat cheese
Nonstick cooking spray

1. Preheat the oven to 375ºF (190ºC). Spray a baking dish with nonstick cooking spray and set aside.
2. Mix the spinach, artichoke hearts, bell peppers, beaten eggs, almond milk, garlic, salt, and pepper in a large bowl, and stir to incorporate.
3. Pour the mixture into the greased baking dish and scatter the goat cheese on top.
4. Bake in the preheated oven for 35 minutes, or until the top is lightly golden around the edges and eggs are set.
5. Remove from the oven and serve warm.

Per Serving
calories: 105 | fat: 4.8g | protein: 8.9g
carbs: 6.1g | fiber: 1.7g | sugar: 1.0g
sodium: 486mg

Simple Cottage Cheese Pancakes

Prep time: 5 minutes | Cook time: 10 minutes | Serves 2

Batter:
½ cup low-fat cottage cheese
¼ cup oats
¹⁄₃ cup egg whites (about 2 egg whites)
1 tablespoon stevia
1 teaspoon vanilla
extract
Olive oil cooking spray
Berries or sugar-free jam, for topping (optional)

1. Add the cottage cheese, oats, egg whites, stevia and vanilla extract to a food processor. Pulse into a smooth and thick batter.
2. Coat a large skillet with cooking spray and place it over medium heat.
3. Slowly pour half of the batter into the pan, tilting the pan to spread it evenly. Cook for about 2 to 3 minutes until the pancake turns golden brown around the edges. Gently flip the pancake with a spatula and cook for 1 to 2 minutes more.
4. Transfer the pancake to a plate and repeat with the remaining batter.
5. Top with the berries or sugar-free jam and serve, if desired.

Per Serving
calories: 188 | fat: 1.6g | protein: 24.6g
carbs: 18.9g | fiber: 1.9g | sugar: 2g
sodium: 258mg

Greek Yogurt and Oat Pancakes

Prep time: 5 minutes | Cook time: 20 minutes | Serves 4

1 cup 2 percent plain Greek yogurt
3 eggs
1½ teaspoons pure vanilla extract
1 cup rolled oats
1 tablespoon granulated sweetener
1 teaspoon baking powder
1 teaspoon ground cinnamon
Pinch ground cloves
Nonstick cooking spray

1. Place the yogurt, eggs, and vanilla in a blender and pulse to combine.
2. Add the oats, sweetener, baking powder, cinnamon, and cloves to the blender and blend until the batter is smooth.
3. Place a large nonstick skillet over medium heat and lightly coat it with cooking spray.
4. Spoon ¼ cup of batter per pancake, 4 at a time, into the skillet. Cook the pancakes until the bottoms are firm and golden, about 4 minutes.
5. Flip the pancakes over and cook the other side until they are cooked through, about 3 minutes.
6. Remove the pancakes to a plate and repeat with the remaining batter.
7. Serve with fresh fruit.

Per Serving
calories: 244 | fat: 8.1g | protein: 13.1g
carbs: 28.1g | fiber: 4.0g | sugar: 3.0g
sodium: 82mg

Super Grain Porridge

Prep time: 5 minutes | Cook time: 40 minutes | Serves 7

½ cup steel cut oats
½ cup short-grain brown rice
½ cup millet
½ cup barley
⅓ cup wild rice
¼ cup corn grits or polenta (not instant)
3 tablespoons ground flaxseed

½ teaspoon salt
Ground cinnamon (optional)
Unsweetened almond milk (optional)
Berries (optional)
Sliced almonds or chopped walnuts (optional)

1. In the electric pressure cooker, combine the oats, brown rice, millet, barley, wild rice, grits, flaxseed, salt, and 8 cups of water.
2. Close and lock the lid of the pressure cooker. Set the valve to sealing.
3. Cook on high pressure for 20 minutes.
4. When the cooking is complete, hit Cancel and allow the pressure to release naturally for 15 minutes, then quick release any remaining pressure.
5. Once the pin drops, unlock and remove the lid. Stir.
6. Serve with any combination of cinnamon, almond milk, berries, and nuts (if using).

Per Serving
calories: 265 | fat: 3.1g | protein: 7.9g
carbs: 50.9g | fiber: 7.1g | sugar: 0.5g
sodium: 141mg

Vanilla Coconut Pancakes

Prep time: 5 minutes | Cook time: 15 minutes | Serves 4

½ cup coconut flour
1 teaspoon baking powder
½ teaspoon ground cinnamon
⅛ teaspoon salt
8 large eggs

⅓ cup unsweetened almond milk
2 tablespoons avocado or coconut oil
1 teaspoon vanilla extract

1. Stir together the flour, baking powder, cinnamon, and salt in a large bowl. Set aside.
2. Beat the eggs with the almond milk, oil, and vanilla in a medium bowl until fully mixed.
3. Heat a large nonstick skillet over medium-low heat.
4. Make the pancakes: Pour ⅓ cup of batter into the hot skillet, tilting the pan to spread it evenly. Cook for 3 to 4 minutes until bubbles form on the surface. Flip the pancake with a spatula and cook for about 3 minutes, or until the pancake is browned around the edges and cooked through. Repeat with the remaining batter.
5. Serve the pancakes on a plate while warm.

Per Serving
calories: 269 | fat: 17.8g | protein: 13.9g
carbs: 10.1g | fiber: 5.1g | sugar: 1.9g
sodium: 324mg

Easy Turkey Breakfast Patties

Prep time: 10 minutes | Cook time: 10 minutes | Serves 8 (1 patty each)

1 pound (454 g) lean ground turkey
½ teaspoon dried thyme
½ teaspoon dried sage
½ teaspoon salt

½ teaspoon freshly ground black pepper
¼ teaspoon ground fennel seeds
1 teaspoon extra-virgin olive oil

1. Mix the ground turkey, thyme, sage, salt, pepper, and fennel in a large bowl, and stir until well combined.
2. Form the turkey mixture into 8 equal-sized patties with your hands.
3. In a skillet, heat the olive oil over medium-high heat. Cook the patties for 3 to 4 minutes per side until cooked through.
4. Transfer the patties to a plate and serve hot.

Per Serving
calories: 91 | fat: 4.8g | protein: 11.2g
carbs: 0.1g | fiber: 0.1g | sugar: 0g
sodium: 155mg

Scrumptious Orange Muffins

Prep time: 15 minutes | Cook time: 15 minutes | Serves 8

Dry Ingredients:
2½ cups finely ground almond flour
½ teaspoon baking powder
½ teaspoon ground cardamom
¾ teaspoon ground cinnamon
¼ teaspoon salt

Wet Ingredients:
2 large eggs
4 tablespoons avocado or coconut oil
1 tablespoon raw honey
¼ teaspoon vanilla extract
Grated zest and juice of 1 medium orange

Special Equipment:
An 8-cup muffin tin

1. Preheat the oven to 375ºF (190ºC) and line an 8-cup muffin tin with paper liners.
2. Stir together the almond flour, baking powder, cardamon, cinnamon, and salt in a large bowl. Set aside.
3. Whisk together the eggs, oil, honey, vanilla, zest and juice in a medium bowl. Pour the mixture into the bowl of dry ingredients and stir with a spatula just until incorporated.
4. Pour the batter into the prepared muffin cups, filling each about three-quarters full.
5. Bake in the preheated oven for 15 minutes, or until the tops are golden and a toothpick inserted in the center comes out clean.
6. Let the muffins cool for 10 minutes before serving.

Per Serving
calories: 287 | fat: 23.5g | protein: 7.9g
carbs: 15.8g | fiber: 3.8g | sugar: 9.8g
sodium: 96mg

Fresh Huevos Rancheros

Prep time: 5 minutes | Cook time: 15 minutes | Serves 4

Huevos Rancheros:
1 cup low-sodium black beans, drained and rinsed
½ cup jarred salsa verde
Avocado oil cooking spray
8 large eggs
1 cup fresh Pico de Gallo (see below)
4 lime wedges

Pico De Gallo:
1 tomato, diced
½ large white onion, diced
½ jalapeño pepper, stemmed, seeded, and diced
2 tablespoons fresh cilantro, chopped
1 tablespoon freshly squeezed lime juice
⅛ teaspoon salt

Make the Huevos Rancheros
1. In a small saucepan, add the black beans and salsa verde. Cover, and cook over low heat for 10 minutes until the black beans are heated through.
2. Meantime, heat a skillet over medium-low heat until hot. Coat the skillet with cooking spray.
3. One at a time, crack the eggs into the skillet and fry about 4 to 5 minutes, or until the eggs white are opaque and the yolks are firm.
4. Remove the black bean and fried eggs from the heat to a plate.
5. To serve, place ¼ of the cooked black beans and pico de gallo on top of two fried eggs, finished by the juice squeezed from the lime wedges.

Make the Pico De Gallo
1. Mix together the tomato, onion, pepper, cilantro, lime juice, and salt in a bowl. Stir well with a fork to incorporate.

Per Serving
calories: 212 | fat: 9.6g | protein: 15.2g
carbs: 18.2g | fiber: 5.2g | sugar: 4.2g
sodium: 440mg

Carrot and Oat Pancakes

Prep time: 10 minutes | Cook time: 8 minutes | Serves 4

¼ cup plain Greek yogurt
1 tablespoon pure maple syrup
1 cup rolled oats
1 cup low-fat cottage cheese
1 cup shredded carrots
½ cup unsweetened plain almond milk
2 eggs
1 teaspoon baking powder
2 tablespoons ground flaxseed
½ teaspoon ground cinnamon
2 teaspoons canola oil, divided

1. Stir together the yogurt and maple syrup in a small bowl and set aside.
2. Grind the oats in a blender, or until they are ground into a flour-like consistency.
3. Make the batter: Add the cheese, carrots, almond milk, eggs, baking powder, flaxseed, and cinnamon to the blender, and process until fully mixed and smooth.
4. Heat 1 teaspoon of canola oil in a large skillet over medium heat.
5. Make the pancakes: Pour ¼ cup of batter into the skillet and swirl the pan so the batter covers the bottom evenly. Cook for 1 to 2 minutes until bubbles form on the surface. Gently flip the pancake with a spatula and cook for 1 to 2 minutes more, or until the pancake turns golden brown around the edges. Repeat with the remaining canola oil and batter.
6. Top the pancakes with the maple yogurt and serve warm.

Per Serving
calories: 227 | fat: 8.1g | protein: 14.9g
carbs: 24.2g | fiber: 4.0g | sugar: 7.0g
sodium: 403mg

Savory Breakfast Egg Bites

Prep time: 10 minutes | Cook time: 20 to 25 minutes | Serves 8 (1 egg bite each)

6 eggs, beaten
¼ cup unsweetened plain almond milk
¼ cup crumbled goat cheese
½ cup sliced brown mushrooms
1 cup chopped spinach
¼ cup sliced sun-dried tomatoes
1 red bell pepper, diced
Salt and freshly ground black pepper, to taste
Nonstick cooking spray

Special Equipment:
An 8-cup muffin tin

1. Preheat the oven to 350ºF (180ºC). Grease an 8-cup muffin tin with nonstick cooking spray.
2. Make the egg bites: Mix together the beaten eggs, almond milk, cheese, mushroom, spinach, tomatoes, bell pepper, salt, and pepper in a large bowl, and whisk to combine.
3. Spoon the mixture into the prepared muffin cups, filling each about three-quarters full.
4. Bake in the preheated oven for 20 to 25 minutes, or until the top is golden brown and a fork comes out clean.
5. Let the egg bites sit for 5 minutes until slightly cooled. Remove from the muffin tin and serve warm.

Per Serving
calories: 68 | fat: 4.1g | protein: 6.2g
carbs: 2.9g | fiber: 1.1g | sugar: 2.0g
sodium: 126mg

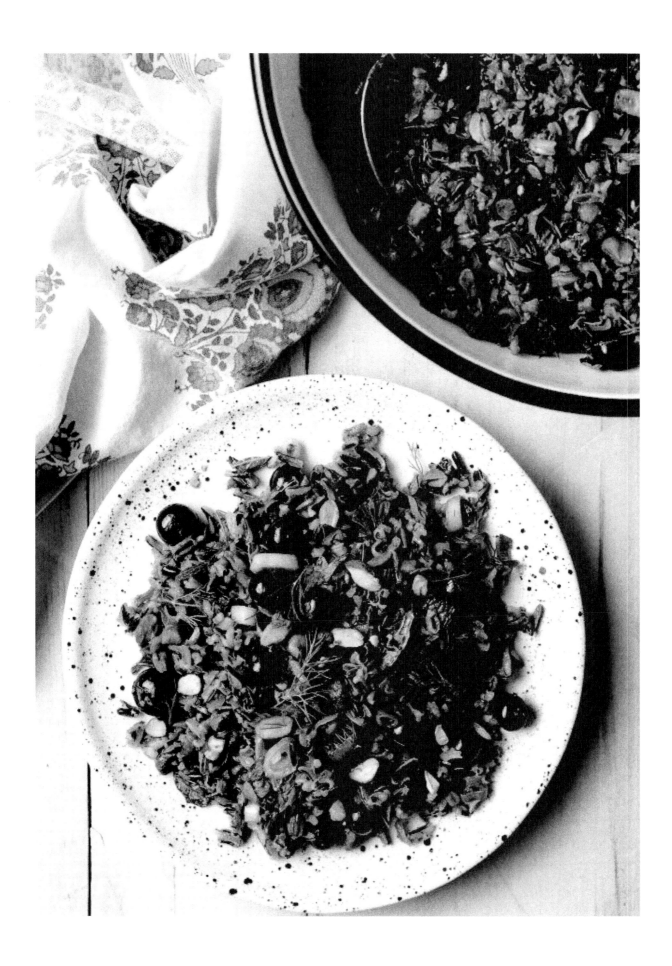

Chapter 5: Grains, Beans, and Legumes

Macaroni and Vegetable Pie

Prep time: 15 minutes | Cook time: 30 minutes | Serves 6

1 (1-pound / 454-g) package whole-wheat macaroni
2 celery stalks, thinly sliced
1 small yellow onion, chopped
2 garlic cloves, minced
Salt, to taste
¼ teaspoon freshly ground black pepper
2 tablespoons chickpea flour
2 cups grated reduced-fat sharp Cheddar cheese
1 cup fat-free milk
2 large zucchini, finely grated and squeezed dry
2 roasted red peppers, chopped into ¼-inch pieces

1. Preheat the oven to 350ºF (180ºC).
2. Bring a pot of water to a boil, then add the macaroni and cook for 4 minutes or until al dente.
3. Drain the macaroni and transfer to a large bowl. Reserve 1 cup of the macaroni water.
4. Pour the macaroni water in an oven-safe skillet and heat over medium heat.
5. Add the celery, onion, garlic, salt, and black pepper to the skillet and sauté for 4 minutes or until tender.
6. Gently mix in the chickpea flour, then fold in the cheese and milk. Keep stirring until the mixture is thick and smooth.
7. Add the cooked macaroni, zucchini, and red peppers. Stir to combine well.
8. Cover the skillet with aluminum foil and transfer it to the preheated oven.
9. Bake for 15 minutes or until the cheese melts, then remove the foil and bake for 5 more minutes or until lightly browned.
10. Remove the pie from the oven and serve immediately.

Per Serving
calories: 378 | fat: 4.0g | protein: 24.0g
carbs: 67.0g | fiber: 8.0g | sugar: 6.0g
sodium: 332mg

Wild Rice, Almonds, and Cranberries Salad

Prep time: 10 minutes | Cook time: 45 minutes | Serves 6 Cups

For the Rice:
2½ cups chicken bone broth, vegetable broth, or water
2 cups wild rice
blend, rinsed
1 teaspoon kosher salt
For the Dressing:
Juice of 1 medium orange (about ¼ cup)
1½ teaspoons grated orange zest
¼ cup white wine
vinegar
1 teaspoon pure maple syrup
¼ cup extra-virgin olive oil
For the Salad:
½ cup sliced almonds, toasted
¾ cup unsweetened
dried cranberries
Freshly ground black pepper, to taste

For the Rice
1. Pour the broth in a pot, then add the rice and sprinkle with salt. Bring to a boil over medium-high heat.
2. Reduce the heat to low. Cover the pot, then simmer for 45 minutes.
3. Turn off the heat and fluff the rice with a fork. Set aside until ready to use.
For the Dressing
1. When cooking the rice, make the dressing: Combine the ingredients for the dressing in a small bowl. Stir to combine well. Set aside until ready to use.
For the Salad
1. Put the cooked rice, almonds, and cranberries in a bowl, then sprinkle with black pepper. Add the dressing, then toss to combine well.
2. Serve immediately.

Per Serving (¹/₃ Cup)
calories: 126 | fat: 5.0g | protein: 3.0g
carbs: 18.0g | fiber: 2.0g | sugar: 2.0g
sodium: 120mg

Linguine with Kale Pesto

Prep time: 10 minutes | Cook time: 20 minutes | Serves 6

½ cup shredded kale
½ cup fresh basil
½ cup sun-dried tomatoes
¼ cup chopped almonds
2 tablespoons extra-virgin olive oil
8 ounces (227 g) dry whole-wheat linguine
½ cup grated Parmesan cheese

1. Place the kale, basil, sun-dried tomatoes, almonds, and olive oil in a food processor or blender, and pulse until a chunky paste forms, about 2 minutes. Scoop the pesto into a bowl and set it aside.
2. Place a large pot filled with water on high heat and bring to a boil.
3. Cook the pasta al dente, according to the package directions.
4. Drain the pasta and toss it with the pesto and the Parmesan cheese.
5. Serve immediately.

Per Serving
calories: 218 | fat: 10.1g | protein: 9.1g
carbs: 25.1g | fiber: 1.1g | sugar: 2.9g
sodium: 195mg

Lemon Wax Beans

Prep time: 5 minutes | Cook time: 15 minutes | Serves 4

2 pounds (907 g) wax beans
2 tablespoons extra-virgin olive oil
Sea salt and freshly ground black pepper, to taste
Juice of ½ lemon

1. Preheat the oven to 400ºF (205ºC).
2. Line a baking sheet with aluminum foil.
3. In a large bowl, toss the beans and olive oil. Season lightly with salt and pepper.
4. Transfer the beans to the baking sheet and spread them out.
5. Roast the beans until caramelized and tender, about 10 to 12 minutes.
6. Transfer the beans to a serving platter and sprinkle with the lemon juice.

Per Serving
calories: 99 | fat: 7.1g | protein: 2.1g
carbs: 8.1g | fiber: 4.2g | sugar: 3.9g
sodium: 814mg

Chickpea Tortillas

Prep time: 5 minutes | Cook time: 10 minutes | Serves 4

1 cup chickpea flour
1 cup water
¼ teaspoon salt
Nonstick cooking spray

1. In a large bowl, whisk all together until no lumps remain.
2. Spray a skillet with cooking spray and place over medium-high heat.
3. Pour batter in, ¼ cup at a time, and tilt pan to spread thinly.
4. Cook until golden brown on each side, about 2 minutes per side.
5. Use for taco shells, enchiladas, quesadillas or whatever you desire.

Per Serving
calories: 90 | fat: 2.0g | protein: 5.1g
carbs: 13.1g | fiber: 3.0g | sugar: 3.0g
sodium: 161mg

Blueberry Wild Rice

Prep time: 15 minutes | Cook time: 45 minutes | Serves 4

1 tablespoon extra-virgin olive oil
½ sweet onion, chopped
2½ cups sodium-free chicken broth
1 cup wild rice,
rinsed and drained
Pinch sea salt
½ cup toasted pumpkin seeds
½ cup blueberries
1 teaspoon chopped fresh basil

1. Place a medium saucepan over medium-high heat and add the oil.
2. Sauté the onion until softened and translucent, about 3 minutes.
3. Stir in the broth and bring to a boil.
4. Stir in the rice and salt and reduce the heat to low. Cover and simmer until the rice is tender, about 40 minutes.
5. Drain off any excess broth, if necessary. Stir in the pumpkin seeds, blueberries, and basil.
6. Serve warm.

Per Serving
calories: 259 | fat: 9.1g | protein: 10.8g
carbs: 37.1g | fiber: 3.9g | sugar: 4.1g
sodium: 543mg

Fried Rice with Snap Peas

Prep time: 5 minutes | Cook time: 15 minutes | Serves 8

2 cups sugar snap peas
2 egg whites
1 egg
1 cup instant

brown rice, cooked according to directions
2 tablespoons lite soy sauce

1. Add the peas to the cooked rice and mix to combine.
2. In a small skillet, scramble the egg and egg whites. Add the rice and peas to the skillet and stir in soy sauce. Cook, stirring frequently, about 2 to 3 minutes, or until heated through. Serve.

Per Serving
calories: 108 | fat: 1.0g | protein: 4.1g
carbs: 20.1g | fiber: 1.0g | sugar: 1.0g
sodium: 151mg

Enchilada Black Bean Casserole

Prep time: 15 minutes | Cook time: 15 minutes | Serves 6

1 tablespoon extra-virgin olive oil
½ onion, chopped
½ red bell pepper, seeded and chopped
½ green bell pepper, seeded and chopped
2 small zucchini, chopped
3 garlic cloves, minced
1 (15-ounce / 425-g) can low-sodium black beans, drained and rinsed
1 (10-ounce / 283-g) can low-sodium

enchilada sauce
1 teaspoon ground cumin
¼ teaspoon salt
¼ teaspoon freshly ground black pepper
½ cup shredded Cheddar cheese, divided
2 (6-inch) corn tortillas, cut into strips
Chopped fresh cilantro, for garnish
Plain yogurt, for serving

1. Heat the broiler to high.
2. In a large oven-safe skillet, heat the oil over medium-high heat.
3. Add the onion, red bell pepper, green bell pepper, zucchini, and garlic to the skillet, and cook for 3 to 5 minutes until the onion softens.
4. Add the black beans, enchilada sauce, cumin, salt, pepper, ¼ cup of cheese, and tortilla strips, and mix together. Top with the remaining ¼ cup of cheese.
5. Put the skillet under the broiler and broil for 5 to 8 minutes until the cheese is melted and bubbly. Garnish with cilantro and serve with yogurt on the side.

Per Serving
calories: 172 | fat: 7.1g | protein: 8.1g
carbs: 20.9g | fiber: 6.9g | sugar: 3.0g
sodium: 566mg

Crispy Parmesan Bean and Veggie Cups

Prep time: 10 minutes | Cook time: 5 minutes | Serves 4

1 cup grated Parmesan cheese, divided
1 (15-ounce / 425-g) can low-sodium white beans, drained and rinsed
1 cucumber, peeled and finely diced
½ cup finely diced red onion
¼ cup thinly sliced

fresh basil
1 garlic clove, minced
½ jalapeño pepper, diced
1 tablespoon extra-virgin olive oil
1 tablespoon balsamic vinegar
¼ teaspoon salt
Freshly ground black pepper, to taste

1. Heat a medium nonstick skillet over medium heat. Sprinkle 2 tablespoons of cheese in a thin circle in the center of the pan, flattening it with a spatula.
2. When the cheese melts, use a spatula to flip the cheese and lightly brown the other side.
3. Remove the cheese "pancake" from the pan and place into the cup of a muffin tin, bending it gently with your hands to fit in the muffin cup.
4. Repeat with the remaining cheese until you have 8 cups.
5. In a mixing bowl, combine the beans, cucumber, onion, basil, garlic, jalapeño, olive oil, and vinegar, and season with the salt and pepper.
6. Fill each cup with the bean mixture just before serving.

Per Serving
calories: 260 | fat: 12.1g | protein: 14.9
carbs: 23.9g | fiber: 8.0g | sugar: 3.9g
sodium: 552mg

Green Lentils with Summer Vegetables

Prep time: 15 minutes | Cook time: 0 minutes | Serves 4

3 tablespoons extra-virgin olive oil
2 tablespoons balsamic vinegar
2 teaspoons chopped fresh basil
1 teaspoon minced garlic
Sea salt and freshly ground black pepper, to taste
2 (15-ounce / 425-g) cans sodium-free green lentils, rinsed and drained
½ English cucumber, diced
2 tomatoes, diced
½ cup halved Kalamata olives
¼ cup chopped fresh chives
2 tablespoons pine nuts

1. Whisk together the olive oil, vinegar, basil, and garlic in a medium bowl. Season with salt and pepper.
2. Stir in the lentils, cucumber, tomatoes, olives, and chives.
3. Top with the pine nuts, and serve.

Per Serving
calories: 400 | fat: 15.1g | protein: 19.8g
carbs: 48.8g | fiber: 18.8g | sugar: 7.1g
sodium: 439mg

Triple Bean Chili

Prep time: 20 minutes | Cook time: 60 minutes | Serves 8

1 teaspoon extra-virgin olive oil
1 sweet onion, chopped
1 red bell pepper, seeded and diced
1 green bell pepper, seeded and diced
2 teaspoons minced garlic
1 (28-ounce / 794-g) can low-sodium diced tomatoes
1 (15-ounce / 425-g) can sodium-free black beans, rinsed and drained
1 (15-ounce / 425-g) can sodium-free red kidney beans, rinsed and drained
1 (15-ounce / 425-g) can sodium-free navy beans, rinsed and drained
2 tablespoons chili powder
2 teaspoons ground cumin
1 teaspoon ground coriander
¼ teaspoon red pepper flakes

1. Place a large saucepan over medium-high heat and add the oil.
2. Sauté the onion, red and green bell peppers, and garlic until the vegetables have softened, about 5 minutes.
3. Add the tomatoes, black beans, red kidney beans, navy beans, chili powder, cumin, coriander, and red pepper flakes to the pan.
4. Bring the chili to a boil, then reduce the heat to low.
5. Simmer the chili, stirring occasionally, for at least 1 hour.
6. Serve hot.

Per Serving
calories: 480 | fat: 28.1g | protein: 15.1g
carbs: 45.1g | fiber: 16.9g | sugar: 4.0g
sodium: 16mg

Eggplant and Bulgur Pilaf

Prep time: 10 minutes | Cook time: 60 minutes | Serves 4

1 tablespoon extra-virgin olive oil
½ sweet onion, chopped
2 teaspoons minced garlic
1 cup chopped eggplant
1½ cups bulgur
4 cups low-sodium chicken broth
1 cup diced tomato
Sea salt and freshly ground black pepper, to taste
2 tablespoons chopped fresh basil

1. Place a large saucepan over medium-high heat. Add the oil and sauté the onion and garlic until softened and translucent, about 3 minutes.
2. Stir in the eggplant and sauté 4 minutes to soften.
3. Stir in the bulgur, broth, and tomatoes. Bring the mixture to a boil.
4. Reduce the heat to low, cover, and simmer until the water has been absorbed, about 50 minutes.
5. Season the pilaf with salt and pepper.
6. Garnish with the basil, and serve.

Per Serving
calories: 300 | fat: 4.0g | protein: 14.0g
carbs: 54.0g | fiber: 12.0g | sugar: 7.0g
sodium: 358mg

Dandelion and Beet Greens with Black Beans

Prep time: 10 minutes | Cook time: 15 minutes | Serves 4

1 tablespoon olive oil
½ Vidalia onion, thinly sliced
1 bunch dandelion greens, cut into ribbons
1 bunch beet greens, cut into ribbons
½ cup low-sodium vegetable broth
1 (15-ounce / 425-g) can no-salt-added black beans
Salt and freshly ground black pepper, to taste

1. Heat the olive oil in a nonstick skillet over low heat until shimmering.
2. Add the onion and sauté for 3 minutes or until translucent.
3. Add the dandelion and beet greens, and broth to the skillet. Cover and cook for 8 minutes or until wilted.
4. Add the black beans and cook for 4 minutes or until soft. Sprinkle with salt and pepper. Stir to mix well.
5. Serve immediately.

Per Serving

calories: 161 | fat: 4.0g | protein: 9.0g
carbs: 26.0g | fiber: 10.0g | sugar: 1.0g
sodium: 224mg

Mexican Black Bean and Chicken Soup

Prep time: 10 minutes | Cook time: 25 minutes | Serves 7

2 tablespoons olive oil
½ onion, diced
1 pound (454 g) boneless and skinless chicken breast, cut into ½-inch cubes
½ teaspoon Adobo seasoning, divided
¼ teaspoon black pepper
1 (15-ounce / 425-g) can no-salt-added black beans, rinsed and drained
1 (14.5-ounce / 411-g) can fire-roasted tomatoes
½ cup frozen corn
½ teaspoon cumin
1 tablespoon chili powder
5 cups low-sodium chicken broth

1. Grease a stockpot with olive oil and heat over medium-high heat until shimmering.
2. Add the onion and sauté for 3 minutes or until translucent.
3. Add the chicken breast and sprinkle with Adobo seasoning and pepper. Put the lid on and cook for 6 minutes or until lightly browned. Shake the pot halfway through the cooking time.
4. Add the remaining ingredients. Reduce the heat to low and simmer for 15 minutes or until the black beans are soft.
5. Serve immediately.

Per Serving

calories: 170 | fat: 3.5g | protein: 20.0g
carbs: 15.0g | fiber: 5.0g | sugar: 3.0g
sodium: 390mg

Mushroom Rice with Hazelnut

Prep time: 20 minutes | Cook time: 35 minutes | Serves 8

1 tablespoon extra-virgin olive oil
1 cup chopped button mushrooms
½ sweet onion, chopped
1 celery stalk, chopped
2 teaspoons minced garlic
2 cups brown basmati rice
4 cups low-sodium chicken broth
1 teaspoon chopped fresh thyme
Sea salt and freshly ground black pepper, to taste
½ cup chopped hazelnuts

1. Place a large saucepan over medium-high heat and add the oil.
2. Sauté the mushrooms, onion, celery, and garlic until lightly browned, about 10 minutes.
3. Add the rice and sauté for an additional minute.
4. Add the chicken broth and bring to a boil.
5. Reduce the heat to low and cover the pot. Simmer until the liquid is absorbed and the rice is tender, about 20 minutes.
6. Stir in the thyme and season with salt and pepper.
7. Top with the hazelnuts, and serve.

Per Serving

calories: 240 | fat: 6.1g | protein: 7.1g
carbs: 38.9g | fiber: 0.9g | sugar: 1.1g
sodium: 388mg

Barley Kale and Squash Risotto

Prep time: 10 minutes | Cook time: 15 minutes | Serves 6

1 teaspoon extra-virgin olive oil	2 cups cooked butternut squash, cut into ½-inch cubes
½ sweet onion, finely chopped	2 tablespoons chopped pistachios
1 teaspoon minced garlic	1 tablespoon chopped fresh thyme
2 cups cooked barley	Sea salt, to taste
2 cups chopped kale	

1. Place a large skillet over medium heat and add the oil.
2. Sauté the onion and garlic until softened and translucent, about 3 minutes.
3. Add the barley and kale, and stir until the grains are heated through and the greens are wilted, about 7 minutes.
4. Stir in the squash, pistachios, and thyme.
5. Cook until the dish is hot, about 4 minutes, and season with salt.

Per Serving
calories: 160 | fat: 1.9g | protein: 5.1g
carbs: 32.1g | fiber: 7.0g | sugar: 2.0g
sodium: 63mg

Quinoa and Lush Vegetable Bowl

Prep time: 15 minutes | Cook time: 15 minutes | Serves 6

2 cups vegetable broth	lengthwise and cut into half disks
1 cup quinoa, well rinsed and drained	1 red bell pepper, seeded and cut into thin strips
1 teaspoon extra-virgin olive oil	1 cup fresh or frozen corn kernels
½ sweet onion, chopped	1 teaspoon chopped fresh basil
2 teaspoons minced garlic	Sea salt and freshly ground black pepper, to taste
½ large green zucchini, halved	

1. Place a medium saucepan over medium heat and add the vegetable broth. Bring the broth to a boil and add the quinoa. Cover and reduce the heat to low.
2. Cook until the quinoa has absorbed all the broth, about 15 minutes. Remove from the heat and let it cool slightly.
3. While the quinoa is cooking, place a large skillet over medium-high heat and add the oil.
4. Sauté the onion and garlic until softened and translucent, about 3 minutes.
5. Add the zucchini, bell pepper, and corn, and sauté until the vegetables are tender-crisp, about 5 minutes.
6. Remove the skillet from the heat. Add the cooked quinoa and the basil to the skillet, stirring to combine. Season with salt and pepper, and serve.

Per Serving
calories: 159 | fat: 3.0g | protein: 7.1g
carbs: 26.1g | fiber: 2.9g | sugar: 3.0g
sodium: 300mg

Couscous with Balsamic Dressing

Prep time: 10 minutes | Cook time: 5 minutes | Serves 6

For the Dressing:

¼ cup extra-virgin olive oil	1 teaspoon honey
2 tablespoons balsamic vinegar	Sea salt and freshly ground black pepper, to taste

For the Couscous:

1¼ cups whole-wheat couscous	green parts, chopped
Pinch sea salt	½ cup chopped pecans
1 teaspoon butter	2 tablespoons chopped fresh parsley
2 cups boiling water	
1 scallion, white and	

To Make the Dressing
1. Whisk together the oil, vinegar, and honey.
2. Season with salt and pepper and set it aside.

To Make the Couscous
1. Put the couscous, salt, and butter in a large heat-proof bowl and pour the boiling water on top. Stir and cover the bowl. Let it sit for 5 minutes. Uncover and fluff the couscous with a fork.
2. Stir in the dressing, scallion, pecans, and parsley.
3. Serve warm.

Per Serving
calories: 250 | fat: 12.9g | protein: 5.1g
carbs: 30.1g | fiber: 2.2g | sugar: 1.1g
sodium: 77mg

Easy Coconut Quinoa

Prep time: 15 minutes | Cook time: 25 minutes | Serves 4

2 teaspoons extra-virgin olive oil
1 sweet onion, chopped
1 tablespoon grated fresh ginger
2 teaspoons minced garlic
1 cup low-sodium chicken broth
1 cup coconut milk
1 cup quinoa, well rinsed and drained
Sea salt, to taste
¼ cup shredded, unsweetened coconut

1. Place a large saucepan over medium-high heat and add the oil.
2. Sauté the onion, ginger, and garlic until softened, about 3 minutes.
3. Add the chicken broth, coconut milk, and quinoa.
4. Bring the mixture to a boil, then reduce the heat to low and cover. Simmer the quinoa, stirring occasionally, until the quinoa is tender and most of the liquid has been absorbed, about 20 minutes.
5. Season the quinoa with salt, and serve topped with the coconut.

Per Serving
calories: 355 | fat: 21.1g | protein: 9.1g
carbs: 35.1g | fiber: 6.1g | sugar: 4.0g
sodium: 33mg

Herbed Beans and Brown Rice Bowl

Prep time: 15 minutes | Cook time: 15 minutes | Serves 8

2 teaspoons extra-virgin olive oil
½ sweet onion, chopped
1 teaspoon minced jalapeño pepper
1 teaspoon minced garlic
1 (15-ounce / 425-g) can sodium-free red kidney beans, rinsed
and drained
1 large tomato, chopped
1 teaspoon chopped fresh thyme
Sea salt and freshly ground black pepper, to taste
2 cups cooked brown rice

1. Place a large skillet over medium-high heat and add the olive oil.
2. Sauté the onion, jalapeño, and garlic until softened, about 3 minutes.
3. Stir in the beans, tomato, and thyme.

4. Cook until heated through, about 10 minutes. Season with salt and pepper.
5. Serve over the warm brown rice.

Per Serving
calories: 200 | fat: 2.1g | protein: 9.1g
carbs: 37.1g | fiber: 6.1g | sugar: 2.0g
sodium: 40mg

Crispy Cowboy Black Bean Fritters

Prep time: 10 minutes | Cook time: 25 minutes | Serves 20 Fritters

1¾ cups all-purpose flour
½ teaspoon cumin
2 teaspoons baking powder
2 teaspoons salt
½ teaspoon black pepper
4 egg whites, lightly
beaten
1 cup salsa
2 (16-ounce / 454-g) cans no-salt-added black beans, rinsed and drained
1 tablespoon canola oil, plus extra if needed

1. Combine the flour, cumin, baking powder, salt, and pepper in a large bowl, then mix in the egg whites and salsa. Add the black beans and stir to mix well.
2. Heat the canola oil in a nonstick skillet over medium-high heat.
3. Spoon 1 teaspoon of the mixture into the skillet to make a fritter. Make more fritters to coat the bottom of the skillet. Keep a little space between each two fritters. You may need to work in batches to avoid overcrowding.
4. Cook for 3 minutes or until the fritters are golden brown on both sides. Flip the fritters and flatten with a spatula halfway through the cooking time. Repeat with the remaining mixture. Add more oil as needed.
5. Serve immediately.

Per Serving
calories: 115 | fat: 1.0g | protein: 6.0g
carbs: 20.0g | fiber: 5.0g | sugar: 2.0g
sodium: 350mg

Brown Rice with Collard and Scrambled Egg

Prep time: 15 minutes | Cook time: 20 minutes | Serves 4

1 tablespoon extra-virgin olive oil
1 bunch collard greens, stemmed and cut into chiffonade
1 carrot, cut into 2-inch matchsticks
1 red onion, thinly sliced
½ cup low-sodium vegetable broth
2 tablespoons coconut aminos
1 garlic clove, minced
1 cup cooked brown rice
1 large egg
1 teaspoon red pepper flakes
1 teaspoon paprika
Salt, to taste

1. Heat the olive oil in a Dutch oven or a nonstick skillet over medium heat until shimmering.
2. Add the collard greens and sauté for 4 minutes or until wilted.
3. Add the carrot, onion, broth, coconut aminos, and garlic to the Dutch oven, then cover and cook 6 minutes or until the carrot is tender.
4. Add the brown rice and cook for 4 minutes. Keep stirring during the cooking.
5. Break the egg over them, then cook and scramble the egg for 4 minutes or until the egg is set.
6. Turn off the heat and sprinkle with red pepper flakes, paprika, and salt before serving.

Per Serving
calories: 154 | fat: 6.0g | protein: 6.0g
carbs: 22.0g | fiber: 6.0g | sugar: 2.0g
sodium: 78mg

Navy Bean Pico de Gallo

Prep time: 20 minutes | Cook time: 0 minutes | Serves 4

2½ cups cooked navy beans
1 tomato, diced
½ red bell pepper, seeded and chopped
¼ jalapeño pepper, chopped
1 scallion, white and green parts, chopped
1 teaspoon minced garlic
1 teaspoon ground cumin
½ teaspoon ground coriander
½ cup low-sodium feta cheese

1. Put the beans, tomato, bell pepper, jalapeño, scallion, garlic, cumin, and coriander in a medium bowl and stir until well mixed.
2. Top with the feta cheese and serve.

Per Serving
calories: 225 | fat: 4.1g | protein: 14.1g
carbs: 34.1g | fiber: 13.1g | sugar: 3.9g
sodium: 165mg

Tomato and Navy Bean Bake

Prep time: 10 minutes | Cook time: 25 minutes | Serves 8

1 teaspoon extra-virgin olive oil
½ sweet onion, chopped
2 teaspoons minced garlic
2 sweet potatoes, peeled and diced
1 (28-ounce / 794-g) can low-sodium diced tomatoes
¼ cup sodium-free tomato paste
2 tablespoons granulated sweetener
2 tablespoons hot sauce
1 tablespoon Dijon mustard
3 (15-ounce / 425-g) cans sodium-free navy or white beans, drained
1 tablespoon chopped fresh oregano

1. Place a large saucepan over medium-high heat and add the oil.
2. Sauté the onion and garlic until translucent, about 3 minutes.
3. Stir in the sweet potatoes, diced tomatoes, tomato paste, sweetener, hot sauce, and mustard and bring to a boil.
4. Reduce the heat and simmer the tomato sauce for 10 minutes.
5. Stir in the beans and simmer for 10 minutes more.
6. Stir in the oregano and serve.

Per Serving
calories: 256 | fat: 2.1g | protein: 15.1g
carbs: 48.1g | fiber: 11.9g | sugar: 8.1g
sodium: 150mg

Farro and Avocado Bowl

Prep time: 5 minutes | Cook time: 25 minutes | Serves 4

3 cups water
1 cup uncooked farro
1 tablespoon extra-virgin olive oil
1 teaspoon ground cumin
½ teaspoon salt
½ teaspoon freshly

ground black pepper
4 hardboiled eggs, sliced
1 avocado, sliced
⅓ cup plain low-fat Greek yogurt
4 lemon wedges

1. In a medium saucepan, bring the water to a boil over high heat.
2. Pour the farro into the boiling water, and stir to submerge the grains. Reduce the heat to medium and cook for 20 minutes. Drain and set aside.
3. Heat a medium skillet over medium-low heat. When hot, pour in the oil, then add the cooked farro, cumin, salt, and pepper. Cook for 3 to 5 minutes, stirring occasionally.
4. Divide the farro into four equal portions, and top each with one-quarter of the eggs, avocado, and yogurt. Add a squeeze of lemon over the top of each portion.

Per Serving
calories: 333 | fat: 16.1g | protein: 15.1g
carbs: 31.9g | fiber: 7.9g | sugar: 2.0g
sodium: 360mg

Black-Eyed Peas Curry

Prep time: 15 minutes | Cook time: 40 minutes | Serves 12

1 pound (454 g) dried black-eyed peas, rinsed and drained
4 cups vegetable broth
1 cup coconut water
1 cup chopped onion
4 large carrots, coarsely chopped
1½ tablespoons curry

powder
1 tablespoon minced garlic
1 teaspoon peeled and minced fresh ginger
1 tablespoon extra-virgin olive oil
Kosher salt (optional)
Lime wedges, for serving

1. In the electric pressure cooker, combine the black-eyed peas, broth, coconut water, onion, carrots, curry powder, garlic, and ginger. Drizzle the olive oil over the top.

2. Close and lock the lid of the pressure cooker. Set the valve to sealing.
3. Cook on high pressure for 25 minutes.
4. When the cooking is complete, hit Cancel and allow the pressure to release naturally for 10 minutes, then quick release any remaining pressure.
5. Once the pin drops, unlock and remove the lid.
6. Season with salt (if using) and squeeze some fresh lime juice on each serving.

Per Serving
calories: 113 | fat: 3.1g | protein: 10.1g
carbs: 30.9g | fiber: 6.1g | sugar: 6.0g
sodium: 672mg

Crispy Baked Flounder with Green Beans

Prep time: 10 minutes | Cook time: 20 minutes | Serves 4

1 pound (454 g) flounder
2 cups green beans
4 tablespoons margarine
8 basil leaves
1.75 ounces (50 g) pork rinds

½ cup reduced fat Parmesan cheese
3 cloves garlic
Salt and ground black pepper, to taste
Nonstick cooking spray

1. Heat oven to 350ºF (180ºC). Spray a baking dish with cooking spray.
2. Steam green beans until they are almost tender, about 15 minutes, less if you use frozen or canned beans. Lay green beans in the prepared dish.
3. Place the fish filets over the green beans and season with salt and pepper.
4. Place the garlic, basil, pork rinds, and Parmesan in a food processor and pulse until mixture resembles crumbs. Sprinkle over fish. Cut margarine into small pieces and place on top.
5. Bake 15 to 20 minutes or until fish flakes easily with a fork. Serve.

Per Serving
calories: 360 | fat: 20.0g | protein: 39.1g
carbs: 5.1g | fiber: 2.0g | sugar: 1.0g
sodium: 322mg

Classic Texas Caviar

Prep time: 10 minutes | Cook time: 0 minutes | Serves 6

For the Salad:

1 ear fresh corn, kernels removed

1 cup cooked lima beans

1 cup cooked black-eyed peas

1 red bell pepper, chopped

2 celery stalks, chopped

½ red onion, chopped

For the Dressing:

3 tablespoons apple cider vinegar

1 teaspoon paprika

2 tablespoons extra-virgin olive oil

1. Combine the corn, beans, peas, bell pepper, celery, and onion in a large bowl. Stir to mix well.
2. Combine the vinegar, paprika, and olive oil in a small bowl. Stir to combine well.
3. Pour the dressing into the salad and toss to mix well. Let sit for 20 minutes to infuse before serving.

Per Serving

calories: 170 | fat: 5.0g | protein: 10.0g carbs: 29.0g | fiber: 10.0g | sugar: 4.0g sodium: 20mg

Black Bean and Tomato Soup with Lime Yogurt

Prep time: 8 hours 10 minutes | Cook time: 1 hour 33 minutes | Serves 8

2 tablespoons avocado oil

1 medium onion, chopped

1 (10-ounce / 284-g) can diced tomatoes and green chilies

1 pound (454 g) dried black beans, soaked in water for at least 8 hours, rinsed

1 teaspoon ground cumin

3 garlic cloves, minced

6 cups chicken bone broth, vegetable broth, or water

Kosher salt, to taste

1 tablespoon freshly squeezed lime juice

¼ cup plain Greek yogurt

1. Heat the avocado oil in a nonstick skillet over medium heat until shimmering.
2. Add the onion and sauté for 3 minutes or until translucent.
3. Transfer the onion to a pot, then add the tomatoes and green chilies and their juices, black beans, cumin, garlic, broth, and salt. Stir to combine well.
4. Bring to a boil over medium-high heat, then reduce the heat to low. Simmer for 1 hour and 30 minutes or until the beans are soft.
5. Meanwhile, combine the lime juice with Greek yogurt in a small bowl. Stir to mix well.
6. Pour the soup in a large serving bowl, then drizzle with lime yogurt before serving.

Per Serving (1 Cup)

calories: 285 | fat: 6.0g | protein: 19.0g carbs: 42.0g | fiber: 10.0g | sugar: 3.0g sodium: 174mg

Red Kidney Beans with Green Beans

Prep time: 10 minutes | Cook time: 8 to 12 minutes | Serves 8

2 tablespoons olive oil

1 medium yellow onion, chopped

1 cup crushed tomatoes

2 garlic cloves, minced

2 cups low-sodium

canned red kidney beans, rinsed

1 cup roughly chopped green beans

¼ cup low-sodium vegetable broth

1 teaspoon smoked paprika

Salt, to taste

1. Heat the olive oil in a nonstick skillet over medium heat until shimmering.
2. Add the onion, tomatoes, and garlic. Sauté for 3 to 5 minutes or until fragrant and the onion is translucent.
3. Add the kidney beans, green beans, and broth to the skillet. Sprinkle with paprika and salt, then sauté to combine well.
4. Cover the skillet and cook for 5 to 7 minutes or until the vegetables are tender. Serve immediately.

Per Serving

calories: 187 | fat: 1.0g | protein: 13.0g carbs: 34.0g | fiber: 10.0g | sugar: 4.0g sodium: 102mg

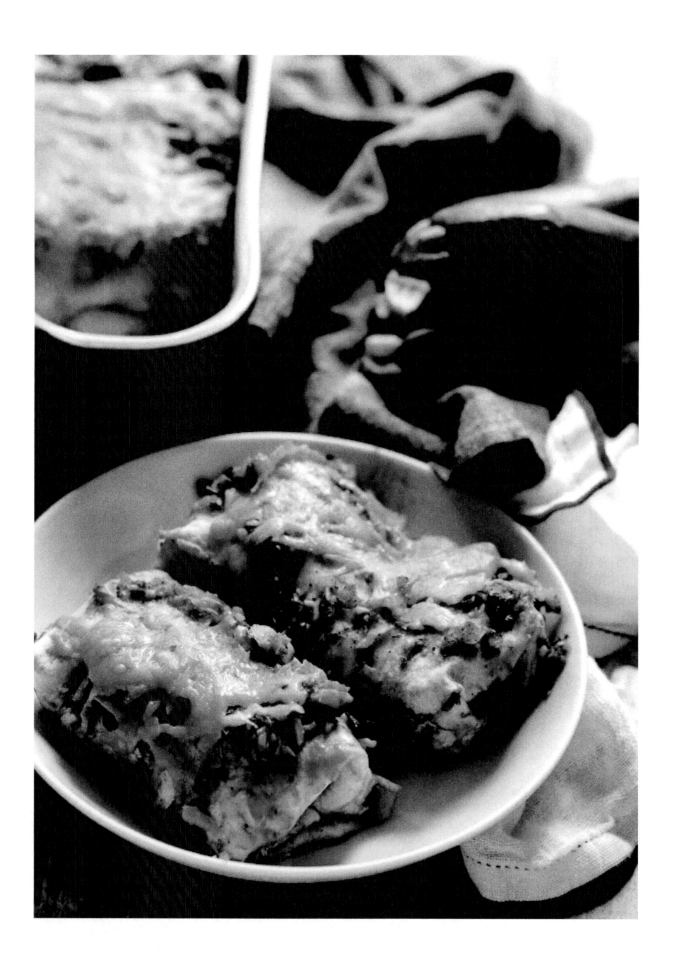

Chapter 6: Meatless Mains

Vegetable Enchilada Casserole

Prep time: 15 minutes | Cook time: 15 minutes | Serves 6

1 tablespoon extra-virgin olive oil
½ onion, chopped
3 garlic cloves, minced
½ green bell pepper, deseeded and chopped
½ red bell pepper, deseeded and chopped
2 small zucchinis, chopped
1 (10-ounce / 284-g) can low-sodium enchilada sauce
1 (15-ounce / 425-g) can low-sodium black beans, drained and rinsed
1 teaspoon ground cumin
½ cup shredded Cheddar cheese, divided
2 (6-inch) corn tortillas, cut into strips
¼ teaspoon salt
¼ teaspoon freshly ground black pepper
Chopped fresh cilantro, for garnish
Plain yogurt, for serving

1. Preheat the broiler to high.
2. Heat the olive oil in a large ovenproof skillet until it shimmers.
3. Stir in the onion, garlic, bell peppers, and zucchinis and sauté for 3 to 5 minutes, or until the onion is translucent.
4. Add the enchilada sauce, black beans, cumin, ¼ cup of cheese, tortilla strips, salt, and pepper and whisk to combine. Scatter the top with the remaining ¼ cup of cheese.
5. Place the skillet under the broiler and broil until the cheese melts, 5 to 8 minutes.
6. Sprinkle the cilantro on top for garnish and serve topped with the yogurt.

Per Serving
calories: 172 | fat: 7.2g | protein: 8.3g
carbs: 21.2g | fiber: 7.2g | sugar: 3.2g
sodium: 563mg

Zucchini and Pinto Bean Casserole

Prep time: 15 minutes | Cook time: 15 minutes | Serves 4

1 (6 to 7-inch) zucchini, trimmed
Nonstick cooking spray
1 (15-ounce / 425-g) can pinto beans
or 1½ cups Salt-Free No-Soak Beans, rinsed and drained
1⅓ cups salsa
1⅓ cups shredded Mexican cheese blend

1. Slice the zucchini into rounds. You'll need at least 16 slices.
2. Spray a 6-inch cake pan with nonstick spray.
3. Put the beans into a medium bowl and mash some of them with a fork.
4. Cover the bottom of the pan with about 4 zucchini slices. Add about ⅓ of the beans, ⅓ cup of salsa, and ⅓ cup of cheese. Press down. Repeat for 2 more layers. Add the remaining zucchini, salsa, and cheese. (There are no beans in the top layer.)
5. Cover the pan loosely with foil.
6. Pour 1 cup of water into the electric pressure cooker.
7. Place the pan on the wire rack and carefully lower it into the pot. Close and lock the lid of the pressure cooker. Set the valve to sealing.
8. Cook on high pressure for 15 minutes.
9. When the cooking is complete, hit Cancel and allow the pressure to release naturally.
10. Once the pin drops, unlock and remove the lid.
11. Carefully remove the pan from the pot, lifting by the handles of the wire rack. Let the casserole sit for 5 minutes before slicing into quarters and serving.

Per Serving
calories: 251 | fat: 12.1g | protein: 16.1g
carbs: 22.9g | fiber: 7.1g | sugar: 4.0g
sodium: 1080mg

Pita Stuffed with Tabbouleh

Prep time: 20 minutes | Cook time: 0 minutes | Serves 4

1 cup cooked bulgur wheat
1 English cucumber, finely chopped
1 yellow bell pepper, deseeded and finely chopped
2 cups halved cherry tomatoes
½ cup fresh parsley, finely chopped

2 scallions, white and green parts, finely chopped
Juice of 1 lemon
2 tablespoons extra-virgin olive oil
Salt and freshly ground black pepper, to taste
4 whole-wheat pitas, cut in half

1. Combine the bulgur wheat, cucumber, bell pepper, tomatoes, parsley, scallions, lemon juice, and olive oil in a large bowl and stir to mix well. Season with salt and pepper to taste.
2. Place the pita halves on a clean work surface. Evenly divide the bulgur mixture among pita halves and serve immediately.

Per Serving
calories: 245 | fat: 8.2g | protein: 7.2g
carbs: 39.2g | fiber: 6.2g | sugar: 4.2g
sodium: 166mg

Egg and Pea Salad in Kale Wraps

Prep time: 10 minutes | Cook time: 0 minutes | Serves 2

4 hard-boiled large eggs, chopped
1 cup fresh peas, shelled
2 tablespoons red onion, finely chopped
½ teaspoon sea salt
¼ teaspoon paprika

1 teaspoon Dijon mustard
1 tablespoon fresh dill, chopped
3 tablespoons mayonnaise
2 large kale leaves

1. Combine all the ingredients, except for the kale leaves, in a bowl. Stir to mix well.
2. Divide and spoon the mixture on the kale leaves, then roll up the leaves to wrap the mixture. Serve immediately.

Per Serving
calories: 296 | fat: 18.2g | protein: 17.2g
carbs: 18.2g | fiber: 4.2g | sugar: 12.3
sodium: 623mg

Crock Pot Stroganoff

Prep time: 10 minutes | Cook time: 2 hours | Serves 2

8 cups mushrooms, cut into quarters
1 onion, halved and sliced thin
4 tablespoons fresh parsley, chopped
1½ tablespoons low fat sour cream

1 cup low sodium vegetable broth
3 cloves garlic, diced fine
2 teaspoons smoked paprika
Salt and ground black pepper, to taste

1. Add all , except sour cream and parsley to crock pot.cover and cook on high 2 hours.
2. Stir in sour cream and serve garnished with parsley.

Per Serving
calories: 113 | fat: 2.0g | protein: 10.1g
carbs: 18.1g | fiber: 4.0g | sugar: 8.0g
sodium: 595mg

Collard Greens with Tomato

Prep time: 10 minutes | Cook time: 20 minutes | Serves 4

1 cup low-sodium vegetable broth, divided
½ onion, thinly sliced
2 garlic cloves, thinly sliced
1 medium tomato, chopped

1 large bunch collard greens including stems, roughly chopped
1 teaspoon ground cumin
½ teaspoon freshly ground black pepper

1. Add ½ cup of vegetable broth to a Dutch oven over medium heat and bring to a simmer.
2. Stir in the onion and garlic and cook for about 4 minutes until tender.
3. Add the remaining broth, tomato, greens, cumin, and pepper, and gently stir to combine.
4. Reduce the heat to low and simmer uncovered for 15 minutes. Serve warm.

Per Serving
calories: 68 | fat: 2.1g | protein: 4.8g
carbs: 13.8g | fiber: 7.1g | sugar: 2.0g
sodium: 67mg

Wilted Dandelion Greens with Sweet Onion

Prep time: 15 minutes | Cook time: 12 minutes | Serves 4

1 tablespoon extra-virgin olive oil
1 Vidalia onion, thinly sliced
2 garlic cloves, minced
2 bunches dandelion greens, roughly chopped
½ cup low-sodium vegetable broth
Freshly ground black pepper, to taste

1. Heat the olive oil in a large skillet over low heat.
2. Cook the onion and garlic for 2 to 3 minutes until tender, stirring occasionally.
3. Add the dandelion greens and broth and cook for 5 to 7 minutes, stirring frequently, or until the greens are wilted.
4. Transfer to a plate and season with black pepper. Serve warm.

Per Serving
calories: 81 | fat: 3.8g | protein: 3.1g
carbs: 10.7g | fiber: 3.8g | sugar: 2.0g
sodium: 72mg

Grilled Tofu and Veggie Skewers

Prep time: 15 minutes | Cook time: 15 minutes | Serves 6

1 block tofu
2 small zucchini, sliced
1 red bell pepper, cut into 1-inch cubes
1 yellow bell pepper, cut into 1-inch cubes
1 red onion, cut into 1-inch cubes
2 cups cherry tomatoes
2 tablespoons lite soy sauce
3 teaspoons barbecue sauce
2 teaspoons sesame seeds
Salt and ground black pepper, to taste
Nonstick cooking spray

1. Press tofu to extract liquid, for about half an hour. Then, cut tofu into cubes and marinate in soy sauce for at least 15 minutes.
2. Heat the grill to medium-high heat. Spray the grill rack with cooking spray.
3. Assemble skewers with tofu alternating with vegetables.
4. Grill for 2 to 3 minutes per side until vegetables start to soften, and tofu is golden brown. At the very end of cooking time, season with salt and pepper and brush with barbecue sauce. Serve garnished with sesame seeds.

Per Serving
calories: 65 | fat: 2.0g | protein: 5.1g
carbs: 10.1g | fiber: 3.0g | sugar: 6.0g
sodium: 237mg

Veggie Fajitas with Guacamole

Prep time: 10 minutes | Cook time: 15 minutes | Serves 4

For the Guacamole:
2 small avocados pitted and peeled
1 teaspoon freshly squeezed lime juice
¼ teaspoon salt
9 cherry tomatoes, halved

For the Fajitas:
1 red bell pepper
1 green bell pepper
1 small white onion
Avocado oil cooking spray
1 cup canned low-sodium black beans, drained and rinsed
½ teaspoon ground cumin
¼ teaspoon chili powder
¼ teaspoon garlic powder
4 (6-inch) yellow corn tortillas

To Make the Guacamole
1. In a medium bowl, use a fork to mash the avocados with the lime juice and salt.
2. Gently stir in the cherry tomatoes.

To Make the Fajitas
1. Cut the red bell pepper, green bell pepper, and onion into ½-inch slices.
2. Heat a large skillet over medium heat. When hot, coat the cooking surface with cooking spray. Put the peppers, onion, and beans into the skillet.
3. Add the cumin, chili powder, and garlic powder, and stir.
4. Cover and cook for 15 minutes, stirring halfway through.
5. Divide the fajita mixture equally between the tortillas, and top with guacamole and any preferred garnishes.

Per Serving
calories: 270 | fat: 15.1g | protein: 8.1g
carbs: 29.9g | fiber: 11.1g | sugar: 5.0g
sodium: 176mg

Spaghetti Squash and Chickpea Bolognese

Prep time: 5 minutes | Cook time: 25 minutes | Serves 4

1 (3- to 4-pound / 1.4- to 1.8-kg) spaghetti squash
½ teaspoon ground cumin
1 cup no-sugar-added spaghetti sauce
1 (15-ounce / 425-g) can low-sodium chickpeas, drained and rinsed
6 ounces (170 g) extra-firm tofu

1. Preheat the oven to 400ºF (205ºC).
2. Cut the squash in half lengthwise. Scoop out the seeds and discard.
3. Season both halves of the squash with the cumin, and place them on a baking sheet cut-side down. Roast for 25 minutes.
4. Meanwhile, heat a medium saucepan over low heat, and pour in the spaghetti sauce and chickpeas.
5. Press the tofu between two layers of paper towels, and gently squeeze out any excess water.
6. Crumble the tofu into the sauce and cook for 15 minutes.
7. Remove the squash from the oven, and comb through the flesh of each half with a fork to make thin strands.
8. Divide the "spaghetti" into four portions, and top each portion with one-quarter of the sauce.

Per Serving
calories: 276 | fat: 7.1g | protein: 14.1g
carbs: 41.9g | fiber: 10.1g | sugar: 7.0g
sodium: 56mg

Chimichurri Dumplings

Prep time: 20 minutes | Cook time: 15 minutes | Serves 8 to 10

4 cups water
4 cups low-sodium vegetable broth
1 cup cassava flour
1 cup gluten-free all-purpose flour
2 teaspoons baking powder
1 teaspoon salt
1 cup fat-free milk
2 tablespoons bottled chimichurri or sofrito

1. In a large pot, bring the water and the broth to a slow boil over medium-high heat.
2. In a large mixing bowl, whisk the cassava flour, all-purpose flour, baking powder, and salt together.
3. In a small bowl, whisk the milk and chimichurri together until combined.
4. Stir the wet ingredients into the dry ingredients a little at a time to create a firm dough.
5. With clean hands, pinch off a small piece of dough. Roll into a ball, and gently flatten in the palm of your hand, forming a disk. Repeat until no dough remains.
6. Carefully drop the dumplings one at a time into the boiling liquid. Cover and simmer for 15 minutes, or until the dumplings are cooked through. You can test by inserting a fork into the dumpling; it should come out clean.
7. Serve warm.

Per Serving
calories: 133 | fat: 1.1g | protein: 4.1g
carbs: 25.9g | fiber: 3.1g | sugar: 2.0g
sodium: 328mg

Cheesy Vegetable and Hummus Pitas

Prep time: 15 minutes | Cook time: 0 minutes | Serves 4

4 whole wheat pitas, sliced into pockets
2 tablespoons light mayonnaise
½ cup hummus
2¼ ounces (64 g) reduced-fat Swiss cheese, cut into 4 slices
¼ cup sunflower seeds
1 large tomato, cut into 4 equal slices
1 medium cucumber, sliced
1 medium red onion, thinly sliced
4 romaine lettuce leaves

1. Smear the insides of the pita pockets with mayo.
2. Divide the hummus on each cheese slice and smear to spread evenly, then sprinkle with sunflower seeds.
3. Sit the tomato slices, cucumber slices, onion slices, and lettuce leaves on top of the hummus alternatively.
4. Then stuff the pitas with these slices and serve immediately.

Per Serving
calories: 170 | fat: 6.0g | protein: 8.0g
carbs: 23.0g | fiber: 4.0g | sugar: 7.0g
sodium: 280mg

Redux Okra Callaloo

Prep time: 15 minutes | Cook time: 25 minutes | Serves 6

3 cups low-sodium vegetable broth
1 (13.5-ounce / 383-g) can light coconut milk
¼ cup coconut cream
1 tablespoon unsalted non-hydrogenated plant-based butter
12 ounces (340 g) okra, cut into 1-inch chunks

1 small onion, chopped
½ butternut squash, peeled, seeded, and cut into 4-inch chunks
1 bunch collard greens, stemmed and chopped
1 hot pepper (Scotch bonnet or habanero)

1. In an electric pressure cooker, combine the vegetable broth, coconut milk, coconut cream, and butter.
2. Layer the okra, onion, squash, collard greens, and whole hot pepper on top.
3. Close and lock the lid, and set the pressure valve to sealing.
4. Select the Manual/Pressure Cook setting, and cook for 20 minutes.
5. Once cooking is complete, quick-release the pressure. Carefully remove the lid.
6. Remove and discard the hot pepper. Carefully transfer the callaloo to a blender, and blend until smooth. Serve spooned over grits.

Per Serving
calories: 174 | fat: 8.1g | protein: 4.1g
carbs: 24.9g | fiber: 5.1g | sugar: 10.0g
sodium: 126mg

Baby Spinach Mini Quiches

Prep time: 10 minutes | Cook time: 15 minutes | Serves 6

Nonstick cooking spray
2 tablespoons extra-virgin olive oil
1 onion, finely chopped
2 cups baby spinach
2 garlic cloves,

minced
8 large eggs, beaten
¼ cup whole milk
½ teaspoon sea salt
¼ teaspoon freshly ground black pepper
1 cup shredded Swiss cheese

1. Preheat the oven to 375ºF (190ºC). Spray a 6-cup muffin tin with nonstick cooking spray.

2. In a large skillet over medium-high heat, heat the olive oil until it shimmers. Add the onion and cook until soft, about 4 minutes. Add the spinach and cook, stirring, until the spinach softens, about 1 minute. Add the garlic. Cook, stirring constantly, for 30 seconds. Remove from heat and let cool.
3. In a medium bowl, beat together the eggs, milk, salt, and pepper.
4. Fold the cooled vegetables and the cheese into the egg mixture. Spoon the mixture into the prepared muffin tins. Bake until the eggs are set, about 15 minutes. Allow to rest for 5 minutes before serving.

Per Serving
calories: 220 | fat: 17.1g | protein: 14.1g
carbs: 3.9g | fiber: 1.0g | sugar: 2.9g
sodium: 238mg

Vegetable Egg Bake with Avocado

Prep time: 5 minutes | Cook time: 25 minutes | Serves 4

2 tablespoons extra-virgin olive oil
1 red onion, chopped
1 green bell pepper, seeded and chopped
1 sweet potato, cut into ½-inch pieces
1 teaspoon chili

powder
½ teaspoon sea salt
4 large eggs
½ cup shredded pepper Jack cheese
1 avocado, cut into cubes

1. Preheat the oven to 350ºF (180ºC).
2. In a large, ovenproof skillet over medium-high heat, heat the olive oil until it shimmers. Add the onion, bell pepper, sweet potato, chili powder, and salt, and cook, stirring occasionally, until the vegetables start to brown, about 10 minutes.
3. Remove from heat. Arrange the vegetables in the pan to form 4 wells. Crack an egg into each well. Sprinkle the cheese on the vegetables, around the edges of the eggs.
4. Bake until the eggs set, about 10 minutes.
5. Top with avocado before serving.

Per Serving
calories: 285 | fat: 21.1g | protein: 12.1g
carbs: 15.9g | fiber: 5.1g | sugar: 10.0g
sodium: 265mg

Tofu and Broccoli Stir-Fry

Prep time: 10 minutes | Cook time: 20 minutes | Serves 4

3 tablespoons extra-virgin olive oil
4 scallions, sliced
12 ounces (340 g) firm tofu, cut into ½-inch pieces
4 cups broccoli, broken into florets
4 garlic cloves, minced
1 teaspoon peeled

and grated fresh ginger
¼ cup vegetable broth
2 tablespoons soy sauce (use gluten-free soy sauce if necessary)
1 cup cooked brown rice

1. In a large skillet over medium-high heat, heat the olive oil until it shimmers. Add the scallions, tofu, and broccoli and cook, stirring, until the vegetables begin to soften, about 6 minutes. Add the garlic and ginger and cook, stirring constantly, for 30 seconds.
2. Add the broth, soy sauce, and rice. Cook, stirring, 1 to 2 minutes more to heat the rice through.

Per Serving
calories: 235 | fat: 13.1g | protein: 11.1g
carbs: 20.9g | fiber: 4.1g | sugar: 12.3g
sodium: 362mg

Mushroom and Broccoli Frittata

Prep time: 5 minutes | Cook time: 10 minutes | Serves 4

2 tablespoons extra-virgin olive oil
½ onion, finely chopped
1 cup broccoli florets
1 cup sliced shiitake

mushrooms
1 garlic clove, minced
8 large eggs, beaten
½ teaspoon sea salt
½ cup grated Parmesan cheese

1. Preheat the oven broiler on high.
2. In a medium ovenproof skillet over medium-high heat, heat the olive oil until it shimmers.
3. Add the onion, broccoli, and mushrooms, and cook, stirring occasionally, until the vegetables start to brown, about 5 minutes. Add the garlic and cook, stirring constantly, for 30 seconds. Arrange the vegetables in an even layer on the bottom of the pan.
4. While the vegetables cook, in a small bowl, whisk together the eggs and salt. Carefully pour the eggs over the vegetables. Cook without stirring, allowing the eggs to set around the vegetables. As the eggs begin to set around the edges, use a spatula to pull the edges away from the sides of the pan. Tilt the pan and allow the uncooked eggs to run into the spaces. Cook 1 to 2 minutes more, until it sets around the edges. The eggs will still be runny on top.
5. Sprinkle with the Parmesan and place the pan in the broiler. Broil until brown and puffy, about 3 minutes.
6. Cut into wedges to serve.

Per Serving
calories: 281 | fat: 21.1g | protein: 19.1g
carbs: 6.9g | fiber: 2.1g | sugar: 4.0g
sodium: 655mg

Sautéed Zucchini and Tomatoes

Prep time: 10 minutes | Cook time: 10 minutes | Serves 4

1 tablespoon vegetable oil
1 sliced onion
2 pounds (907 g) zucchini, peeled and cut into 1-inch-thick slices

2 tomatoes, chopped
1 green bell pepper, chopped
Salt and freshly ground black pepper, to taste

1. Heat the vegetable oil in a nonstick skillet until it shimmers.
2. Sauté the onion slices in the oil for about 3 minutes until translucent, stirring occasionally.
3. Add the zucchini, tomatoes, bell pepper, salt, and pepper to the skillet and stir to combine.
4. Reduce the heat, cover, and continue cooking for about 5 minutes, or until the veggies are tender.
5. Remove from the heat to a large plate and serve hot.

Per Serving
calories: 110 | fat: 4.4g | protein: 6.9g
carbs: 10.7g | fiber: 3.4g | sugar: 2.2g
sodium: 11mg

Tomato, Lentil and Chickpea Curry

Prep time: 10 minutes | Cook time: 25 minutes | Serves 6

1 tablespoon extra-virgin olive oil
1 sweet onion, chopped
1 teaspoon minced garlic
1 tablespoon grated fresh ginger
2 tablespoons red curry paste
½ teaspoon turmeric
1 teaspoon ground cumin
Pinch cayenne pepper
2 cups cooked lentils
1 (28-ounce / 794-g) can low-sodium diced tomatoes
1 (15-ounce / 425-g) can water-packed chickpeas, rinsed and drained
¼ cup coconut milk
2 tablespoons chopped fresh cilantro

1. Heat the olive oil in a large saucepan over medium-high heat.
2. Add the onion, garlic, and ginger and sauté for about 3 minutes until tender, stirring occasionally.
3. Stir in the red curry paste, turmeric, cumin, and cayenne pepper and sauté for another 1 minute.
4. Add the cooked lentils, tomatoes, chickpeas, and coconut milk and stir to combine, then bring the curry to a boil.
5. Once it starts to boil, reduce the heat to low and bring to a simmer for 20 minutes.
6. Serve garnished with the cilantro.

Per Serving
calories: 340 | fat: 8.2g | protein: 18.2g
carbs: 50.2g | fiber: 20.2g | sugar: 9.2g
sodium: 25mg | Cholesterol: 0mg

Cheesy Quinoa Casserole

Prep time: 20 minutes | Cook time: 30 minutes | Serves 4

1 teaspoon extra-virgin olive oil
½ sweet onion, chopped
2 teaspoons minced garlic
2 eggs, whisked
2 cups cooked quinoa
2 cups cherry tomatoes
½ cup low-fat ricotta cheese
Salt and freshly ground black pepper, to taste
1 zucchini, cut into thin ribbons
⅛ cup toasted pine nuts

1. Preheat the oven to 350ºF (180ºC).
2. Heat the olive oil in a medium skillet over medium-high heat.
3. Sauté the onion and garlic for 3 minutes, stirring occasionally, or until softened.
4. Remove the skillet from the heat. Add the whisked eggs, cooked quinoa, cherry tomatoes, and cheese and stir to incorporate. Sprinkle with salt and pepper. Transfer the mixture to a baking dish.
5. Sprinkle the top with the zucchini ribbons and pine nuts. Bake in the preheated oven for about 25 minutes, or until the casserole is heated through.
6. Cool for 5 to 10 minutes before serving.

Per Serving
calories: 305 | fat: 9.3g | protein: 17.2g
carbs: 38.2g | fiber: 4.2g | sugar: 5.2g
sodium: 236mg | cholesterol: 122mg

Chili Relleno Casserole

Prep time: 5 minutes | Cook time: 35 minutes | Serves 8

3 eggs
1 cup Monterey jack pepper cheese, grated
¾ cup half-and-half
½ cup cheddar cheese, grated
2 (7-ounce / 198-g) cans whole green chilies, drain well
½ teaspoon salt
Nonstick cooking spray

1. Heat oven to 350ºF (180ºC). Spray a baking pan with cooking spray.
2. Slice each chili down one long side and lay flat.
3. Arrange half the chilies in the prepared baking pan, skin side down, in single layer.
4. Sprinkle with the pepper cheese and top with remaining chilies, skin side up.
5. In a small bowl, beat eggs, salt, and half-and-half. Pour over chilies. Top with cheddar cheese.
6. Bake 35 minutes, or until top is golden brown. Let rest 10 minutes before serving.

Per Serving
calories: 296 | fat: 13.0g | protein: 13.1g
carbs: 36.1g | fiber: 14.0g | sugar: 21.0g
sodium: 463mg

Scrambled Egg Whites with Bell Pepper

Prep time: 5 minutes | Cook time: 10 minutes | Serves 2

2 tablespoons extra-virgin olive oil
1 green bell pepper, deseeded and finely chopped
½ red onion, finely chopped
4 eggs whites
½ teaspoon sea salt
2 ounces (57 g) pepper Jack cheese, grated

1. Heat the olive oil in a nonstick skillet over medium-high heat..
2. Add the bell pepper and onion to the skillet and sauté for 5 minutes or until tender.
3. Sprinkle the egg white with salt in a bowl, then pour the egg whites in the skillet. Cook for 3 minutes or until the egg whites are scrambled. Stir the egg whites halfway through.
4. Scatter with cheese and cook for an additional 1 minutes until the cheese melts.
5. Divide them onto two serving plates and serve warm.

Per Serving
calories: 316 | fat: 23.3g | protein: 22.3g
carbs: 6.2g | fiber: 1.1g | sugar: 4.2g
sodium: 975mg

Cheesy Mushroom and Pesto Flatbreads

Prep time: 5 minutes | Cook time: 13 to 17 minutes | Serves 2

1 teaspoon extra-virgin olive oil
½ red onion, sliced
½ cup sliced mushrooms
Salt and freshly ground black pepper,
to taste
¼ cup store-bought pesto sauce
2 whole-wheat flatbreads
¼ cup shredded Mozzarella cheese

1. Preheat the oven to 350ºF (180ºC).
2. Heat the olive oil in a small skillet over medium heat. Add the onion slices and mushrooms to the skillet, and sauté for 3 to 5 minutes, stirring occasionally, or until they start to soften. Season with salt and pepper.
3. Meanwhile, spoon 2 tablespoons of pesto sauce onto each flatbread and spread it all over. Evenly divide the mushroom mixture between two flatbreads, then scatter each top with 2 tablespoons of shredded cheese.
4. Transfer the flatbreads to a baking sheet and bake until the cheese melts and bubbles, about 10 to 12 minutes.
5. Let the flatbreads cool for 5 minutes and serve warm.

Per Serving
calories: 346 | fat: 22.8g | protein: 14.2g
carbs: 27.6g | fiber: 7.3g | sugar: 4.0g
sodium: 790mg

Zoodles with Beet and Walnut Pesto

Prep time: 20 minutes | Cook time: 40 minutes | Serves 2

1 medium red beet, peeled, chopped
½ cup walnut pieces, toasted
½ cup crumbled goat cheese
3 garlic cloves
2 tablespoons freshly
squeezed lemon juice
2 tablespoons plus 2 teaspoons extra-virgin olive oil, divided
¼ teaspoon salt
4 small zucchini, spiralized

1. Preheat the oven to 375ºF (190ºC).
2. Wrap the red beet in aluminum foil, making sure to seal the foil completely.
3. Roast in the preheated oven for 30 to 40 minutes until tender.
4. When ready, transfer the red beet to a food processor. Fold in the toasted walnut, goat cheese, garlic, lemon juice, 2 tablespoons of olive oil, and salt and pulse until smooth. Transfer the beet mixture to a small bowl.
5. Heat the remaining 2 teaspoons of olive oil in a large skillet over medium heat. Add the zucchini, tossing to coat in the oil. Cook for 2 to 3 minutes, stirring constantly, or until the zucchini is softened.
6. Remove the zucchini from the heat to a plate and top with the beet mixture. Toss well and serve warm.

Per Serving
calories: 424 | fat: 39.3g | protein: 8.1g
carbs: 17.2g | fiber: 6.2g | sugar: 10.1g
sodium: 340mg

Homemade Vegetable Chili

Prep time: 10 minutes | Cook time: 15 minutes | Serves 4

2 tablespoons extra-virgin olive oil
1 onion, finely chopped
1 green bell pepper, deseeded and chopped
1 (14-ounce / 397-g) can kidney beans, drained and rinsed

2 (14-ounce / 397-g) cans crushed tomatoes
2 cups veggie crumbles
1 teaspoon garlic powder
1 tablespoon chili powder
½ teaspoon sea salt

1. Heat the olive oil in a large skillet over medium-high heat until shimmering.
2. Add the onion and bell pepper and sauté for 5 minutes, stirring occasionally.
3. Fold in the beans, tomatoes, veggie crumbles, garlic powder, chili powder, and salt. Stir to incorporate and bring them to a simmer.
4. Reduce the heat and cook for an additional 5 minutes, stirring occasionally, or until the mixture is heated through.
5. Allow the mixture to cool for 5 minutes and serve warm.

Per Serving
calories: 282 | fat: 10.1g | protein: 16.7g
carbs: 38.2g | fiber: 12.9g | sugar: 7.2g
sodium: 1128mg

Cheesy Summer Squash and Quinoa Casserole

Prep time: 15 minutes | Cook time: 27 to 30 minutes | Serves 8

1 tablespoon extra-virgin olive oil
1 Vidalia onion, thinly sliced
1 large portobello mushroom, thinly sliced
6 yellow summer squash, thinly sliced
1 cup shredded

Parmesan cheese, divided
1 cup shredded Cheddar cheese
½ cup tri-color quinoa
½ cup whole-wheat bread crumbs
1 tablespoon Creole seasoning

1. Preheat the oven to 350ºF (180ºC).
2. Heat the olive oil in a large cast iron pan over medium heat.
3. Sauté the onion, mushroom, and squash in the oil for 7 to 10 minutes, stirring occasionally, or until the vegetables are softened.
4. Remove from the heat and add ½ cup of Parmesan cheese and the Cheddar cheese to the vegetables. Stir well.
5. Mix together the quiona, bread crumbs, the remaining Parmesan cheese, Creole seasoning in a small bowl, then scatter the mixture over the vegetables.
6. Place the cast iron pan in the preheated oven and bake until browned and cooked through, about 20 minutes.
7. Cool for 10 minutes and serve on plates while warm.

Per Serving
calories: 184 | fat: 8.9g | protein: 11.7g
carbs: 17.6g | fiber: 3.2g | sugar: 3.8g
sodium: 140mg

Tofu Curry

Prep time: 10 minutes | Cook time: 2 hours | Serves 4

2 cup green bell pepper, diced
1 cup firm tofu, cut into cubes
1 onion, peeled and diced
1½ cups canned coconut milk
1 cup tomato paste

2 cloves garlic, diced fine
2 tablespoons raw peanut butter
1 tablespoon garam masala
1 tablespoon curry powder
1½ teaspoons salt

1. Add all , except the tofu to a blender or food processor. Process until thoroughly combined.
2. Pour into a crock pot and add the tofu. Cover and cook on high 2 hours.
3. Stir well and serve over cauliflower rice.

Per Serving
calories: 390 | fat: 28.0g | protein: 13.1g
carbs: 28.1g | fiber: 8.0g | sugar: 16.0g
sodium: 1004mg

Pizza Stuffed Portobello's

Prep time: 5 minutes | Cook time: 10 minutes | Serves 4

8 Portobello mushrooms, stems removed
1 cup Mozzarella cheese, grated
1 cup cherry tomatoes, sliced
½ cup crushed tomatoes
½ cup fresh basil, chopped

2 tablespoons balsamic vinegar
1 tablespoon olive oil
1 tablespoon oregano
1 tablespoon red pepper flakes
½ tablespoon garlic powder
¼ teaspoon pepper
Pinch salt

1. Heat oven to broil. Line a baking sheet with foil.
2. Place mushrooms, stem side down, on foil and drizzle with oil. Sprinkle with garlic powder, salt and pepper. Broil for 5 minutes.
3. Flip mushrooms over and top with crushed tomatoes, oregano, parsley, pepper flakes, cheese and sliced tomatoes. Broil another 5 minutes.
4. Top with basil and drizzle with balsamic. Serve.

Per Serving
calories: 115 | fat: 5.0g | protein: 9.1g
carbs: 11.1g | fiber: 4.0g | sugar: 3.0g
sodium: 257mg

Tempeh Lettuce Wraps

Prep time: 5 minutes | Cook time: 5 minutes | Serves 2

1 package tempeh, crumbled
1 head butter-leaf lettuce
½ red bell pepper, diced
½ onion, diced
1 tablespoon garlic, diced fine

1 tablespoon olive oil
1 tablespoon low-sodium soy sauce
1 teaspoon ginger,
1 teaspoon onion powder
1 teaspoon garlic powder

1. Heat oil and garlic in a large skillet over medium heat.
2. Add onion, tempeh, and bell pepper and sauté for 3 minutes.

3. Add soy sauce and spices and cook for another 2 minutes.
4. Spoon mixture into lettuce leaves.

Per Serving
calories: 131 | fat: 5.0g | protein: 8.1g
carbs: 14.1g | fiber: 4.0g | sugar: 2.0g
sodium: 268mg

Roasted Brussels Sprouts with Wild Rice Bowl

Prep time: 15 minutes | Cook time: 12 minutes | Serves 4

2 cups sliced Brussels sprouts
2 teaspoons plus 2 tablespoons extra-virgin olive oil
1 teaspoon Dijon mustard
Juice of 1 lemon

1 garlic clove, minced
½ teaspoon salt
¼ teaspoon freshly ground black pepper
1 cup sliced radishes
1 cup cooked wild rice
1 avocado, sliced

1. Preheat the oven to 400ºF (205ºC). Line a baking sheet with parchment paper and set aside.
2. Add 2 teaspoons of olive oil and Brussels sprouts to a medium bowl, and toss to coat well.
3. Spread out the oiled Brussels sprouts on the prepared baking sheet. Roast in the preheated oven for 12 minutes, or until the Brussels sprouts are browned and crisp. Stir the Brussels sprouts once during cooking to ensure even cooking.
4. Meanwhile, Make the dressing by whisking together the remaining olive oil, mustard, lemon juice, garlic, salt, and pepper in a small bowl.
5. Remove the Brussels sprouts from the oven to a large bowl. Add the radishes and cooked wild rice to the bowl. Drizzle with the prepared dressing and gently toss to coat everything evenly.
6. Divide the mixture into four bowls and scatter each bowl evenly with avocado slices. Serve immediately.

Per Serving
calories: 177 | fat: 10.7g | protein: 2.3g
carbs: 17.6g | fiber: 5.1g | sugar: 2.0g
sodium: 297mg

Faux Chow Mein

Prep time: 10 minutes | Cook time: 20 minutes | Serves 4

1 large spaghetti squash, halved and seeds removed
3 stalks celery, sliced diagonally
1 onion, diced fine
2 cup Cole slaw mix
2 teaspoons fresh ginger, grated
¼ cup Tamari
3 cloves garlic, diced fine
3-4 tablespoons water
2 tablespoons olive oil
1 tablespoon Splenda
¼ teaspoon pepper

1. Place squash, cut side down, in shallow glass dish and add water. Microwave on high 8 to 10 minutes, or until squash is soft. Use a fork to scoop out the squash into a bowl.
2. In a small bowl, whisk together Tamari, garlic, sugar, ginger and pepper.
3. Heat oil in large skillet over medium-high heat. Add onion and celery and cook, stirring frequently, 3 to 4 minutes. Add Cole slaw and cook until heated through, about 1 minute.
4. Add the squash and sauce mixture and stir well. Cook 2 minutes, stirring frequently. Serve.

Per Serving
calories: 130 | fat: 7.0g | protein: 3.1g
carbs: 13.1g | fiber: 2.0g | sugar: 6.0g
sodium: 1028mg

Butternut Noodles With Mushroom Sauce

Prep time: 10 minutes | Cook time: 15 minutes | Serves 4

¼ cup extra-virgin olive oil
½ red onion, finely chopped
1 pound (454 g) cremini mushrooms, sliced
1 teaspoon dried thyme
½ teaspoon sea salt
3 garlic cloves, minced
½ cup dry white wine
Pinch red pepper flakes
4 cups butternut noodles
4 ounces (113 g) Parmesan cheese, grated (optional)

1. Heat the olive oil in a large skillet over medium-high heat until shimmering.

2. Add the onion, mushrooms, thyme, and salt to the skillet. Sauté for 6 minutes, stirring occasionally, or until the mushrooms begin to brown.
3. Stir in the garlic and cook for 30 seconds until fragrant.
4. Fold in the wine and red pepper flakes and whisk to combine.
5. Add the butternut noodles to the skillet and continue cooking for 5 minutes, stirring occasionally, or until the noodles are softened.
6. Divide the mixture among four bowls. Sprinkle the grated Parmesan cheese on top, if desired.

Per Serving
calories: 243 | fat: 14.2g | protein: 3.7g
carbs: 21.9g | fiber: 4.1g | sugar: 2.1g
sodium: 157mg

Teriyaki Tofu Burger

Prep time: 15 minutes | Cook time: 15 minutes | Serves 2

2 (3-ounce / 85-g) tofu portions, extra firm, pressed between paper towels 15 minutes
¼ red onion, sliced
2 tablespoons carrot, grated
1 teaspoon margarine
Butter leaf lettuce, for serving
2 whole wheat sandwich thins
1 tablespoon teriyaki marinade
1 tablespoon Sriracha
1 teaspoon red chili flakes

1. Heat grill, or charcoal, to a medium heat.
2. Marinate tofu in teriyaki marinade, red chili flakes and Sriracha.
3. Melt margarine in a small skillet over medium-high heat. Add onions and cook until caramelized, about 5 minutes.
4. Grill tofu for 3 to 4 minutes per side.
5. To assemble, place tofu on bottom roll. Top with lettuce, carrot, and onion. Add top of the roll and serve.

Per Serving
calories: 180 | fat: 5.0g | protein: 12.1g
carbs: 27.1g | fiber: 7.0g | sugar: 5.0g
sodium: 580mg

Fiesta Casserole

Prep time: 15 minutes | Cook time: 30 minutes | Serves 12

1 head cauliflower, grated	1½ cups cheddar cheese, grated
1 red bell pepper, diced fine	1 teaspoon cilantro, diced fine
1 green bell pepper, diced fine	½ cup salsa
1 jalapeno pepper, seeded and diced fine	3 tablespoons water
½ white onion, diced fine	1 teaspoon chili powder
	Nonstick cooking spray

1. Heat oven to 350ºF (180ºC). Spray a 7x11x2-inch baking pan with cooking spray.
2. In a large skillet, over medium heat, cook onions and peppers until soft, about 5 minutes. Add cilantro and chili powder and stir.
3. Place the cauliflower and water in a glass bowl and microwave on high for 3 minutes. Stir in 1 cup cheese and the salsa.
4. Stir the pepper mixture into the cauliflower and combine. Spread in prepared pan. Sprinkle the remaining cheese over the top and bake 30 to 35 minutes.
5. Let rest 5 minutes before cutting into 12 squares and serving.

Per Serving
calories: 75 | fat: 5.0g | protein: 4.1g
carbs: 4.1g | fiber: 1.0g | sugar: 2.0g
sodium: 206mg

Spaghetti Puttanesca

Prep time: 20 minutes | Cook time: 35 minutes | Serves 6

1 tablespoon extra-virgin olive oil	diced tomatoes
3 teaspoons minced garlic	1 tablespoon chopped fresh oregano
1 sweet onion, chopped	2 tablespoons chopped fresh basil
2 celery stalks, chopped	½ teaspoon red pepper flakes
2 (28-ounce / 794-g) cans sodium-free	½ cup quartered, pitted Kalamata olives
¼ cup freshly squeezed lemon juice 8 ounces (227 g)	cooked whole-wheat spaghetti

1. Heat the olive oil in a large saucepan over medium-high heat.
2. Add the garlic, onion, and celery to the saucepan and sauté for about 3 minutes, stirring occasionally, or until softened.
3. Toss in the tomatoes, oregano, basil, and pepper flakes and stir to combine. Allow the sauce to boil, stirring often to prevent from sticking to the bottom of the pan.
4. Reduce the heat to low and bring the sauce to a simmer, stirring occasionally, about 20 minutes.
5. Add the olives and lemon juice to the sauce and mix well.
6. Remove from the heat and spoon the sauce over the spaghetti. Toss well and serve warm.

Per Serving
calories: 199 | fat: 4.7g | protein: 7.2g
carbs: 34.9g | fiber: 3.9g | sugar: 8.1g
sodium: 89mg

Grilled Portobello and Zucchini Burger

Prep time: 5 minutes | Cook time: 10 minutes | Serves 2

2 large portabella mushroom caps	2 whole wheat sandwich thins
½ small zucchini, sliced	2 teaspoons roasted red bell peppers
2 slices low fat cheese	2 teaspoons olive oil

1. Heat grill, or charcoal, to medium-high heat.
2. Lightly brush mushroom caps with olive oil. Grill mushroom caps and zucchini slices until tender, about 3 to 4 minutes per side.
3. Place on sandwich thin. Top with sliced cheese and roasted red bell pepper. Serve.

Per Serving
calories: 178 | fat: 3.0g | protein: 15.1g
carbs: 26.1g | fiber: 8.0g | sugar: 3.0g
sodium: 520mg

Tex Mex Veggie Bake

Prep time: 10 minutes | Cook time: 35 minutes | Serves 8

2 cup cauliflower, grated
1 cup fat free sour cream
1 cup reduced fat cheddar cheese, grated
1 cup reduced fat Mexican cheese blend, grated
½ cup red onion, diced
1 (11-ounce / 312-g)
can Mexicorn, drain
10 ounces (283 g) tomatoes and green chilies
2.25 ounces (64 g) black olives, drain
1 cup black beans, rinsed
1 cup salsa
¼ teaspoon pepper
Nonstick cooking spray

1. Heat oven to 350ºF (180ºC). Spray a 2½-quart baking dish with cooking spray.
2. In a large bowl, combine beans, corn, tomatoes, salsa, sour cream, cheddar cheese, pepper, and cauliflower. Transfer to baking dish. Sprinkle with onion and olives.
3. Bake 30 minutes. Sprinkle with Mexican blend cheese and bake another 5 to 10 minutes, or until cheese is melted and casserole is heated through. Let rest 10 minutes before serving.

Per Serving
calories: 267 | fat: 8.0g | protein: 16.1g
carbs: 33.1g | fiber: 6.0g | sugar: 8.0g
sodium: 812mg

Cauliflower Mushroom Risotto

Prep time: 10 minutes | Cook time: 30 minutes | Serves 2

1 medium head cauliflower, grated
8 ounces (227 g) Porcini mushrooms, sliced
1 yellow onion, diced fine
2 cup low sodium vegetable broth
2 teaspoons garlic, diced fine
2 teaspoons white wine vinegar
Salt and ground black pepper, to taste
Olive oil cooking spray

1. Heat oven to 350ºF (180ºC). Line a baking sheet with foil.
2. Place the mushrooms on the prepared pan and spray with cooking spray. Sprinkle with salt and toss to coat. Bake 10 to 12 minutes, or until golden brown and the mushrooms start to crisp.
3. Spray a large skillet with cooking spray and place over medium-high heat. Add onion and cook, stirring frequently, until translucent, about 3 to 4 minutes. Add garlic and cook 2 minutes, until golden.
4. Add the cauliflower and cook 1 minute, stirring.
5. Place the broth in a saucepan and bring to a simmer. Add to the skillet, ¼ cup at a time, mixing well after each addition.
6. Stir in vinegar. Reduce heat to low and let simmer, 4 to 5 minutes, or until most of the liquid has evaporated.
7. Spoon cauliflower mixture onto plates, or in bowls, and top with mushrooms. Serve.

Per Serving
calories: 135 | fat: 0g | protein: 10.1g
carbs: 22.1g | fiber: 2.0g | sugar: 5.0g
sodium: 1105mg

Eggplant-Zucchini Parmesan

Prep time: 10 minutes | Cook time: 2 hours | Serves 6

1 medium eggplant, peeled and cut into 1-inch cubes
1 medium zucchini, cut into 1-inch pieces
1 medium onion, cut
into thin wedges
1½ cups purchased light spaghetti sauce
²/₃ cup reduced fat Parmesan cheese, grated

1. Place the vegetables, spaghetti sauce and ¹/₃ cup Parmesan in the crock pot. Stir to combine. Cover and cook on high for 2 to 2 ½ hours, or on low 4 to 5 hours.
2. Sprinkle remaining Parmesan on top before serving.

Per Serving
calories: 82 | fat: 2.0g | protein: 5.1g
carbs: 12.1g | fiber: 5.0g | sugar: 7.0g
sodium: 456mg

Mexican Scrambled Eggs and Greens

Prep time: 15 minutes | Cook time: 5 minutes | Serves 4

8 egg whites
4 egg yolks
3 tomatoes, cut in ½-inch pieces
1 jalapeno pepper, slice thin
½ avocado, cut in ½-inch pieces
½ red onion, diced fine
½ head Romaine lettuce, torn
½ cup cilantro, chopped
2 tablespoons fresh lime juice
12 tortilla chips, broken into small pieces
2 tablespoons water
1 tablespoon olive oil
¾ teaspoon pepper, divided
½ teaspoon salt, divided

1. In a medium bowl, combine tomatoes, avocado, onion, jalapeno, cilantro, lime juice, ¼ teaspoon salt, and ¼ teaspoon pepper.
2. In a large bowl, whisk egg whites, egg yolks, water, and remaining salt and pepper. Stir in tortilla chips.
3. Heat oil in a large skillet over medium heat. Add egg mixture and cook, stirring frequently, 3 to 5 minutes, or desired doneness.
4. To serve, divide lettuce leaves among 4 plates. Add scrambled egg mixture and top with salsa.

Per Serving
calories: 281 | fat: 21.0g | protein: 15.1g
carbs: 10.1g | fiber: 4.0g | sugar: 4.0g
sodium: 441mg

Florentine Pizza

Prep time: 15 minutes | Cook time: 20 minutes | Serves 2

1¾ cup grated Mozzarella cheese
½ cup frozen spinach, thaw
1 egg
2 tablespoons reduced fat Parmesan cheese, grated
2 tablespoons cream cheese, soft
¾ cup almond flour
¼ cup light Alfredo sauce
½ teaspoon Italian seasoning
¼ teaspoon red pepper flakes
Pinch of salt

1. Heat oven to 400ºF (205ºC).
2. Squeeze all the excess water out of the spinach.
3. In a glass bowl, combine Mozzarella and almond flour. Stir in cream cheese. Microwave 1 minute on high, then stir. If the mixture is not melted, microwave another 30 seconds.
4. Stir in the egg, seasoning, and salt. Mix well. Place dough on a piece of parchment paper and press into a 10-inch circle.
5. Place directly on the oven rack and bake 8 to 10 minutes or until lightly browned.
6. Remove the crust and spread with the Alfredo sauce, then add spinach, Parmesan and red pepper flakes evenly over top. Bake another 8 to 10 minutes. Slice and serve.

Per Serving
calories: 442 | fat: 35.0g | protein: 24.1g
carbs: 14.1g | fiber: 5.0g | sugar: 4.0g
sodium: 1178mg

Tofu Salad Sandwiches

Prep time: 15 minutes | Cook time: 20 minutes | Serves 4

1 package silken firm tofu, pressed
4 lettuce leaves
2 green onions, diced
¼ cup celery, diced
8 slices whole-wheat bread
¼ cup lite mayonnaise
2 tablespoons sweet pickle relish
1 tablespoon Dijon mustard
¼ teaspoon turmeric
¼ teaspoon salt
⅛ teaspoon cayenne pepper

1. Press tofu between layers of paper towels for 15 minutes to remove excess moisture. Cut into small cubes.
2. In a medium bowl, stir together remaining . Fold in tofu. Spread over 4 slices of bread. Top with a lettuce leaf and another slice of bread. Serve.

Per Serving
calories: 380 | fat: 20.0g | protein: 24.1g
carbs: 15.1g | fiber: 2.0g | sugar: 2.0g
sodium: 575mg

Tofu Bento

Prep time: 15 minutes | Cook time: 10 minutes | Serves 4

1 package extra firm tofu
1 red bell pepper, sliced
1 orange bell pepper, sliced
2 cup cauliflower rice, cooked
2 cups broccoli, chopped
¼ cup green onion, sliced
2 tablespoons low-sodium soy sauce
1 tablespoon olive oil
1 teaspoon ginger,
1 teaspoon garlic powder
1 teaspoon onion powder
1 teaspoon chili paste

1. Remove tofu from package and press with paper towels to absorb all excess moisture, let set for 15 minutes.
2. Chop tofu into cubes. Add tofu and seasonings to a large Ziploc bag and shake to coat.
3. Heat oil in a large skillet over medium heat. Add tofu and vegetables and cook, stirring frequently, 5 to 8 minutes, until tofu is browned on all sides and vegetables are tender.
4. To serve, place ½ cup cauliflower rice on 4 plates and top evenly with tofu mixture.

Per Serving
calories: 95 | fat: 3.0g | protein: 7.1g
carbs: 12.1g | fiber: 4.0g | sugar: 5.0g
sodium: 310mg

Creamy Macaroni and Cheese

Prep time: 10 minutes | Cook time: 25 minutes | Serves 6

1 cup fat-free evaporated milk
½ cup skim milk
½ cup low-fat Cheddar cheese
½ cup low-fat cottage cheese
1 teaspoon nutmeg
Pinch cayenne pepper
Sea salt and freshly ground black pepper, to taste
6 cups cooked whole-wheat elbow macaroni
2 tablespoons grated Parmesan cheese

1. Preheat the oven to 350ºF (180ºC).
2. Heat the milk in a large saucepan over low heat until it steams.
3. Add the Cheddar cheese and cottage cheese to the milk, and keep whisking, or until the cheese is melted.

4. Add the nutmeg and cayenne pepper and stir well. Sprinkle the salt and pepper to season.
5. Remove from the heat. Add the cooked macaroni to the cheese mixture and stir until well combined. Transfer the macaroni and cheese to a large casserole dish and top with the grated Parmesan cheese.
6. Bake in the preheated oven for about 20 minutes, or until bubbly and lightly browned.
7. Divide the macaroni and cheese among six bowls and serve.

Per Serving
calories: 245 | fat: 2.1g | protein: 15.7g
carbs: 43.8g | fiber: 3.8g | sugar: 6.8g
sodium: 186mg

Pad Thai

Prep time: 15 minutes | Cook time: 30 minutes | Serves 6

12 ounces (340 g) extra firm tofu organic, cut into 1-inch cubes
2 zucchini, shredded into long zoodles
1 carrot, grated
3 cups bean sprouts
2 Green onions sliced
1 cup red cabbage, shredded
¼ cup cilantro, chopped
¼ cup lime juice
2 cloves garlic, diced fine
2 tablespoons reduced fat peanut butter
2 tablespoons tamari
1 tablespoon sesame seeds
½ tablespoon sesame oil
2 teaspoons red chili flakes

1. Heat half the oil in a saucepan over medium heat. Add tofu and cook until it starts to brown, about 5 minutes. Add garlic and stir until light brown.
2. Add zucchini, carrot, cabbage, lime juice, peanut butter, tamari, and chili flakes. Stir to combine all . Cook, stirring frequently, until vegetables are tender, about 5 minutes. Add bean sprouts and remove from heat.
3. Serve topped with green onions, sesame seeds and cilantro.

Per Serving
calories: 135 | fat: 6.0g | protein: 12.1g
carbs: 13.1g | fiber: 2.0g | sugar: 3.0g
sodium: 450mg

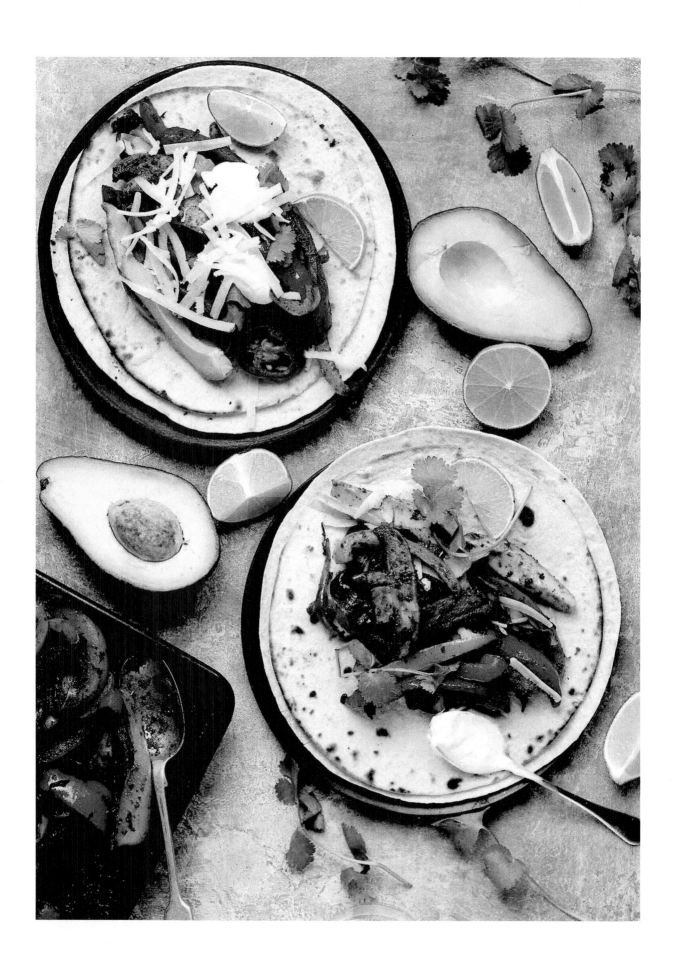

Chapter 7: Vegetable Sides

Lemony Brussels Sprouts

Prep time: 10 minutes | Cook time: 20 minutes | Serves 4

1 pound (454 g) Brussels sprouts
2 tablespoons avocado oil, divided
1 cup vegetable broth or chicken bone broth
1 tablespoon minced garlic
½ teaspoon kosher salt
Freshly ground black pepper, to taste
½ medium lemon
½ tablespoon poppy seeds

1. Trim the Brussels sprouts by cutting off the stem ends and removing any loose outer leaves. Cut each in half lengthwise (through the stem).
2. Set the electric pressure cooker to the Sauté/More setting. When the pot is hot, pour in 1 tablespoon of the avocado oil.
3. Add half of the Brussels sprouts to the pot, cut-side down, and let them brown for 3 to 5 minutes without disturbing. Transfer to a bowl and add the remaining tablespoon of avocado oil and the remaining Brussels sprouts to the pot. Hit Cancel and return all of the Brussels sprouts to the pot.
4. Add the broth, garlic, salt, and a few grinds of pepper. Stir to distribute the seasonings.
5. Close and lock the lid of the pressure cooker. Set the valve to sealing.
6. Cook on high pressure for 2 minutes.
7. While the Brussels sprouts are cooking, zest the lemon, then cut it into quarters.
8. When the cooking is complete, hit Cancel and quick release the pressure.
9. Once the pin drops, unlock and remove the lid.
10. Using a slotted spoon, transfer the Brussels sprouts to a serving bowl. Toss with the lemon zest, a squeeze of lemon juice, and the poppy seeds. Serve immediately.

Per Serving
calories: 126 | fat: 8.1g | protein: 4.1g
carbs: 12.9g | fiber: 4.9g | sugar: 3.0g
sodium: 500mg

Orange Tofu

Prep time: 15 minutes | Cook time: 2 hours | Serves 4

1 package extra firm tofu, pressed for at least 15 minutes, cut into cubes
2 cups broccoli florets, fresh
1 tablespoon margarine
¼ cup orange juice
¼ cup reduced sodium soy sauce
¼ cup honey
2 cloves garlic, diced fine

1. Melt butter in a medium skillet, over medium high heat. Add tofu and garlic and cook, stirring occasionally until tofu starts to brown, about 5 to 10 minutes. Transfer to crock pot.
2. Whisk the wet together in a small bowl. Pour over tofu and add the broccoli.
3. Cover and cook on high 90 minutes, or on low 2 hours.
4. Serve warm.

Per Serving
calories: 138 | fat: 4.0g | protein: 4.1g
carbs: 24.1g | fiber: 2.0g | sugar: 20.0g
sodium: 592mg

Sauteed Green Beans with Nutmeg

Prep time: 15 minutes | Cook time: 5 minutes | Serves 4

1 tablespoon butter
1½ pounds (680 g) green beans, trimmed
1 teaspoon ground nutmeg
Sea salt, to taste

1. Melt the butter in a large skillet over medium heat.
2. Sauté the green beans in the melted butter for 5 minutes until tender but still crisp, stirring frequently.
3. Season with nutmeg and salt and mix well.
4. Remove from the heat and cool for a few minutes before serving.

Per Serving
calories: 83 | fat: 3.2g | protein: 3.2g
carbs: 12.2g | fiber: 6.1g | sugar: 3.2g
sodium: 90mg

Bread Pudding with Kale and Mushrooms

Prep time: 20 minutes | Cook time: 20 minutes | Serves 2

1 large egg
½ cup 2% milk
½ teaspoon Dijon mustard
Pinch freshly grated nutmeg
Pinch kosher salt
Pinch freshly ground black pepper
1 slice sourdough bread (about 1 ounce / 28 g), cut into 1-inch cubes
1 tablespoon avocado oil
¼ cup chopped onion
2 ounces (57 g) mushrooms, sliced (about 3 creminis)
¼ teaspoon dried thyme
1 cup chopped lacinato kale, stems and ribs removed (from 2 stems)
Nonstick cooking spray
¼ cup grated Gruyère cheese
1 tablespoon shredded Parmesan

1. In a 2-cup measuring cup with a spout, whisk together the egg, milk, mustard, nutmeg, salt, and pepper. Add the bread and submerge it in the liquid.
2. Set the electric pressure cooker to the Sauté setting. When the pot is hot, pour in the avocado oil.
3. Add the onion, mushrooms, and thyme to the pot and sauté for 3 to 5 minutes or until the onion begins to soften. Stir in the kale and cook for about 2 minutes or until it wilts. Hit Cancel.
4. Spray the ramekins with cooking spray. Divide the mushroom mixture between the ramekins. Top each with 2 tablespoons Gruyère. Pour half of the egg mixture into each ramekin and stir. Make sure the bread stays submerged. Cover with foil.
5. Pour 1 cup of water into the electric pressure cooker and insert a wire rack or trivet. Place the ramekins on the rack.
6. Close and lock the lid of the pressure cooker. Set the valve to sealing.
7. Cook on high pressure for 8 minutes.
8. When the cooking is complete, hit Cancel. Allow the pressure to release naturally for 10 minutes, then quick release any remaining pressure.
9. Using tongs or the handles of the rack, transfer the ramekins to a cutting board. Carefully lift the foil and sprinkle the Parmesan on top. Replace the foil for about 5 minutes or until the cheese melts.
10. Remove the foil and serve immediately.

Per Serving
calories: 296 | fat: 17.1g | protein: 13.1g
carbs: 22.9g | fiber: 2.9g | sugar: 7.0g
sodium: 312mg

Vegetarian Fajitas

Prep time: 10 minutes | Cook time: 15 minutes | Serves 4

Guacamole:
2 small avocados, pitted and peeled
1 teaspoon freshly squeezed lime juice
¼ teaspoon salt
9 halved cherry tomatoes

Fajitas:
1 red bell pepper, cut into into ½-inch slices
1 green bell pepper, cut into into ½-inch slices
1 small white onion, cut into into ½-inch slices
1 cup canned low-sodium black beans, drained and rinsed
¼ teaspoon garlic powder
¼ teaspoon chili powder
½ teaspoon ground cumin
4 (6-inch) yellow corn tortillas
Avocado oil cooking spray

1. Make the guacamole: In a bowl, add the avocados and lime juice. Using a fork to mash until a uniform consistency is achieved. Season with salt and fold in the cherry tomatoes. Stir well and set aside.
2. Make the fajitas: Heat a large skillet over medium heat until hot. Cover the bottom with cooking spray.
3. Add the bell peppers, white onion, black beans, garlic powder, chili powder, and cumin to the skillet. Stir and cook for about 15 minutes until the beans are tender.
4. Remove from the heat to a plate. Arrange the corn tortillas on a clean work surface and evenly divide the fajita mixture among the tortillas. Serve topped with the guacamole.

Per Serving
calories: 273 | fat: 15.2g | protein: 8.1g
carbs: 30.1g | fiber: 11.2g | sugar: 5.2g
sodium: 176mg

Hearty Corn on the Cob

Prep time: 10 minutes | Cook time: 20 minutes | Serves 12

6 ears corn

1. Remove the husks and silk from the corn. Cut or break each ear in half.
2. Pour 1 cup of water into the bottom of the electric pressure cooker. Insert a wire rack or trivet.
3. Place the corn upright on the rack, cut-side down. Close and lock the lid of the pressure cooker. Set the valve to sealing.
4. Cook on high pressure for 5 minutes.
5. When the cooking is complete, hit Cancel and quick release the pressure.
6. Once the pin drops, unlock and remove the lid.
7. Use tongs to remove the corn from the pot. Season as desired and serve immediately.

Per Serving
calories: 64 | fat: 1.1g | protein: 2.1g
carbs: 13.9g | fiber: 0.9g | sugar: 5.0g
sodium: 12mg

Simple Parmesan Acorn Squash

Prep time: 10 minutes | Cook time: 20 minutes | Serves 4

1 acorn squash (about 1 pound / 454 g)
1 tablespoon extra-virgin olive oil
1 teaspoon dried sage leaves, crumbled
¼ teaspoon freshly grated nutmeg
⅛ teaspoon kosher salt
⅛ teaspoon freshly ground black pepper
2 tablespoons freshly grated Parmesan cheese

1. Cut the acorn squash in half lengthwise and remove the seeds. Cut each half in half for a total of 4 wedges. Snap off the stem if it's easy to do.
2. In a small bowl, combine the olive oil, sage, nutmeg, salt, and pepper. Brush the cut sides of the squash with the olive oil mixture.
3. Pour 1 cup of water into the electric pressure cooker and insert a wire rack or trivet.
4. Place the squash on the trivet in a single layer, skin-side down.
5. Close and lock the lid of the pressure cooker. Set the valve to sealing.
6. Cook on high pressure for 20 minutes.
7. When the cooking is complete, hit Cancel and quick release the pressure.
8. Once the pin drops, unlock and remove the lid.
9. Carefully remove the squash from the pot, sprinkle with the Parmesan, and serve.

Per Serving
calories: 86 | fat: 4.1g | protein: 2.1g
carbs: 11.9g | fiber: 2.1g | sugar: 0g
sodium: 283mg

Jicama with Guacamole

Prep time: 5 minutes | Cook time: 0 minutes | Serves 4

1 avocado, cut into cubes
Juice of ½ lime
2 tablespoons finely chopped red onion
2 tablespoons chopped fresh cilantro
1 garlic clove, minced
¼ teaspoon sea salt
1 cup sliced jicama

1. In a small bowl, combine the avocado, lime juice, onion, cilantro, garlic, and salt. Mash lightly with a fork.
2. Serve with the jicama for dipping.

Per Serving
calories: 74 | fat: 5.1g | protein: 1.1g
carbs: 7.9g | fiber: 4.9g | sugar: 3.0g
sodium: 80mg

Peppers with Zucchini Dip

Prep time: 10 minutes | Cook time: 0 minutes | Serves 4

2 zucchini, chopped
3 garlic cloves
2 tablespoons extra-virgin olive oil
2 tablespoons tahini
Juice of 1 lemon
½ teaspoon sea salt
1 red bell pepper, seeded and cut into sticks

1. In a blender or food processor, combine the zucchini, garlic, olive oil, tahini, lemon juice, and salt. Blend until smooth.
2. Serve with the red bell pepper for dipping.

Per Serving
calories: 120 | fat: 11.1g | protein: 2.1g
carbs: 6.9g | fiber: 2.9g | sugar: 4.0g
sodium: 155mg

Garlicky Broccoli Florets

Prep time: 10 minutes | Cook time: 25 minutes | Serves 8

2 large broccoli heads, cut into florets
2 tablespoons extra-virgin olive oil
3 garlic cloves, minced
¼ teaspoon salt
¼ teaspoon ground black pepper
2 tablespoons freshly squeezed lemon juice

1. Preheat the oven to 425ºF (220ºC) and line a large baking sheet with parchment paper.
2. In a large bowl, add the broccoli, olive oil, garlic, salt, and pepper. Toss well until the broccoli is coated completely. Transfer the broccoli to the prepared baking sheet.
3. Roast in the preheated oven for about 25 minutes, flipping the broccoli halfway through, or until the broccoli is browned and fork-tender.
4. Remove from the oven to a plate and let cool for 5 minutes. Serve drizzled with the lemon juice.

Per Serving
calories: 33 | fat: 2.1g | protein: 1.2g
carbs: 3.1g | fiber: 1.1g | sugar: 1.1g
sodium: 85mg

Roasted Cauliflower with Lime Juice

Prep time: 5 minutes | Cook time: 25 minutes | Serves 4

1 cauliflower head, broken into small florets
2 tablespoons extra-virgin olive oil
½ teaspoon salt, or more to taste
½ teaspoon ground chipotle chili powder
Juice of 1 lime

1. Preheat the oven to 450ºF (235ºC) and line a large baking sheet with parchment paper. Set aside.
2. Toss the cauliflower florets in the olive oil in a large bowl. Season with salt and chipotle chili powder.
3. Arrange the cauliflower florets on the baking sheet.
4. Roast in the preheated oven for 15 minutes until lightly browned. Flip the cauliflower and continue to roast until crisp and tender, about 10 minutes.

5. Remove from the oven and season as needed with salt.
6. Cool for 6 minutes and drizzle with the lime juice, then serve.

Per Serving
calories: 100 | fat: 7.1g | protein: 3.2g
carbs: 8.1g | fiber: 3.2g | sugar: 3.2g
sodium: 285mg

Mini Spinach Quiches

Prep time: 10 minutes | Cook time: 15 minutes | Serves 6

2 tablespoons olive oil, divided
1 onion, finely chopped
2 garlic cloves, minced
2 cups baby spinach
8 large eggs
¼ cup whole milk
½ teaspoon sea salt
¼ teaspoon freshly ground black pepper
1 cup Swiss cheese, shredded

Special Equipment:
A 6-cup muffin tin

1. Preheat the oven to 375ºF (190ºC). Grease a 6-cup muffin tin with 1 tablespoon olive oil.
2. Heat the olive oil in a nonstick skillet over medium-high heat.
3. Add the onion and garlic to the skillet and sauté for 4 minutes until translucent.
4. Add the spinach to the skillet and sauté for 1 minute until tender. Transfer them to a plate and set aside.
5. Whisk together the eggs, milk, salt, and black pepper in a bowl.
6. Dunk the cooked vegetables in the bowl of egg mixture, then scatter with the cheese.
7. Divide the mixture among the muffin cups. Bake in the preheated oven for 15 minutes until puffed and the edges are golden brown.
8. Transfer the quiches to six small plates and serve warm.

Per Serving
calories: 220 | fat: 17.2g | protein: 14.3g
carbs: 4.2g | fiber: 0.8g | saturated fat: 6g
sodium: 235mg

Vegetable Stuffed Portobello Mushrooms

Prep time: 5 minutes | Cook time: 20 minutes | Serves 4

8 large portobello mushrooms
3 teaspoons extra-virgin olive oil, divided
4 cups fresh spinach
1 medium red bell pepper, diced
¼ cup feta cheese, crumbled

1. Preheat the oven to 450°F (235°C).
2. On your cutting board, remove the mushroom stems. Scoop out the gills with a spoon and discard. Grease the mushrooms with 2 tablespoons olive oil.
3. Arrange the mushrooms, cap-side down, on a baking sheet. Roast in the preheated oven for 20 minutes until browned on top.
4. Meanwhile, in a skillet, heat the remaining olive oil over medium heat until shimmering.
5. Add the spinach and red bell pepper to the skillet and sauté for 8 minutes until the vegetables are tender, stirring occasionally. Remove from the heat to a bowl.
6. Remove the mushrooms from the oven to a plate. Using a spoon to stuff the mushrooms with the vegetables and sprinkle with the feta cheese. Serve warm.

Per Serving
calories: 118 | fat: 6.3g | protein: 7.2g
carbs: 12.2g | fiber: 4.1g | sugar: 6.1g
sodium: 128mg

Minestrone

Prep time: 10 minutes | Cook time: 20 minutes | Serves 4

2 tablespoons extra-virgin olive oil
1 chopped onion
1 red bell pepper, seeded and chopped
2 minced garlic cloves
1 (14-ounce / 397-g) can crushed tomatoes
2 cups green beans (fresh or frozen;
halved if fresh)
6 cups low-sodium vegetable broth
1 tablespoon Italian seasoning
½ cup dried whole-wheat elbow macaroni
Pinch red pepper flakes (or to taste)
½ teaspoon sea salt

1. Heat the olive oil in a large saucepan over medium-high heat until shimmering.

2. Sauté the onion and bell pepper for about 3 minutes, stirring frequently, or until they start to soften.
3. Add the garlic and cook for 30 seconds until fragrant, stirring occasionally.
4. Stir in the tomatoes, green beans, vegetable broth, and Italian seasoning, then bring the mixture to a boil.
5. Add the elbow macaroni, red pepper flakes, and salt. Continue to cook for 8 minutes, stirring occasionally, or until the macaroni is cooked through.
6. Remove from the heat to a large bowl and cool for 6 minutes before serving.

Per Serving
calories: 202 | fat: 7.2g | protein: 5.2g
carbs: 29.2g | fiber: 7.2g | saturated fat: 1g
sodium: 479mg

Veggie and Tofu Stir-Fry

Prep time: 10 minutes | Cook time: 10 minutes | Serves 4

3 tablespoons extra-virgin olive oil
12 ounces (340 g) firm tofu, cut into ½-inch pieces
4 cups broccoli, broken into florets
4 scallions, sliced
1 teaspoon peeled and grated fresh ginger
4 garlic cloves, minced
2 tablespoons soy sauce (use gluten-free soy sauce if necessary)
¼ cup vegetable broth
1 cup cooked brown rice

1. Heat the olive oil in a large skillet over medium-high heat until simmering.
2. Add the tofu, broccoli, and scallions and stir fry for 6 minutes, or until the vegetables start to become tender.
3. Add the ginger and garlic and cook for about 30 seconds, stirring constantly.
4. Fold in the soy sauce, vegetable broth, and brown rice. Stir to combine and cook for an additional 1 to 2 minutes until the rice is heated through.
5. Let it cool for 5 minutes before serving.

Per Serving
calories: 238 | fat: 13.2g | protein: 11.1g
carbs: 21.2g | fiber: 4.2g | saturated fat: 2g
sodium:360 mg

Honey Roasted Pumpkin Seeds

Prep time: 10 minutes | Cook time: 30 minutes | Serves 8

2 cup raw fresh pumpkin seeds, wash and pat dry
1 tablespoon butter

3 tablespoons honey
1 tablespoon coconut oil
1 teaspoon cinnamon

1. Heat oven to 275ºF (135ºC). Line a baking sheet with parchment paper, making sure it hangs over both ends.
2. Place the pumpkin seeds in a medium bowl.
3. In a small microwave safe bowl, add butter, coconut oil, and honey. Microwave until the butter melts and the honey is runny. Pour the honey mixture over the pumpkin seeds and stir. Add the cinnamon and stir again.
4. Dump the pumpkin seeds into the middle of the paper and place it in the oven. Bake for 30 to 40 minutes until the seeds and honey are a deep golden brown, stirring every 10 minutes.
5. When the seeds are roasted, remove from the oven and stir again. Stir a few times as they cool to keep them from sticking in one big lump. Enjoy the seeds once they are cool enough to eat. Store uncovered for up to one week. Serving size is ¼ cup.

Per Serving
calories: 270 | fat: 22.0g | protein: 8.2g
carbs: 13.1g | fiber: 1.0g | sugar: 7.0g
sodium: 87mg

Roasted Tomato Brussels Sprouts

Prep time: 15 minutes | Cook time: 20 minutes | Serves 4

1 pound (454 g) Brussels sprouts, trimmed and halved
1 tablespoon extra-virgin olive oil
Sea salt and freshly ground black pepper,

to taste
½ cup sun-dried tomatoes, chopped
2 tablespoons freshly squeezed lemon juice
1 teaspoon lemon zest

1. Preheat the oven to 400ºF (205ºC). Line a large baking sheet with aluminum foil.
2. Toss the Brussels sprouts in the olive oil in a large bowl until well coated. Sprinkle with salt and pepper.
3. Spread out the seasoned Brussels sprouts on the prepared baking sheet in a single layer.
4. Roast in the preheated oven for 20 minutes, shaking the pan halfway through, or until the Brussels sprouts are crispy and browned on the outside.
5. Remove from the oven to a serving bowl. Add the tomatoes, lemon juice, and lemon zest, and stir to incorporate. Serve immediately.

Per Serving
calories: 111 | fat: 5.8g | protein: 5.0g
carbs: 13.7g | fiber: 4.9g | sugar: 2.7g
sodium: 103mg

Vegetable Baked Eggs

Prep time: 5 minutes | Cook time: 25 minutes | Serves 4

2 tablespoons extra-virgin olive oil
1 red onion, chopped
1 sweet potato, cut into ½-inch pieces
1 green bell pepper, seeded and chopped
½ teaspoon sea salt

1 teaspoon chili powder
4 large eggs
½ cup shredded pepper Jack cheese
1 avocado, cut into cubes

1. Preheat the oven to 350ºF (180ºC).
2. Heat the olive oil in a large skillet over medium-high heat until shimmering.
3. Add the onion, sweet potato, bell pepper, salt, and chili powder. Cook for about 10 minutes, stirring constantly, or until the vegetables are lightly browned.
4. Remove from the heat. With the back of a spoon, make 4 wells in the vegetables, then crack an egg into each well. Scatter the shredded cheese over the vegetables.
5. Bake in the preheated oven for about 10 minutes until the cheese is melted and eggs are set.
6. Remove from the heat and sprinkle the avocado on top before serving.

Per Serving
calories: 286 | fat: 21.3g | protein: 12.3g
carbs: 16.2g | fiber: 5.2g | saturated fat g
sodium: 266mg

Roasted Delicata Squash with Thyme

Prep time: 10 minutes | Cook time: 20 minutes | Serves 4

1 (1- to 1½-pound) delicata squash, halved, seeded, and cut into ½-inch-thick strips
1 tablespoon extra-
virgin olive oil
½ teaspoon dried thyme
¼ teaspoon salt
¼ teaspoon freshly ground black pepper

1. Preheat the oven to 400ºF (205ºC). Line a baking sheet with parchment paper and set aside.
2. Add the squash strips, olive oil, thyme, salt, and pepper in a large bowl, and toss until the squash strips are fully coated.
3. Place the squash strips on the prepared baking sheet in a single layer. Roast for about 20 minutes until lightly browned, flipping the strips halfway through.
4. Remove from the oven and serve on plates.

Per Serving
calories: 78 | fat: 4.2g | protein: 1.1g
carbs: 11.8g | fiber: 2.1g | sugar: 2.9g
sodium: 122mg

Asian Fried Eggplant

Prep time: 10 minutes | Cook time: 40 minutes | Serves 4

1 large eggplant, sliced into fourths
3 green onions, diced, green tips only
1 teaspoon fresh ginger, peeled and diced fine
¼ cup plus 1 teaspoon cornstarch
1½ tablespoons soy
sauce
1½ tablespoons sesame oil
1 tablespoon vegetable oil
1 tablespoon fish sauce
2 teaspoons Splenda
¼ teaspoon salt

1. Place eggplant on paper towels and sprinkle both sides with salt. Let for 1 hour to remove excess moisture. Pat dry with more paper towels.
2. In a small bowl, whisk together soy sauce, sesame oil, fish sauce, Splenda, and 1 teaspoon cornstarch.
3. Coat both sides of the eggplant with the ¼ cup cornstarch, use more if needed.

4. Heat oil in a large skillet, over medium-high heat. Add ½ the ginger and 1 green onion, then lay 2 slices of eggplant on top. Use ½ the sauce mixture to lightly coat both sides of the eggplant. Cook 8 to 10 minutes per side. Repeat.
5. Serve garnished with remaining green onions.

Per Serving
calories: 156 | fat: 9.0g | protein: 2.1g
carbs: 18.1g | fiber: 5.0g | sugar: 6.0g
sodium: 719mg

Butter-Orange Yams

Prep time: 7 minutes | Cook time: 45 minutes | Serves 8 (½ cup each)

2 medium jewel yams, cut into 2-inch dices
2 tablespoons unsalted butter
Juice of 1 large orange
1½ teaspoons ground
cinnamon
¼ teaspoon ground ginger
¾ teaspoon ground nutmeg
⅛ teaspoon ground cloves

1. Preheat the oven to 350ºF (180ºC).
2. Arrange the yam dices on a rimmed baking sheet in a single layer. Set aside.
3. Add the butter, orange juice, cinnamon, ginger, nutmeg, and garlic cloves to a medium saucepan over medium-low heat. Cook for 3 to 5 minutes, stirring continuously, or until the sauce begins to thicken and bubble.
4. Spoon the sauce over the yams and toss to coat well.
5. Bake in the preheated oven for 40 minutes until tender.
6. Let the yams cool for 8 minutes in the baking sheet before removing and serving.

Per Serving
calories: 129 | fat: 2.8g | protein: 2.1g
carbs: 24.7g | fiber: 5.0g | sugar: 2.9g
sodium: 28mg

Lime Asparagus with Cashews

Prep time: 10 minutes | Cook time: 15 to 20 minutes | Serves 4

2 pounds (907 g) asparagus, woody ends trimmed	ground black pepper, to taste
1 tablespoon extra-virgin olive oil	½ cup chopped cashews
Sea salt and freshly	Zest and juice of 1 lime

1. Preheat the oven to 400ºF (205ºC). Line a baking sheet with aluminum foil.
2. Toss the asparagus with the olive oil in a medium bowl. Sprinkle the salt and pepper to season.
3. Arrange the asparagus on the baking sheet and bake for 15 to 20 minutes, or until lightly browned and tender.
4. Remove the asparagus from the oven to a serving bowl. Add the cashews, lime zest and juice, and toss to coat well. Serve immediately.

Per Serving

calories: 173 | fat: 11.8g | protein: 8.0g
carbs: 43.7g | fiber: 4.9g | sugar: 5.0g
sodium: 65mg

Popcorn Style Cauliflower

Prep time: 5 minutes | Cook time: 20 minutes | Serves 4

1 head cauliflower, separated into bite-sized florets	¼ teaspoon salt
¼ teaspoon garlic powder	⅛ teaspoon black pepper
	Butter-flavored cooking spray

1. Heat oven to 400ºF (205ºC).
2. Place cauliflower in a large bowl and spray with cooking spray, making sure to coat all sides. Sprinkle with seasonings and toss to coat.
3. Place in a single layer on a cookie sheet. Bake for 20 to 25 minutes or until cauliflower starts to brown. Serve warm.

Per Serving

calories: 55 | fat: 0g | protein: 4.2g
carbs: 11.1g | fiber: 5.0g | sugar: 5.0g
sodium: 165mg

Sesame Bok Choy with Almonds

Prep time: 15 minutes | Cook time: 7 minutes | Serves 4

2 teaspoons sesame oil	sodium soy sauce
2 pounds (907 g) bok choy, cleaned and quartered	Pinch red pepper flakes
2 teaspoons low-	½ cup toasted sliced almonds

1. Heat the sesame oil in a large skillet over medium heat until hot.
2. Sauté the bok choy in the hot oil for about 5 minutes, stirring occasionally, or until tender but still crisp.
3. Add the soy sauce and red pepper flakes and stir to combine. Continue sautéing for 2 minutes.
4. Transfer to a plate and serve topped with sliced almonds.

Per Serving

calories: 118 | fat: 7.8g | protein: 6.2g
carbs: 7.9g | fiber: 4.1g | sugar: 3.0g
sodium: 293mg

Roasted Asparagus and Red Peppers

Prep time: 5 minutes | Cook time: 15 minutes | Serves 4

1 pound (454 g) asparagus, woody ends trimmed, cut into 2-inch segments	1-inch pieces
	1 small onion, quartered
2 red bell peppers, seeded, cut into	2 tablespoons Italian dressing

1. Preheat the oven to 400ºF (205ºC). Line a baking sheet with parchment paper and set aside.
2. Combine the asparagus with the peppers, onion, and dressing in a large bowl, and toss well.
3. Arrange the vegetables on the baking sheet and roast for about 15 minutes until softened. Flip the vegetables with a spatula once during cooking.
4. Transfer to a large platter and serve.

Per Serving

calories: 92 | fat: 4.8g | protein: 2.9g
carbs: 10.7g | fiber: 4.0g | sugar: 5.7g
sodium: 31mg

Zucchini Chips

Prep time: 5 minutes | Cook time: 10 minutes | Serves 6

1 large zucchini, sliced into ¼-inch circle
¼ cup reduced fat, Parmesan cheese, grated fine
3 tablespoons low-fat milk
¹/₃ cup whole wheat

breadcrumbs
½ teaspoon garlic powder
⅛ teaspoon cayenne pepper
Nonstick cooking spray

1. After slicing zucchini pat dry with paper towels. Let sit for 60 minutes before using. Then pat dry again.
2. Heat oven to 425°F (220°C). Spray a wire rack with cooking spray and place on cookie sheet.
3. In a medium bowl combine all except milk and zucchini. Pour milk into a shallow bowl.
4. Dip zucchini into milk the coat with bread crumb mixture. Place on wire rack and bake 10 to 15 minutes or until browned and crisp. Serve immediately.

Per Serving
calories: 30 | fat: 1.0g | protein: 2.1g
carbs: 3.1g | fiber: 0g | sugar: 1.0g
sodium: 111mg

Cauliflower Purée

Prep time: 10 minutes | Cook time: 15 minutes | Serves 6

2½ pounds (1.1 kg) cauliflower florets
½ leek, white and pale green part, halved
4 tablespoons butter
2 teaspoons fresh parsley, diced

2 tablespoons low sodium chicken broth
2 teaspoons extra virgin olive oil
4 cloves garlic, diced fine
¼ teaspoon salt
¼ teaspoon pepper

1. Place the cauliflower in a steamer basket over boiling water. Cover and steam 10 to 15 minutes or until fork tender.
2. Rinse the leek under water and pat dry. Chop into thin slices.

3. Heat oil in a large skillet over medium-low heat. Add the leek and cook 2 to 3 minutes, or until soft. Add the garlic and cook 1 minute more.
4. Add all to a food processor and pulse until almost smooth. Serve warm, or refrigerate for a later use.

Per Serving
calories: 147 | fat: 9.0g | protein: 5.1g
carbs: 14.1g | fiber: 6.0g | sugar: 6.0g
sodium: 218mg

Onion Rings

Prep time: 5 minutes | Cook time: 15 minutes | Serves 4

1 large onion, slice ½-inch thick
1 egg
¼ cup sunflower oil
2 tablespoons coconut flour
2 tablespoons reduced fat Parmesan cheese

¼ teaspoon parsley flakes
⅛ teaspoon garlic powder
⅛ teaspoon cayenne pepper
Salt, to taste
Ketchup, for serving

1. Heat oil in a large skillet over medium-high heat.
2. In a shallow bowl, combine flour, Parmesan, and seasonings.
3. Beat the egg.
4. Separate onion slices into individual rings and place in large bowl, add beaten egg and toss to coat well. Let rest 1 to 2 minutes.
5. In small batches, coat onion in flour mixture and add to skillet. Cook 1 to 2 minutes per side, or until golden brown. Transfer to paper towel lined cookie sheet.
6. Serve with ketchup.

Per Serving
calories: 185 | fat: 16.0g | protein: 3.2g
carbs: 8.1g | fiber: 3.0g | sugar: 2.0g
sodium: 95mg

Sautéed Collard Greens and Cabbage

Prep time: 10 minutes | Cook time: 10 minutes | Serves 8

2 tablespoons extra-virgin olive oil
1 collard greens bunch, stemmed and thinly sliced
½ small green

cabbage, thinly sliced
6 garlic cloves, minced
1 tablespoon low-sodium soy sauce

1. Heat the olive oil in a large skillet over medium-high heat.
2. Sauté the collard greens in the oil for about 2 minutes, or until the greens start to wilt.
3. Toss in the cabbage and mix well. Reduce the heat to medium-low, cover, and cook for 5 to 7 minutes, stirring occasionally, or until the greens are softened.
4. Fold in the garlic and soy sauce and stir to combine. Cook for about 30 seconds more until fragrant.
5. Remove from the heat to a plate and serve.

Per Serving
calories: 73 | fat: 4.1g | protein: 3.2g
carbs: 5.9g | fiber: 2.9g | sugar: 0g
sodium: 128mg

Pesto Stuffed Mushrooms

Prep time: 5 minutes | Cook time: 20 minutes | Serves 4

12 cremini mushrooms, stems removed
4 ounces (113 g) low fat cream cheese, soft
½ cup Mozzarella cheese, grated

⅓ cup reduced fat Parmesan cheese
6 tablespoons basil pesto
Nonstick cooking spray

1. Heat oven to 375ºF (190ºC). Line a square baking dish with foil and spray with cooking spray. Arrange the mushrooms in the baking pan. Set aside.
2. In a medium bowl, beat cream cheese, pesto and Parmesan until smooth and creamy. Spoon mixture into mushroom caps. Top with a heaping teaspoon of Mozzarella.

3. Bake 20 to 23 minutes or until cheese is melted and golden brown. Let cook 5 to 10 minutes before serving.

Per Serving
calories: 77 | fat: 3.0g | protein: 8.2g
carbs: 4.1g | fiber: 0g | sugar: 1.0g
sodium: 541mg

Parmesan Truffle Chips

Prep time: 10 minutes | Cook time: 20 minutes | Serves 4

4 egg whites
½ teaspoon fresh parsley, diced fine
3 tablespoons reduced fat Parmesan cheese, divided

2 teaspoons water
½ teaspoon salt
Truffle oil to taste
Nonstick cooking spray

1. Heat oven to 400ºF (205ºC). Spray two muffin pans with cooking spray.
2. In a small bowl, whisk together egg whites, water, and salt until combined.
3. Spoon just enough egg white mixture into each muffin cup to barely cover the bottom. Sprinkle a small pinch of Parmesan on each egg white.
4. Bake 10 to 15 minutes or until the edges are dark brown, be careful not to burn them.
5. Let cool in the pans 3 to 4 minutes then transfer to a small bowl and drizzle lightly with truffle oil. Add parsley and ½ tablespoon Parmesan and toss to coat. Serve.

Per Serving
calories: 47 | fat: 3.0g | protein: 4.1g
carbs: 0g | fiber: 0g | sugar: 0g
sodium: 671mg

Pickled Cucumbers

Prep time: 15 minutes | Cook time: 5 minutes | Serves 10

2 cucumbers, cut into ¼-inch slices
½ onion, sliced thin
1½ cups vinegar
2 tablespoons stevia
1 tablespoon dill
2 cloves garlic, sliced thin

1 teaspoon peppercorns
1 teaspoon coriander seeds
½ teaspoon salt
¼ teaspoon red pepper flakes

1. In a medium saucepan, combine vinegar and spices. Bring to a boil over high heat. Set aside.
2. Place the cucumbers, onions, and garlic into a quart-sized jar, or plastic container, with an air tight lid. Pour hot liquid over the vegetables, making sure they are completely covered.
3. Add the lid and chill at least a day before serving.

Per Serving
calories: 35 | fat: 0g | protein: 0g
carbs: 6.1g | fiber: 0g | sugar: 4.0g
sodium: 124mg

Fried Zucchini

Prep time: 10 minutes | Cook time: 10 minutes | Serves 4

3 zucchini, slice ¼- to ⅛-inch thick
2 eggs
½ cup sunflower oil

⅓ cup coconut flour
¼ cup reduced fat Parmesan cheese
1 tablespoon water

1. Heat oil in a large skillet over medium heat.
2. In a shallow bowl whisk the egg and water together.
3. In another shallow bowl, stir flour and Parmesan together.
4. Coat zucchini in the egg then flour mixture. Add, in a single layer, to the skillet. Cook 2 minutes per side until golden brown. Transfer to paper towel lined plate. Repeat.
5. Serve immediately with your favorite dipping sauce.

Per Serving
calories: 140 | fat: 11.0g | protein: 6.2g
carbs: 6.1g | fiber: 2.0g | sugar: 3.0g
sodium: 139mg

Tarragon Spring Peas

Prep time: 10 minutes | Cook time: 12 minutes | Serves 6 (½ cup each)

1 tablespoon unsalted butter
½ Vidalia onion, thinly sliced
1 cup low-sodium

vegetable broth
3 cups fresh shelled peas
1 tablespoon minced fresh tarragon

1. Melt the butter in a skillet over medium heat.
2. Sauté the onion in the melted butter for about 3 minutes until translucent, stirring occasionally.
3. Pour in the vegetable broth and whisk well. Add the peas and tarragon to the skillet and stir to combine.
4. Reduce the heat to low, cover, and cook for about 8 minutes more, or until the peas are tender.
5. Let the peas cool for 5 minutes and serve warm.

Per Serving
calories: 82 | fat: 2.1g | protein: 4.2g
carbs: 12.0g | fiber: 3.8g | sugar: 4.9g
sodium: 48mg

Garlicky Mushrooms

Prep time: 10 minutes | Cook time: 12 minutes | Serves 4

1 tablespoon butter
2 teaspoons extra-virgin olive oil
2 pounds (907 g) button mushrooms, halved
2 teaspoons minced

fresh garlic
1 teaspoon chopped fresh thyme
Sea salt and freshly ground black pepper, to taste

1. Heat the butter and olive oil in a large skillet over medium-high heat.
2. Add the mushrooms and sauté for 10 minutes, stirring occasionally, or until the mushrooms are lightly browned and cooked though.
3. Stir in the garlic and thyme and cook for an additional 2 minutes.
4. Season with salt and pepper and serve on a plate.

Per Serving
calories: 96 | fat: 6.1g | protein: 6.9g
carbs: 8.2g | fiber: 1.7g | sugar: 3.9g
sodium: 91mg

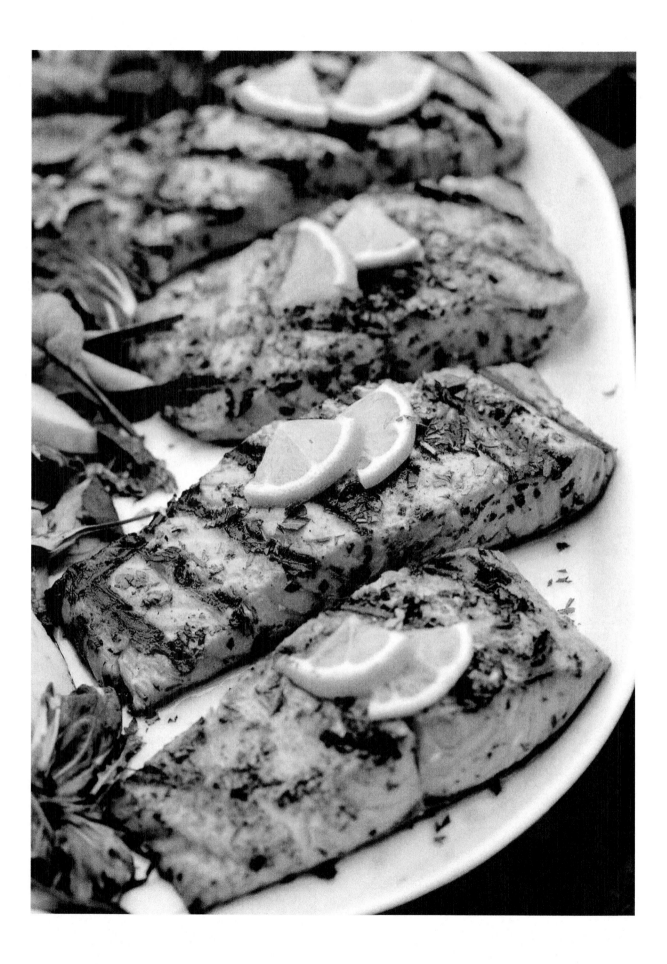

Chapter 8: Fish and Seafood

Mexican Ceviche

Prep time: 10 minutes | Cook time: 0 minutes | Serves 4

½ pound (227 g) fresh skinless, white, ocean fish fillet (halibut, mahi mahi, etc.), diced
1 cup freshly squeezed lime juice, divided
2 tablespoons chopped fresh cilantro, divided
1 serrano pepper, sliced
1 garlic clove, crushed
¾ teaspoon salt, divided
½ red onion, thinly sliced
2 tomatoes, diced
1 red bell pepper, seeded and diced
1 tablespoon extra-virgin olive oil

1. In a large mixing bowl, combine the fish, ¾ cup of lime juice, 1 tablespoon of cilantro, serrano pepper, garlic, and ½ teaspoon of salt. The fish should be covered or nearly covered in lime juice. Cover the bowl and refrigerate for 4 hours.
2. Sprinkle the remaining ¼ teaspoon of salt over the onion in a small bowl, and let sit for 10 minutes. Drain and rinse well.
3. In a large bowl, combine the tomatoes, bell pepper, olive oil, remaining ¼ cup of lime juice, and onion. Let rest for at least 10 minutes, or as long as 4 hours, while the fish "cooks."
4. When the fish is ready, it will be completely white and opaque. At this time, strain the juice, reserving it in another bowl. If desired, remove the serrano pepper and garlic.
5. Add the vegetables to the fish, and stir gently. Taste, and add some of the reserved lime juice to the ceviche as desired. Serve topped with the remaining 1 tablespoon of cilantro.

Per Serving
calories: 122 | fat: 4.1g | protein: 11.9g
carbs: 11.1g | fiber: 2.1g | sugar: 4.9g
sodium: 404mg

Creamy Tuna and Zoodle Casserole

Prep time: 10 minutes | Cook time: 40 minutes | Serves 4

1 tablespoon avocado oil
1 medium yellow onion, diced
2 tablespoons whole-wheat flour
2 cups low-sodium chicken broth
1 cup unsweetened almond milk
1 (10-ounce / 284-g) package zucchini noodles
1 cup fresh or frozen broccoli, cut into florets
2 (5-ounce / 142-g) cans chunk-light tuna, drained
1 cup Cheddar cheese, shredded

1. Preheat the oven to 375ºF (190ºC).
2. Heat the avocado oil in a nonstick skillet over medium heat until shimmering.
3. Add the onion to the skillet and cook for 3 minutes or until translucent.
4. Add the flour to the skillet and cook for 2 minutes. Stir constantly.
5. Gently fold in the chicken broth and almond milk, then turn up the heat to high and bring the mixture to a boil.
6. Add the zucchini noodles and broccoli to the skillet. Reduce the heat to medium and cook for 6 minutes until the mixture is lightly thickened. Add the tuna to the skillet.
7. Pour the mixture in a casserole dish, and spread the cheese on top. Cover the casserole dish with aluminum foil.
8. Bake in the preheated oven for 20 minutes or until the tuna is opaque.
9. Remove the aluminum foil and broil for an additional 2 minutes.
10. Remove the casserole from the oven. Allow to cool for a few minutes and serve warm.

Per Serving
calories: 273 | fat: 11.8g | protein: 29.1g
carbs: 11.1g | fiber: 3.2g | sugar: 2.8g
sodium: 349mg

Crab Cakes with Salsa

Prep time: 30 minutes | Cook time: 10 minutes | Serves 4

For the Salsa:
1 cup finely chopped honeydew melon
1 scallion, white and green parts, finely chopped
1 red bell pepper, seeded, finely chopped
1 teaspoon chopped fresh thyme
Pinch sea salt
Pinch freshly ground black pepper

For the Crab Cakes:
1 pound (454 g) lump crabmeat, drained and picked over
¼ cup finely chopped red onion
¼ cup panko bread crumbs
1 tablespoon chopped fresh parsley
1 teaspoon lemon zest
1 egg
¼ cup whole-wheat flour
Nonstick cooking spray

To Make the Salsa
1. In a small bowl, stir together the melon, scallion, bell pepper, and thyme.
2. Season the salsa with salt and pepper and set aside.

To Make the Crab Cakes
1. In a medium bowl, mix together the crab, onion, bread crumbs, parsley, lemon zest, and egg until very well combined.
2. Divide the crab mixture into 8 equal portions and form them into patties about ¾-inch thick.
3. Chill the crab cakes in the refrigerator for at least 1 hour to firm them up.
4. Dredge the chilled crab cakes in the flour until lightly coated, shaking off any excess flour.
5. Place a large skillet over medium heat and lightly coat it with cooking spray.
6. Cook the crab cakes until they are golden brown, turning once, about 5 minutes per side.
7. Serve warm with the salsa.

Per Serving
calories: 233 | fat: 3.1g | protein: 31.9g carbs: 18.1g | fiber: 2.1g | sugar: 6.1g sodium: 770mg

Jambalaya

Prep time: 10 minutes | Cook time: 40 minutes | Serves 6

1 pound (454 g) raw shrimp, peel and devein
14 ounces (397 g) Andouille sausage, cut into 1-inch pieces
1 medium cauliflower, riced
4 stalks celery, diced
½ white onion, diced
½ red bell pepper, diced
4 tablespoons margarine
2 cups low sodium chicken broth
½ can tomatoes and green chilies
3 cloves garlic, diced fine
2 teaspoons garlic powder
2 teaspoons Old Bay
1½ teaspoons onion powder
1 teaspoon thyme
1 teaspoon oregano
1 teaspoon basil
½ teaspoons cayenne pepper

1. Place large stock pot over medium-high heat.
2. In a small bowl, stir together garlic powder, onion powder, thyme, oregano, basil, Old Bay, and cayenne until combined.
3. Add 2 tablespoons margarine to the stock pot and let melt.
4. Add the riced cauliflower with 2 teaspoons of the spice mixture. Cook, stirring frequently, about 5 minutes. Transfer to a bowl.
5. Add the remaining margarine to the stock pot and melt. Then add the sausage and cook 5 minutes, stirring to brown all sides.
6. Add onion, celery, and pepper and stir to combine. Cook about 3 minutes until vegetables start to get soft.
7. Add the garlic and cook, stirring, 1 minute. Add the cauliflower and combine then add half the spice mixture and tomatoes, simmer 2 to 3 minutes.
8. Pour in the broth and bring to a boil, cook 8 to 10 minutes.
9. Season shrimp with remaining spice mixture and add to the pot, cook 3 to 4 minutes just until shrimp turn pink. Serve.

Per Serving
calories: 429 | fat: 27.0g | protein: 33.2g carbs: 13.1g | fiber: 3.0g | sugar: 4.0g sodium: 753mg

Chard Cod in Paper

Prep time: 10 minutes | Cook time: 15 minutes | Serves 4

1 chard bunch, stemmed, leaves and stems cut into thin strips
1 red bell pepper, seeded and cut into strips
1 pound (454 g) cod fillets cut into 4 pieces
1 tablespoon grated

fresh ginger
3 garlic cloves, minced
2 tablespoons white wine vinegar
2 tablespoons low-sodium tamari or gluten-free soy sauce
1 tablespoon honey

1. Preheat the oven to 425ºF (220ºC).
2. Cut four pieces of parchment paper, each about 16 inches wide. Lay the four pieces out on a large workspace.
3. On each piece of paper, arrange a small pile of chard leaves and stems, topped by several strips of bell pepper. Top with a piece of cod.
4. In a small bowl, mix the ginger, garlic, vinegar, tamari, and honey. Top each piece of fish with one-fourth of the mixture.
5. Fold the parchment paper over so the edges overlap. Fold the edges over several times to secure the fish in the packets. Carefully place the packets on a large baking sheet.
6. Bake for 12 minutes. Carefully open the packets, allowing steam to escape, and serve.

Per Serving
calories: 120 | fat: 1.0g | protein: 19.1g
carbs: 8.9g | fiber: 1.1g | sugar: 6.1g
sodium: 716mg

Roasted Halibut with Vegetables

Prep time: 10 minutes | Cook time: 15 minutes | Serves 4

1 pound (454 g) green beans, trimmed
2 red bell peppers, seeded and cut into strips
1 onion, sliced
Zest and juice of 2 lemons
3 garlic cloves, minced

2 tablespoons extra-virgin olive oil
1 teaspoon dried dill
1 teaspoon dried oregano
4 (4-ounce / 113-g) halibut fillets
½ teaspoon salt
¼ teaspoon freshly ground black pepper

1. Preheat the oven to 400ºF (205ºC). Line a baking sheet with parchment paper.
2. In a large bowl, toss the green beans, bell peppers, onion, lemon zest and juice, garlic, olive oil, dill, and oregano.
3. Use a slotted spoon to transfer the vegetables to the prepared baking sheet in a single layer, leaving the juice behind in the bowl.
4. Gently place the halibut fillets in the bowl, and coat in the juice. Transfer the fillets to the baking sheet, nestled between the vegetables, and drizzle them with any juice left in the bowl. Sprinkle the vegetables and halibut with the salt and pepper.
5. Bake for 15 to 20 minutes until the vegetables are just tender and the fish flakes apart easily.

Per Serving
calories: 235 | fat: 9.1g | protein: 23.9g
carbs: 16.1g | fiber: 4.9g | sugar: 8.1g
sodium: 350mg

Marinated Grilled Salmon with Lemongrass

Prep time: 10 minutes | Cook time: 8 to 12 minutes | Serves 4

1 tablespoon olive oil
1 tablespoon grated fresh ginger
1 small hot chili pepper
1 tablespoon

lemongrass, minced
2 tablespoons low-sodium soy sauce
1 tablespoon Splenda
4 (4-ounce / 113-g) skinless salmon fillets

1. Except for the salmon, stir together all the ingredients in a medium bowl. Brush the salmon fillets generously with the marinade and place in the fridge to marinate for 30 minutes.
2. Preheat the grill to medium heat.
3. Discard the marinade and transfer the salmon to the preheated grill.
4. Grill each side for 4 to 6 minutes, or until the fish is almost completely cooked through at the thickest part. Serve hot.

Per Serving
calories: 223 | fat: 12.2g | protein: 25.7g
carbs: 2.0g | fiber: 0g | sugar: 2.9g
sodium: 203mg

Broiled Cod with Mango Salsa

Prep time: 10 minutes | Cook time: 5 to 10 minutes | Serves 4

Cod:
1 pound (454 g) cod, cut into 4 fillets, pin bones removed
2 tablespoons extra-virgin olive oil
¾ teaspoon sea salt, divided

Mango Salsa:
1 mango, pitted, peeled, and cut into cubes
¼ cup chopped cilantro
1 jalapeño, deseeded and finely chopped
½ red onion, finely chopped
Juice of 1 lime
1 garlic clove, minced

1. Preheat the broiler to high.
2. Place the cod fillets on a rimmed baking sheet. Brush both sides of the fillets with the olive oil. Sprinkle with ½ teaspoon of the salt.
3. Broil in the preheated broiler for 5 to 10 minutes until the flesh flakes easily with a fork.
4. Meanwhile, make the mango salsa by stirring together the mango, cilantro, jalapeño, red onion, lime juice, garlic, and remaining salt in a small bowl.
5. Serve the cod warm topped with the mango salsa.

Per Serving
calories: 198 | fat: 8.1g | protein: 21.2g
carbs: 13.2g | fiber: 2.2g | saturated fat: 1g
sodium: 355mg

Butter Cod with Asparagus

Prep time: 5 minutes | Cook time: 10 minutes | Serves 4

4 (4-ounce / 113-g) cod fillets
¼ teaspoon garlic powder
¼ teaspoon salt
¼ teaspoon freshly ground black pepper
2 tablespoons
unsalted butter
24 asparagus spears, woody ends trimmed
½ cup brown rice, cooked
1 tablespoon freshly squeezed lemon juice

1. In a large bowl, season the cod fillets with the garlic powder, salt, and pepper. Set aside.

2. Melt the butter in a skillet over medium-low heat.
3. Place the cod fillets and asparagus in the skillet in a single layer. Cook covered for 8 minutes, or until the cod is cooked through.
4. Divide the cooked brown rice, cod fillets, and asparagus among four plates. Serve drizzled with the lemon juice.

Per Serving
calories: 233 | fat: 8.2g | protein: 22.1g
carbs: 20.1g | fiber: 5.2g | sugar: 2.2g
sodium: 275mg

Creamy Cod Fillet with Quinoa and Asparagus

Prep time: 5 minutes | Cook time: 15 minutes | Serves 4

½ cup uncooked quinoa
4 (4-ounce / 113-g) cod fillets
½ teaspoon garlic powder, divided
¼ teaspoon salt
¼ teaspoon freshly
ground black pepper
24 asparagus spears, cut the bottom 1½ inches off
1 tablespoon avocado oil
1 cup half-and-half

1. Put the quinoa in a pot of salted water. Bring to a boil. Reduce the heat to low and simmer for 15 minutes or until the quinoa is soft and has a white "tail". Cover and turn off the heat. Let sit for 5 minutes.
2. On a clean work surface, rub the cod fillets with ¼ teaspoon of garlic powder, salt, and pepper.
3. Heat the avocado oil in a nonstick skillet over medium-low heat.
4. Add the cod fillets and asparagus in the skillet and cook for 8 minutes or until they are tender. Flip the cod and shake the skillet halfway through the cooking time.
5. Pour the half-and-half in the skillet, and sprinkle with remaining garlic powder. Turn up the heat to high and simmer for 2 minutes until creamy.
6. Divide the quinoa, cod fillets, and asparagus in four bowls and serve warm.

Per Serving
calories: 258 | fat: 7.9g | protein: 25.2g
carbs: 22.7g | fiber: 5.2g | sugar: 3.8g
sodium: 410mg

Seafood Enchiladas

Prep time: 20 minutes | Cook time: 1 hour | Serves 8

1¼ pounds (567 g) medium shrimp, raw, peel and devein
8 ounces (227 g) fresh halibut, cod, tilapia, or sea bass
2 poblano peppers, stemmed, seeded, and diced
1 red bell pepper, diced
1 onion, diced
1 cup light sour cream
¾ cup skim milk
½ cup reduced fat cream cheese, soft

½ cup green onions, sliced thin
8 (6-inch) low-carb whole wheat flour tortillas
5 cups water
2 cloves garlic, diced fine
2 tablespoons flour
2 teaspoons sunflower oil
¼ teaspoon salt
¼ teaspoon black pepper
Nonstick cooking spray

1. Rinse shrimp and fish then pat dry with paper towels.
2. Heat oven to 350ºF (180ºC). Spry a 3-quart rectangular baking dish with cooking spray.
3. Add water to a large saucepan and bring to boiling over medium-high heat. Add shrimp and cook until shrimp turn pink, 1 to 3 minutes. Drain, rinse with cold water, and chop.
4. Place a steamer insert into a deep skillet with a tight fitting lid. Add water to just below the insert and bring to a boil. Place fish in the insert, cover and steam 4 to 6 minutes, or until fish flakes easily with a fork.
5. Flake the fish into bite-size pieces and set aside.
6. Heat oil in a large nonstick skillet over medium heat. Add bell pepper, poblanos, and onion. Cook 5 to 10 minutes, or until vegetables are tender. Stir in garlic and 1 minute more. Remove from heat and add shrimp and fish.
7. Wrap tortillas in foil, making sure it's tight, and place in the oven until heated through, about 10 minutes.
8. In a medium bowl, beat cream cheese until smooth. Beat in sour cream, ¼ teaspoon salt and pepper. Slowly beat in the milk until smooth. Stir ½ cup sauce into the fish and shrimp mixture.
9. To assemble, spoon shrimp mixture on one side of the tortillas and roll up. Place, seam side down, in prepare baking dish. Pour remaining sauce over the top.
10. Cover with foil, and bake 35 minutes, or until heated through. Let rest 5 minutes before serving. Garnish with chopped green onions.

Per Serving
calories: 459 | fat: 17.0g | protein: 34.2g
carbs: 38.1g | fiber: 21.0g | sugar: 4.0g
sodium: 470mg

Asparagus with Scallops

Prep time: 10 minutes | Cook time: 15 minutes | Serves 4

3 teaspoons extra-virgin olive oil, divided
1 pound (454 g) asparagus, trimmed and cut into 2-inch segments
1 tablespoon butter
1 pound (454 g) sea

scallops
¼ cup dry white wine
Juice of 1 lemon
2 garlic cloves, minced
¼ teaspoon freshly ground black pepper

1. In a large skillet, heat 1½ teaspoons of oil over medium heat.
2. Add the asparagus and sauté for 5 to 6 minutes until just tender, stirring regularly. Remove from the skillet and cover with aluminum foil to keep warm.
3. Add the remaining 1½ teaspoons of oil and the butter to the skillet. When the butter is melted and sizzling, place the scallops in a single layer in the skillet. Cook for about 3 minutes on one side until nicely browned. Use tongs to gently loosen and flip the scallops, and cook on the other side for another 3 minutes until browned and cooked through. Remove and cover with foil to keep warm.
4. In the same skillet, combine the wine, lemon juice, garlic, and pepper. Bring to a simmer for 1 to 2 minutes, stirring to mix in any browned pieces left in the pan.
5. Return the asparagus and the cooked scallops to the skillet to coat with the sauce. Serve warm.

Per Serving
calories: 253 | fat: 7.1g | protein: 26.1g
carbs: 14.9g | fiber: 2.1g | sugar: 3.1g
sodium: 494mg

Cod Fillet with Quinoa and Asparagus

Prep time: 5 minutes | Cook time: 15 minutes | Serves 4

½ cup uncooked quinoa
4 (4-ounce / 113-g) cod fillets
½ teaspoon garlic powder, divided
¼ teaspoon salt
¼ teaspoon freshly

ground black pepper
24 asparagus spears, cut the bottom 1½ inches off
1 tablespoon avocado oil
1 cup half-and-half

1. Put the quinoa in a pot of salted water. Bring to a boil. Reduce the heat to low and simmer for 15 minutes or until the quinoa is soft and has a white "tail". Cover and turn off the heat. Let sit for 5 minutes.
2. On a clean work surface, rub the cod fillets with ¼ teaspoon of garlic powder, salt, and pepper.
3. Heat the avocado oil in a nonstick skillet over medium-low heat.
4. Add the cod fillets and asparagus in the skillet and cook for 8 minutes or until they are tender. Flip the cod and shake the skillet halfway through the cooking time.
5. Pour the half-and-half in the skillet, and sprinkle with remaining garlic powder. Turn up the heat to high and simmer for 2 minutes until creamy.
6. Divide the quinoa, cod fillets, and asparagus in four bowls and serve warm.

Per Serving
calories: 258 | fat: 7.9g | protein: 25.2g
carbs: 22.7g | fiber: 5.2g | sugar: 3.8g
sodium: 410mg

Tartar Tuna Patties

Prep time: 5 minutes | Cook time: 8 to 10 minutes | Serves 4

1 pound (454 g) canned tuna, drained
1 cup whole-wheat bread crumbs
2 large eggs, lightly beaten
Juice and zest of 1 lemon

½ onion, grated
1 tablespoon chopped fresh dill
3 tablespoons extra-virgin olive oil
½ cup tartar sauce, for topping

1. Mix together the tuna with the bread crumbs, beaten eggs, lemon juice and zest, onion, and dill in a large bowl, and stir until well incorporated.
2. Scoop out the tuna mixture and shape into 4 equal-sized patties with your hands.
3. Transfer the patties to a plate and chill in the refrigerator for 10 minutes.
4. Once chilled, heat the olive oil in a large nonstick skillet over medium-high heat.
5. Add the patties to the skillet and cook each side for 4 to 5 minutes, or until nicely browned on both sides.
6. Remove the patties from the heat and top with the tartar sauce.

Per Serving
calories: 529 | fat: 33.6g | protein: 34.9g
carbs: 18.3g | fiber: 2.1g | sugar: 3.8g
sodium: 673mg

Broiled Teriyaki Salmon

Prep time: 5 minutes | Cook time: 3 to 5 minutes | Serves 4

$^1/_3$ cup low-sodium soy sauce
$^1/_3$ cup pineapple juice
¼ cup water
2 tablespoons rice vinegar
1 garlic clove, minced
1 tablespoon honey

1 teaspoon peeled and grated fresh ginger
Pinch red pepper flakes
1 pound (454 g) salmon fillet, cut into 4 pieces

1. Preheat the oven broiler on high.
2. Stir together the soy sauce, pineapple juice, water, vinegar, garlic, honey, ginger, and red pepper flakes in a small bowl.
3. Marinate the fillets (flesh-side down) in the sauce for about 5 minutes.
4. Transfer the fillets (flesh-side up) to a rimmed baking sheet and brush them generously with any leftover sauce.
5. Broil the fish until it flakes apart easily and reaches an internal temperature of 145ºF (63ºC), about 3 to 5 minutes.
6. Let the fish cool for 5 minutes before serving.

Per Serving
calories: 201 | fat: 6.8g | protein: 23.7g
carbs: 8.9g | fiber: 1.0g | sugar: 10.2g
sodium: 750mg

Cajun Flounder and Tomatoes

Prep time: 10 minutes | Cook time: 15 minutes | Serves 4

4 flounder fillets
2½ cups tomatoes, diced
¾ cup onion, diced
¾ cup green bell pepper, diced
2 cloves garlic, diced fine
1 tablespoon Cajun seasoning
1 teaspoon olive oil

1. Heat oil in a large skillet over medium-high heat. Add onion and garlic and cook 2 minutes, or until soft. Add tomatoes, peppers and spices, and cook 2 to 3 minutes until tomatoes soften.
2. Lay fish over top. Cover, reduce heat to medium and cook, 5 to 8 minutes, or until fish flakes easily with a fork. Transfer fish to serving plates and top with sauce.

Per Serving
calories: 195 | fat: 3.0g | protein: 32.2g
carbs: 8.1g | fiber: 2.0g | sugar: 5.0g
sodium: 1278mg

Blackened Shrimp

Prep time: 5 minutes | Cook time: 5 minutes | Serves 4

1½ pounds (680 g) shrimp, peel and devein
4 lime wedges
4 tablespoons cilantro, chopped
4 cloves garlic, diced
1 tablespoon chili powder
1 tablespoon paprika
1 tablespoon olive oil
2 teaspoons Splenda brown sugar
1 teaspoon cumin
1 teaspoon oregano
1 teaspoon garlic powder
1 teaspoon salt
½ teaspoon pepper

1. In a small bowl combine seasonings and Splenda brown sugar.
2. Heat oil in a skillet over medium-high heat. Add shrimp, in a single layer, and cook 1 to 2 minutes per side.
3. Add seasonings, and cook, stirring, 30 seconds. Serve garnished with cilantro and a lime wedge.

Per Serving
calories: 253 | fat: 7.0g | protein: 39.2g
carbs: 7.1g | fiber: 1.0g | sugar: 2.0g
sodium: 846mg

Paella

Prep time: 25 minutes | Cook time: 35 minutes | Serves 6

1 pound (454 g) chicken thighs, skinless and boneless
1 pound (454 g) medium shrimp, raw, peel and devein
1 dozen mussels, cleaned
2 chorizo sausages, cut into pieces
1 medium head cauliflower, grated
1 yellow onion, diced fine
1 green bell pepper,
sliced into strips
1 cup frozen peas
1 (15-ounce / 425-g) can tomatoes, diced, drain well
2 tablespoons extra-virgin olive oil
2 teaspoons garlic, diced fine
2 teaspoons salt
1 teaspoon saffron
½ teaspoon pepper
¼ teaspoon paprika
Nonstick cooking spray

1. Heat the oven to broil. Spray a baking dish with cooking spray.
2. Sprinkle salt and pepper on both sides of the chicken and place in baking dish. Bake, about 4 minutes per side, until no longer pink in the middle. Let cool completely.
3. Heat 1 tablespoon of the oil in a medium skillet over medium heat. Add onion, pepper, and garlic. Cook, about 4 to 5 minutes, stirring frequently, until peppers start to get soft. Transfer to a bowl.
4. Add chorizo to the skillet and cook 2 minutes, stirring frequently. Drain off the fat and add to the vegetables.
5. Once the chicken has cooled, cut into small pieces and add it to the vegetables.
6. In a large saucepot, over medium heat, add the remaining oil. Once it is hot, add the cauliflower and seasonings. Cook 8 to 10 minutes, until cauliflower is almost tender, stirring frequently.
7. Add the mussels and shrimp and cook until mussels open and shrimp start to turn pink.
8. Add the mixture in the bowl with the tomatoes and peas and stir to combine everything together. Cook another 5 minutes until everything is heated through and all of the mussels have opened. Serve.

Per Serving
calories: 424 | fat: 18.0g | protein: 46.2g
carbs: 21.1g | fiber: 6.0g | sugar: 9.0g
sodium: 1371mg

Garlic Shrimp with Sun Dried Tomatoes

Prep time: 10 minutes | Cook time: 30 minutes | Serves 4

½ pound (227 g) shrimp, peeled and deveined
4 ounces (113 g) sun-dried tomatoes
1 cup half-and-half
1 cup reduced fat Parmesan cheese
4 cloves garlic, diced
fine
2 tablespoons olive oil
1 teaspoon dried basil
¼ teaspoon salt
¼ teaspoon paprika
¼ teaspoon crushed red pepper
1 cup corn pasta, cooked and drained

1. Heat oil in a large skillet over medium heat. Add garlic and tomatoes and cook 1 minute.
2. Add shrimp, sprinkle with salt and paprika, and cook about 2 minutes.
3. Add half-and-half, basil, and crushed red pepper and bring to boil. Reduce heat to simmer. Whisk the Parmesan cheese into the hot cream and stir to melt cheese, on low heat.
4. Remove from heat. Add pasta and stir to coat. Serve.

Per Serving
calories: 354 | fat: 22.0g | protein: 37.2g
carbs: 23.1g | fiber: 3.0g | sugar: 3.0g
sodium: 724mg

Grilled Tuna Steaks

Prep time: 5 minutes | Cook time: 10 minutes | Serves 6

6 (6-ounce / 170-g) tuna steaks
3 tablespoons fresh basil, diced
4½ teaspoon olive oil
¾ teaspoon salt
¼ teaspoon pepper
Nonstick cooking spray

1. Heat grill to medium heat. Spray rack with cooking spray.
2. Drizzle both sides of the tuna with oil. Sprinkle with basil, salt and pepper.
3. Place on grill and cook 5 minutes per side, tuna should be slightly pink in the center. Serve.

Per Serving
calories: 344 | fat: 14.0g | protein: 51.2g
carbs: 0g | fiber: 0g | sugar: 0g
sodium: 367mg

Salmon Milano

Prep time: 10 minutes | Cook time: 20 minutes | Serves 6

2½ pound (1.1 kg) salmon filet
2 tomatoes, sliced
½ cup margarine
½ cup basil pesto

1. Heat the oven to 400ºF (205ºC). Line a baking sheet with foil, making sure it covers the sides. Place another large piece of foil onto the baking sheet and place the salmon filet on top of it.
2. Place the pesto and margarine in blender or food processor and pulse until smooth. Spread evenly over salmon. Place tomato slices on top.
3. Wrap the foil around the salmon, tenting around the top to prevent foil from touching the salmon as much as possible. Bake 15 to 25 minutes, or salmon flakes easily with a fork. Serve.

Per Serving
calories: 445 | fat: 24.0g | protein: 55.2g
carbs: 2.1g | fiber: 0g | sugar: 1.0g
sodium: 288mg

Cajun Catfish

Prep time: 5 minutes | Cook time: 15 minutes | Serves 4

4 (8-ounce / 227-g) catfish fillets
2 tablespoons olive oil
2 teaspoons garlic salt
2 teaspoons thyme
2 teaspoons paprika
½ teaspoon cayenne
pepper
½ teaspoon red hot sauce
¼ teaspoon black pepper
Nonstick cooking spray

1. Heat oven to 450ºF (235ºC). Spray a baking dish with cooking spray.
2. In a small bowl whisk together everything but catfish. Brush both sides of fillets, using all the spice mix.
3. Bake 10 to 13 minutes or until fish flakes easily with a fork. Serve.

Per Serving
calories: 367 | fat: 24.0g | protein: 35.2g
carbs: 0g | fiber: 0g | sugar: 0g
sodium: 70mg

Hearty Faux Conch Fritters

Prep time: 15 minutes | Cook time: 20 minutes | Serves 4

4 medium egg whites
½ cup fat-free milk
1 cup chickpea crumbs
¼ teaspoon freshly ground black pepper
½ teaspoon ground cumin
3 cups frozen chopped scallops, thawed
1 small onion, finely chopped
1 small green bell pepper, finely chopped
2 celery stalks, finely chopped
2 garlic cloves, minced
Juice of 2 limes

1. Preheat the oven to 350ºF (180ºC).
2. In a large bowl, combine the egg whites, milk, and chickpea crumbs.
3. Add the black pepper and cumin and mix well.
4. Add the scallops, onion, bell pepper, celery, and garlic.
5. Form golf ball–size patties and place on a rimmed baking sheet 1 inch apart.
6. Transfer the baking sheet to the oven and cook for 5 to 7 minutes, or until golden brown.
7. Flip the patties, return to the oven, and bake for 5 to 7 minutes, or until golden brown.
8. Top with the lime juice, and serve.

Per Serving
calories: 338 | fat: 0g | protein: 50.1g
carbs: 24.1g | fiber: 5.9g | sugar: 4.0g
sodium: 465mg

BBQ Oysters with Bacon

Prep time: 20 minutes | Cook time: 10 minutes | Serves 2

1 dozen fresh oysters, shucked and left on the half shell
3 slices thick cut bacon, cut into thin strips
Juice of ½ lemon
1/3 cup low-sodium ketchup
¼ cup Worcestershire sauce
1 teaspoon horseradish
Dash of hot sauce
Lime wedges, for garnish
Rock salt, to taste

1. Heat oven to broil. Line a shallow baking dish with rock salt. Place the oysters snugly into the salt.
2. In a large bowl, combine remaining and mix well.
3. Add a dash of Worcestershire to each oyster then top with bacon mixture. Cook 10 minutes, or until bacon is crisp. Serve with lime wedges.

Per Serving
calories: 235 | fat: 13.0g | protein: 13.2g
carbs: 10.1g | fiber: 0g | sugar: 9.0g
sodium: 1310mg

Asparagus and Scallop Skillet with Lemony

Prep time: 10 minutes | Cook time: 15 minutes | Serves 4

3 teaspoons extra-virgin olive oil, divided
1 pound (454 g) asparagus, trimmed and cut into 2-inch segments
1 tablespoon butter
1 pound (454 g) sea
scallops
¼ cup dry white wine
2 garlic cloves, minced
Juice of 1 lemon
¼ teaspoon freshly ground black pepper

1. Heat half of olive oil in a nonstick skillet over medium heat until shimmering.
2. Add the asparagus to the skillet and sauté for 6 minutes until soft. Transfer the cooked asparagus to a large plate and cover with aluminum foil.
3. Heat the remaining half of olive oil and butter in the skillet until the butter is melted.
4. Add the scallops to the skillet and cook for 6 minutes or until opaque and browned. Flip the scallops with tongs halfway through the cooking time. Transfer the scallops to the plate and cover with aluminum foil.
5. Combine the wine, garlic, lemon juice, and black pepper in the skillet. Simmer over medium-low heat for 2 minutes. Keep stirring during the simmering.
6. Pour the sauce over the asparagus and scallops to coat well, then serve warm.

Per Serving
calories: 256 | fat: 6.9g | protein: 26.1g
carbs: 14.9g | fiber: 2.1g | sugar: 2.9g
sodium: 491mg

Shrimp with Pumpkin Risotto

Prep time: 5 minutes | Cook time: 15 minutes | Serves 3

½ pound (227 g) raw shrimp, peel and deveined
2 cups cauliflower, grated
¼ cup half-and-half
2 tablespoons margarine
½ cup low sodium
vegetable broth
¼ cup pumpkin purée
¼ cup reduced fat Parmesan cheese
2 cloves garlic, diced fine
¼ teaspoon sage
¼ teaspoon salt
¼ teaspoon pepper

1. Melt margarine in a large skillet over medium-high heat. Add garlic and cook 1 to 2 minutes.
2. Add the broth, pumpkin, and half-and-half and whisk until smooth.
3. Add cauliflower and Parmesan and cook 5 minutes, or until cauliflower is tender. Stir in shrimp and cook until they turn pink. Season with salt and pepper and serve.

Per Serving
calories: 237 | fat: 13.0g | protein: 21.2g
carbs: 9.1g | fiber: 2.0g | sugar: 3.0g
sodium: 618mg

Tangy Orange Roughy

Prep time: 5 minutes | Cook time: 15 minutes | Serves 4

4 orange roughy filets
¼ cup fresh lemon juice
¼ cup reduced sodium soy sauce
1 tablespoon Splenda
½ teaspoon ginger
½ teaspoon lemon pepper
Nonstick cooking spray

1. In a large Ziploc bag combine lemon juice, soy sauce, Splenda, and ginger. Add fish, seal, and turn to coat. Refrigerate 30 minutes.
2. Heat oven to 350ºF (180ºC). Spray a large baking sheet with cooking spray.
3. Place filets on prepared pan and sprinkle with lemon pepper. Bake 12 to 15 minutes, or until fish flakes easily with fork.

Per Serving
calories: 238 | fat: 12.0g | protein: 25.2g
carbs: 4.1g | fiber: 1.0g | sugar: 4.0g
sodium: 656mg

Oysters with Artichoke Heats

Prep time: 30 minutes | Cook time: 15 minutes | Serves 2

2 cups coarse salt, for holding the oysters
1 dozen fresh oysters, scrubbed
1 tablespoon butter
½ cup artichoke hearts, finely chopped
¼ cup red bell pepper, finely chopped
¼ cup finely chopped scallions, both white
and green parts
1 tablespoon fresh parsley, finely chopped
Zest and juice of ½ lemon
1 garlic clove, minced
Salt and freshly ground black pepper, to taste

1. Spread the coarse salt in the bottom of a baking dish.
2. Shuck the oyster with a shucking knife, then discard the empty half and loose the oyster with the knife. Arrange the oyster on the shells with juices, then place them on the coarse salt in the baking dish. Set aside.
3. Preheat the oven to 425ºF (220ºC).
4. Put the butter in a nonstick skillet, and melt over medium heat.
5. Add the artichokes hearts, bell pepper, and scallions to the skillet and sauté for 6 minutes or until soft.
6. Add the garlic to the skillet and sauté for 1 minutes more until fragrant.
7. Remove them from the skillet in a large bowl, then spread the parsley and lemon zest on top, and drizzle with lemon juice, and then sprinkle with salt and black pepper.
8. Spoon the vegetable mixture in each oyster. Bake in the preheated oven for 12 minutes or until the vegetables are lightly wilted.
9. Remove them from the oven and serve warm.

Per Serving
calories: 136 | fat: 6.9g | protein: 6.1g
carbs: 10.8g | fiber: 2.1g | sugar: 6.7g
sodium: 276mg

Shrimp Cocktail

Prep time: 15 minutes | Cook time: 3 minutes | Serves 4

1 pound (454 g) medium shrimp, peeled and deveined
1 cup diced mango
2 ripe avocados, diced
¼ cup finely diced red onion
2 Roma tomatoes, diced
¼ cup chopped fresh cilantro
2 tablespoons low-carb tomato ketchup
Juice of 1 lime
Juice of 1 orange
1 tablespoon extra-virgin olive oil
1 jalapeño pepper, seeded and minced
Lime wedges, for serving

1. Fill a large pot about halfway with water and bring to a boil. Meanwhile, fill a large bowl ⅔ of the way with ice and about 1 cup of cold water.
2. Add the shrimp to the boiling water and cook for 3 minutes until they are opaque and firm. Drain and quickly transfer to the ice water bath for 3 minutes to stop the cooking and cool them. Drain and pat the shrimp dry with a clean paper towel.
3. In a large bowl, mix together the shrimp, mango, avocado, red onion, tomatoes, and cilantro.
4. In a small bowl, combine the ketchup, lime juice, orange juice, oil, and jalapeño. Mix well and gently fold the sauce into the shrimp mixture.
5. Divide among 4 glasses or small dishes, with a lime wedge on the rim of each.

Per Serving
calories: 278 | fat: 16.1g | protein: 17.9g
carbs: 20.1g | fiber: 6.1g | sugar: 9.9g
sodium: 675mg

Mango Salsa Cod

Prep time: 10 minutes | Cook time: 10 minutes | Serves 4

1 pound (454 g) cod, cut into 4 fillets, pin bones removed
2 tablespoons extra-virgin olive oil
¾ teaspoon sea salt, divided
1 mango, pitted, peeled, and cut into cubes
¼ cup chopped cilantro
½ red onion, finely chopped
1 jalapeño, seeded and finely chopped
1 garlic clove, minced
Juice of 1 lime

1. Preheat the oven broiler on high.
2. On a rimmed baking sheet, brush the cod with the olive oil and season with ½ teaspoon of the salt. Broil until the fish is opaque, 5 to 10 minutes.
3. Meanwhile, in a small bowl, combine the mango, cilantro, onion, jalapeño, garlic, lime juice, and remaining ¼ teaspoon of salt.
4. Serve the cod with the salsa spooned over the top.

Per Serving
calories: 200 | fat: 8.0g | protein: 21.1g
carbs: 12.9g | fiber: 1.9g | sugar: 7.6g
sodium: 355mg

Sole Piccata with Capers

Prep time: 10 minutes | Cook time: 20 minutes | Serves 4

1 teaspoon extra-virgin olive oil
4 (5-ounce / 142-g) sole fillets, patted dry
3 tablespoons butter
2 teaspoons minced garlic
2 tablespoons all-purpose flour
2 cups low-sodium chicken broth
Juice and zest of ½ lemon
2 tablespoons capers

1. Heat the olive oil in a large skillet over medium heat.
2. Add the sole fillets to the skillet and sear each side for about 4 minutes, or until the fish is opaque and flakes easily.
3. Remove from the heat to a plate and set aside.
4. Melt the butter in the skillet and sauté the garlic for 3 minutes until fragrant.
5. Add the flour and cook for about 2 minutes, stirring frequently, or until the mixture is bubbly and foamy. It should look like a thick paste.
6. Stir in the chicken broth, lemon juice and zest and cook for 4 minutes, whisking constantly, or until the sauce is thickened.
7. Scatter with the capers and spoon the sauce over the fish. Serve immediately.

Per Serving
calories: 273 | fat: 13.3g | protein: 30.3g
carbs: 7.1g | fiber: 0g | sugar: 2.2g
sodium: 414mg

Haddock with Cucumber Sauce

Prep time: 10 minutes | Cook time: 10 minutes | Serves 4

Cucumber Sauce:

½ English cucumber, grated and liquid squeezed out
¼ cup plain Greek yogurt
½ scallion, white and

green parts, finely chopped
2 teaspoons chopped fresh mint
1 teaspoon honey
A pinch of salt

Fish:

4 (5-ounce / 142-g) haddock fillets, patted dry
Sea salt and freshly

ground black pepper, to taste
Nonstick cooking spray

1. Whisk together all the ingredients for the cucumber sauce in a small bowl and set aside.
2. On a clean work surface, lightly season the haddock fillets with salt and pepper.
3. Heat a large skillet over medium-high heat and spritz with nonstick cooking spray.
4. Cook the haddock fillets for 10 minutes, flipping them halfway through, or until the fish is lightly browned and cooked through.
5. Divide the haddock fillets among four plates and top with the cucumber sauce. Serve warm.

Per Serving
calories: 165 | fat: 2.2g | protein: 27.3g
carbs: 4.2g | fiber: 0g | sugar: 3.2g
sodium: 105mg

Air-Fried Flounder

Prep time: 5 minutes | Cook time: 12 minutes | Serves 4

2 cups low-fat buttermilk
½ teaspoon onion powder
½ teaspoon garlic powder
4 (4-ounce / 113-g) flounder fillets

½ cup chickpea flour
½ cup plain yellow cornmeal
¼ teaspoon cayenne pepper
Freshly ground black pepper, to taste

1. Whisk together the buttermilk, onion powder, and garlic powder in a large bowl.
2. Add the flounder fillets, coating well on

both sides. Let the fish marinate for 20 minutes.
3. Thoroughly combine the chickpea flour, cornmeal, cayenne pepper, and pepper in a shallow bowl.
4. Dredge each fillet in the flour mixture until they are completely coated.
5. Preheat the air fryer to 380ºF (190ºC).
6. Arrange the fish in the air fryer basket and bake for 12 minutes, flipping the fish halfway through, or until the fish is cooked through.
7. Serve warm.

Per Serving
calories: 231 | fat: 6.2g | protein: 28.2g
carbs: 16.2g | fiber: 2.2g | sugar: 7.1g
sodium: 240mg

Easy Fish Tacos with Yogurt Sauce

Prep time: 5 minutes | Cook time: 10 minutes | Serves 4

Yogurt Sauce:

½ cup plain low-fat Greek yogurt
⅓ cup low-fat mayonnaise

½ teaspoon ground cumin
½ teaspoon garlic powder

Tacos:

2 tablespoons extra-virgin olive oil
4 (6-ounce / 170-g) cod fillets
8 (10-inch) yellow corn tortillas

2 cups packaged shredded cabbage
¼ cup chopped fresh cilantro
4 lime wedges

1. Whisk together all the ingredients for the yogurt sauce in a small bowl. Set aside.
2. Make the tacos: Heat the olive oil in a medium skillet over medium-low heat.
3. Add the fish and cook each side for 4 minutes until flaky.
4. Arrange the tortillas on a clean work surface. Top each tortilla evenly with the shredded cabbage, cooked fish, cilantro, yogurt sauce, finished by a squeeze of lime.
5. Serve immediately.

Per Serving
calories: 375 | fat: 13.2g | protein: 36.2g
carbs: 30.2g | fiber: 4.2g | sugar: 4.1g
sodium: 340mg

Seared Scallops with Orange Sauce

Prep time: 10 minutes | Cook time: 10 minutes | Serves 4

2 pounds (907 g) sea scallops, patted dry
Sea salt and freshly ground black pepper, to taste
2 tablespoons extra-virgin olive oil
1 tablespoon minced garlic
¼ cup freshly squeezed orange juice
1 teaspoon orange zest
2 teaspoons chopped fresh thyme, for garnish

1. In a bowl, season the scallops with salt and pepper. Set aside.
2. Heat the olive oil in a large skillet over medium-high heat until shimmering.
3. Add the garlic and sauté for about 3 minutes, stirring occasionally, or until the garlic is softened.
4. Add the scallops and cook each side for about 4 minutes, or until the scallops are lightly browned and firm.
5. Remove the scallops from the heat to a plate and cover with foil to keep warm. Set aside.
6. Pour the orange juice and zest into the skillet and stir, scraping up any cooked bits.
7. Drizzle the scallops with the orange sauce and sprinkle the thyme on top for garnish before serving.

Per Serving
calories: 268 | fat: 8.2g | protein: 38.2g
carbs: 8.3g | fiber: 0g | sugar: 1.1g
sodium: 360mg

Breaded Scallop Patties

Prep time: 15 minutes | Cook time: 10 to 14 minutes | Serves 4

4 medium egg whites
1 cup chickpea crumbs
½ cup fat-free milk
½ teaspoon ground cumin
¼ teaspoon freshly ground black pepper
3 cups frozen chopped scallops, thawed
1 small onion, finely chopped
2 garlic cloves, minced
2 celery stalks, finely chopped
1 small green bell pepper, finely chopped
Juice of 2 limes

1. Preheat the oven to 350ºF (180ºC).
2. Whisk together the egg whites, chickpea crumbs, milk, cumin, and black pepper in a large bowl until well combined.
3. Stir in the scallops, onion, garlic, celery, and bell pepper. Shape the mixture into golf ball-sized balls and flatten them into patties with your hands.
4. Arrange the patties on a rimmed baking sheet, spacing them 1 inch apart.
5. Bake in the preheated oven for 10 to 14 minutes until golden brown. Flip the patties halfway through the cooking time.
6. Serve drizzled with the lime juice.

Per Serving
calories: 338 | fat: 0g | protein: 50.2g
carbs: 24.2g | fiber: 6.2g | sugar: 4.2g
sodium: 465mg

Lemon Parsley White Fish Fillets

Prep time: 10minutes | Cook time: 10 minutes | Serves 4

4 (6-ounce / 170-g) lean white fish fillets, rinsed and patted dry
Cooking spray
Paprika, to taste
Salt and pepper, to taste
2 tablespoons parsley, finely chopped
½ teaspoon lemon zest
¼ cup extra virgin olive oil
¼ teaspoon dried dill
1 medium lemon, halved

1. Preheat the oven to 400ºF (205ºC). Line a baking sheet with aluminum foil and spray with cooking spray.
2. Place the fillets on the foil and scatter with the paprika. Season as desired with salt and pepper.
3. Bake in the preheated oven for 10 minutes, or until the flesh flakes easily with a fork.
4. Meanwhile, stir together the parsley, lemon zest, olive oil, and dill in a small bowl.
5. Remove the fish from the oven to four plates. Squeeze the lemon juice over the fish and serve topped with the parsley mixture.

Per Serving
calories: 283 | fat: 17.2g | protein: 33.3g
carbs: 1.0g | fiber: 0g | sugar: 0g
sodium: 74mg

Fresh Rosemary Trout

Prep time: 5 minutes | Cook time: 7 to 8 minutes | Serves 2

4 to 6 fresh rosemary sprigs
8 ounces (227 g) trout fillets, about ¼ inch thick; rinsed and patted dry
½ teaspoon olive oil
⅛ teaspoon salt
⅛ teaspoon pepper
1 teaspoon fresh lemon juice

1. Preheat the oven to 350ºF (180ºC).
2. Put the rosemary sprigs in a small baking pan in a single row. Spread the fillets on the top of the rosemary sprigs.
3. Brush both sides of each piece of fish with the olive oil. Sprinkle with the salt, pepper, and lemon juice.
4. Bake in the preheated oven for 7 to 8 minutes, or until the fish is opaque and flakes easily.
5. Divide the fillets between two plates and serve hot.

Per Serving
calories: 180 | fat: 9.1g | protein: 23.8g
carbs: 0g | fiber: 0g | sugar: 0g
sodium: 210mg

Shrimp and Vegetable Stir-Fry

Prep time: 5 minutes | Cook time: 15 minutes | Serves 4

Sauce:
½ cup water
2½ tablespoons low-sodium soy sauce
2 tablespoons honey
1 tablespoon rice vinegar
¼ teaspoon garlic powder
Pinch ground ginger
1 tablespoon cornstarch

Stir-Fry:
8 cups frozen vegetable stir-fry mix
2 tablespoons sesame oil
40 medium fresh shrimp, peeled and deveined

1. Make the sauce: Mix together the water, soy sauce, honey, vinegar, garlic powder, and ginger in a small saucepan and stir to combine. Fold in the cornstarch and whisk constantly until everything is incorporated.
2. Let the sauce boil over medium heat for 1 minute. Remove from the heat and set aside in a bowl.
3. Make the stir-fry: Heat a large saucepan over medium-high heat until hot. Add the vegetable stir-fry mix and cook for 8 to 10 minutes, stirring occasionally, or until the water has evaporated.
4. Reduce the heat, pour in the sesame oil and add the shrimp. Stir well and cook for 3 minutes, stirring occasionally, or until the shrimp are pink and cooked through.
5. Stir in the prepared sauce and cook for another 2 minutes.
6. Remove from the heat and let cool for 5 minutes before serving.

Per Serving
calories: 299 | fat: 17.3g | protein: 24.3g
carbs: 14.2g | fiber: 2.2g | sugar: 9.1g
sodium: 453mg

Butter-Lemon Grilled Cod on Asparagus

Prep time: 5 minutes | Cook time: 9 to 12 minutes | Serves 4

1 pound (454 g) asparagus spears, ends trimmed
Cooking spray
4 (4-ounce / 113-g) cod fillets, rinsed and patted dry
¼ teaspoon black
pepper (optional)
¼ cup light butter with canola oil
Juice and zest of 1 medium lemon
¼ teaspoon salt (optional)

1. Heat a grill pan over medium-high heat.
2. Spray the asparagus spears with cooking spray. Cook the asparagus for 6 to 8 minutes until fork-tender, flipping occasionally.
3. Transfer to a large platter and keep warm.
4. Spray both sides of fillets with cooking spray. Season with ¼ teaspoon black pepper, if needed. Add the fillets to the pan and sear each side for 3 minutes until opaque.
5. Meantime, in a small bowl, whisk together the light butter, lemon zest, and ¼ teaspoon salt (if desired).
6. Spoon and spread the mixture all over the asparagus. Place the fish on top and squeeze the lemon juice over the fish. Serve immediately.

Per Serving
calories: 158 | fat: 6.4g | protein: 23.0g
carbs: 6.1g | fiber: 3.0g | sugar: 2.8g
sodium: 212mg

Grilled Shrimp Skewers

Prep time: 10 minutes | Cook time: 12 minutes | Serves 4

1 pound (454 g) shrimp, shelled and deveined
½ cup plain Greek yogurt
½ tablespoon chili paste
½ tablespoon lime juice
Chopped green onions, for garnish

Special Equipment:
Wooden skewers, soaked in water for at least 30 minutes

1. Thread the shrimp onto skewers, piercing once near the tail and once near the head. You can place about 5 shrimps on each skewer.
2. Preheat the grill to medium.
3. Place the shrimp skewers on the grill and cook for about 6 minutes, flipping the shrimp halfway through, or until the shrimp are totally pink and opaque.
4. Meanwhile, make the yogurt and chili sauce: In a small bowl, stir together the yogurt, chili paste, and lime juice.
5. Transfer the shrimp skewers to a large plate. Scatter the green onions on top for garnish and serve with the yogurt and chili sauce on the side.

Per Serving
calories: 122 | fat: 0.8g | protein: 26.1g
carbs: 2.9g | fiber: 0.5g | sugar: 1.3g
sodium: 175mg

Cioppino (Seafood and Tomato Stew)

Prep time: 10 minutes | Cook time: 15 minutes | Serves 4

2 tablespoons extra-virgin olive oil
1 onion, chopped finely
1 garlic clove, minced
½ cup dry white wine
1 (14-ounce / 397-g) can tomato sauce
8 ounces (227 g) shrimp, peeled and
deveined
8 ounces (227 g) cod, pin bones removed and cut into 1-inch pieces
1 tablespoon Italian seasoning
½ teaspoon sea salt
Pinch red pepper flakes

1. Heat the olive oil in a large skillet over medium-high heat until it shimmers.
2. Toss in the onion and cook for 3 minutes, stirring occasionally, or until the onion is translucent. Stir in the garlic and cook for 30 seconds until fragrant.
3. Add the wine and cook for 1 minute, stirring continuously.
4. Stir in the tomato sauce and bring the mixture to a simmer.
5. Add the shrimp and cod, Italian seasoning, salt, and red pepper flakes, and whisk to combine. Continue simmering for about 5 minutes, or until the fish is cooked through.
6. Remove from the heat and serve on plates.

Per Serving
calories: 242 | fat: 7.8g | protein: 23.2g
carbs: 10.7g | fiber: 2.1g | sugar: 7.7g
sodium:270mg

Cilantro Lime Shrimp

Prep time: 15 minutes | Cook time: 8 minutes | Serves 4

1 teaspoon extra virgin olive oil
½ teaspoon garlic clove, minced
1 pound (454 g) large shrimp, peeled and deveined
¼ cup chopped fresh
cilantro, or more to taste
1 lime, zested and juiced
¼ teaspoon salt
⅛ teaspoon black pepper

1. In a large heavy skillet, heat the olive oil over medium-high heat.
2. Add the minced garlic and cook for 30 seconds until fragrant.
3. Toss in the shrimp and cook for about 5 to 6 minutes, stirring occasionally, or until they turn pink and opaque.
4. Remove from the heat to a bowl. Add the cilantro, lime zest and juice, salt, and pepper to the shrimp, and toss to combine. Serve immediately.

Per Serving
calories: 133 | fat: 3.5g | protein: 24.3g
carbs: 1.0g | fiber: 0g | sugar: 0g
sodium: 258mg

Panko Coconut Shrimp

Prep time: 12 minutes | Cook time: 6 to 8 minutes | Serves 4

2 egg whites
1 tablespoon water
½ cup whole-wheat panko bread crumbs
¼ cup unsweetened coconut flakes
½ teaspoon turmeric
½ teaspoon ground coriander
½ teaspoon ground cumin
⅛ teaspoon salt
1 pound large raw shrimp, peeled, deveined, and patted dry
Nonstick cooking spray

1. Preheat the air fry to 400ºF (205ºC).
2. In a shallow dish, beat the egg whites and water until slightly foamy. Set aside.
3. In a separate shallow dish, mix the bread crumbs, coconut flakes, turmeric, coriander, cumin, and salt, and stir until well combined.
4. Dredge the shrimp in the egg mixture, shaking off any excess, then coat them in the crumb-coconut mixture.
5. Spritz the air fryer basket with nonstick cooking spray and arrange the coated shrimp in the basket.
6. Air fry for 6 to 8 minutes, flipping the shrimp once during cooking, or until the shrimp are golden brown and cooked through.
7. Let the shrimp cool for 5 minutes before serving.

Per Serving
calories: 181 | fat: 4.2g | protein: 27.8g
carbs: 9.0g | fiber: 2.3g | sugar: 0.8g
sodium: 227mg

Italian Steamed Mussels

Prep time: 10 minutes | Cook time: 10 minutes | Serves 4

2 pounds (907 g) mussels, cleaned
2 plum tomatoes, peeled, seeded and diced
1 cup onion, diced
2 tablespoons fresh parsley, diced
¼ cup dry white wine
3 cloves garlic, diced fine
3 tablespoons olive oil
2 tablespoons fresh breadcrumbs
¼ teaspoon crushed red pepper flakes

1. Heat oil in a large sauce pot over medium heat. Add the onions and cook until soft, about 2 to 3 minutes. Add garlic and cook 1 minute more.
2. Stir in wine, tomatoes, and pepper flakes. Bring to a boil, stirring occasionally. Add the mussels and cook 3 to 4 minutes, or until all the mussels have opened. Discard any mussels that do not open.
3. Once mussels open, transfer them to a serving bowl. Add bread crumbs to the sauce and continue to cook, stirring frequently, until mixture thickens. Stir in parsley and pour evenly over mussels. Serve.

Per Serving
calories: 341 | fat: 16.0g | protein: 29.2g
carbs: 18.1g | fiber: 2.0g | sugar: 4.0g
sodium: 682mg

Pan Seared Trout and Salsa

Prep time: 5 minutes | Cook time: 10 minutes | Serves 6

6 (6-ounce / 170-g) trout filets
6 lemon slices
4 tablespoons olive oil
¾ teaspoon salt
½ teaspoon pepper
Italian Salsa:
4 plum tomatoes, diced
½ red onion, diced fine
2 tablespoons fresh
parsley, diced
12 Kalamata olives, pitted and chopped
2 cloves garlic, diced fine
1 tablespoon balsamic vinegar
1 tablespoon olive oil
2 teaspoons capers, drained
¼ teaspoon salt
¼ teaspoon pepper

1. Sprinkle filets with salt and pepper.
2. Heat oil in a large nonstick skillet over medium-high heat. Cook trout, 3 filets at a time, 2 to 3 minutes per side, or fish flakes easily with a fork. Repeat with remaining filets.
3. Meanwhile, combine the ingredients for the salsa in a small bowl.
4. Serve the trout topped with salsa and a slice of lemon.

Per Serving
calories: 321 | fat: 21.0g | protein: 30.2g
carbs: 2.1g | fiber: 0g | sugar: 1.0g
sodium: 634mg

Baked Seafood Casserole

Prep time: 20 minutes | Cook time: 30 minutes | Serves 6

12 ounces (340 g) shrimp, peeled and deveined	1 cup water
12 ounces (340 g) cod, cut into 1-inch squares	½ cup reduced fat Parmesan cheese, grated
2 medium leeks, white part only, cut into matchstick pieces	¼ cup super fine almond flour
2 stalks celery, diced	2 small bay leaves whole
1 cup half-and-half	2½ teaspoon Old Bay Seasoning
4 tablespoons margarine	½ teaspoon xanthan gum
1 cup dry white wine	¼ teaspoon sea salt

1. Heat oven to 400ºF (205ºC).
2. Poach the seafood: In a large, heavy pot, combine wine, water, bay leaves, and ½ teaspoon Old bay. Bring just to boiling over medium-high heat. Reduce heat to low and simmer 3 minutes.
3. Add shrimp and cook until they start to turn pink. Transfer to a bowl. Repeat for cod.
4. Turn heat back to medium-high heat and continue simmering poaching liquid until it is reduced to about 1 cup. Remove from heat, strain and save for later.
5. In a separate large sauce pan melt 2 tablespoons margarine over medium-high heat. Add leeks and celery and season with salt. Cook, stirring occasionally, until vegetables are soft.
6. In a square baking dish, layer vegetables and seafood.
7. In the same saucepan you used for the vegetables, melt 1 tablespoon of margarine. Stir in xanthan gum and stir to coat. After xanthan is coated gradually stir in reserved poaching liquid. Bring to a simmer scraping up the browned bits on the bottom of the pan.
8. When sauce starts to thicken, stir in half-and-half. Bring back to a simmer and cook, stirring frequently, until the sauce has the same texture as gravy. Taste and adjust seasoning as desired. Pour over seafood in the baking dish.
9. In a food processor, or blender, combine the almond flour, Parmesan, 2 teaspoons Old Bay, and 1 tablespoon margarine. Process until thoroughly combined. Sprinkle over casserole and bake 20 minutes or until topping is brown and crisp. Serve.

Per Serving
calories: 345 | fat: 17.0g | protein: 30.2g
carbs: 9.1g | fiber: 1.0g | sugar: 2.0g
sodium: 601mg

Monterey Crab Quiche

Prep time: 20 minutes | Cook time: 45 minutes | Serves 16

½ pound (227 g) lump crab meat	2 (9-inch) pie crusts
8 egg whites, dived	2 (4-ounce / 113-g) cans green chilies, chopped
4 eggs	$1/3$ cup flour
2 cup low fat cottage cheese	2 cloves garlic, diced fine
2 cup Monterey Jack cheese, grated	¾ teaspoon baking powder
½ cup onion, diced	¼ teaspoon salt
1 tablespoon margarine	

1. Heat oven to 400ºF (205ºC).
2. Melt margarine in a small skillet over medium-low heat. Add onion and cook until tender. Add garlic and cook 1 minute more.
3. In a large bowl, combine 6 egg whites, eggs, cottage cheese, 1½ cups cheese, chilies, crab, flour, baking powder, onion mixture, and salt.
4. In a separate large bowl, beat remaining egg whites until stiff peaks form. Fold into crab mixture. Pour into pie crusts.
5. Bake 10 minutes, reduce heat to 350ºF (180ºC) and bake 30 minutes. Sprinkle with remaining cheese and bake 5 minutes more, or a knife inserted in centers comes out clean.
6. Let cool 10 minutes before slicing and serving.

Per Serving
calories: 252 | fat: 13.0g | protein: 14.2g
carbs: 22.1g | fiber: 4.0g | sugar: 7.0g
sodium: 735mg

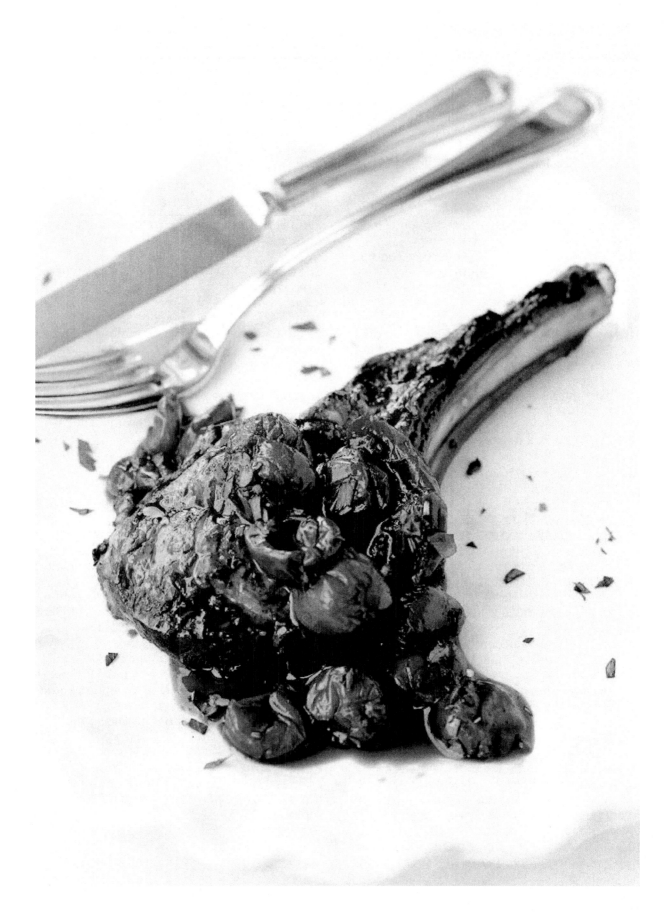

Chapter 9: Pork, Beef, and Lamb

Lamb and Mushroom CheeseBurgers

Prep time: 15 minutes | Cook time: 15 minutes | Serves 4

8 ounces (227 g) grass-fed ground lamb
8 ounces (227 g) brown mushrooms, finely chopped
¼ teaspoon salt
¼ teaspoon freshly ground black pepper
¼ cup crumbled goat cheese
1 tablespoon minced fresh basil

1. In a large mixing bowl, combine the lamb, mushrooms, salt, and pepper, and mix well.
2. In a small bowl, mix the goat cheese and basil.
3. Form the lamb mixture into 4 patties, reserving about ½ cup of the mixture in the bowl. In each patty, make an indentation in the center and fill with 1 tablespoon of the goat cheese mixture. Use the reserved meat mixture to close the burgers. Press the meat firmly to hold together.
4. Heat the barbecue or a large skillet over medium-high heat. Add the burgers and cook for 5 to 7 minutes on each side, until cooked through. Serve.

Per Serving
calories: 172 | fat: 13.1g | protein: 11.1g
carbs: 2.9g | fiber: 0g | sugar: 1.0g
sodium: 155mg

Cherry-Glazed Lamb Chops

Prep time: 10 minutes | Cook time: 20 minutes | Serves 4

4 (4-ounce / 113-g) lamb chops
1½ teaspoons chopped fresh rosemary
¼ teaspoon salt
¼ teaspoon freshly ground black pepper
1 cup frozen cherries, thawed
¼ cup dry red wine
2 tablespoons orange juice
1 teaspoon extra-virgin olive oil

1. Season the lamb chops with the rosemary, salt, and pepper.
2. In a small saucepan over medium-low heat, combine the cherries, red wine, and orange juice, and simmer, stirring regularly, until the sauce thickens, 8 to 10 minutes.
3. Heat a large skillet over medium-high heat. When the pan is hot, add the olive oil to lightly coat the bottom.
4. Cook the lamb chops for 3 to 4 minutes on each side until well-browned yet medium rare.
5. Serve, topped with the cherry glaze.

Per Serving
calories: 355 | fat: 27.1g | protein: 19.8g
carbs: 5.9g | fiber: 1.0g | sugar: 4.0g
sodium: 200mg

Pork Loin, Carrot, and Gold Tomato Roast

Prep time: 5 minutes | Cook time: 40 minutes | Serves 4

1 pound (454 g) pork loin
2 teaspoons honey
½ teaspoon dried rosemary
¼ teaspoon freshly ground black pepper
1 tablespoon extra-virgin olive oil, divided
4 (6-inch) carrots, chopped into ½-inch rounds
2 small gold potatoes, chopped into 2-inch cubes

1. Preheat the oven to 350ºF (180ºC).
2. On a clean work surface, rub the pork with honey, rosemary, black pepper, and ½ tablespoon of olive oil. Brush the carrots and gold potatoes with remaining olive oil.
3. Place the pork, carrots, and potatoes in s single layer on a baking sheet.
4. Roast in the preheated oven for 40 minutes or until the pork is lightly browned and the vegetables are soft.
5. Remove them from the oven. Allow to cool for 10 minutes before serving.

Per Serving
calories: 346 | fat: 9.9g | protein: 26.1g
carbs: 25.9g | fiber: 4.1g | sugar: 5.9g
sodium: 107mg

Lamb Kofta with Cucumber Salad

Prep time: 10 minutes | Cook time: 15 minutes | Serves 4

¼ cup red wine vinegar
Pinch red pepper flakes
1 teaspoon sea salt, divided
2 cucumbers, peeled and chopped
½ red onion, finely chopped
1 pound (454 g) ground lamb
2 teaspoons ground coriander
1 teaspoon ground cumin
3 garlic cloves, minced
1 tablespoon fresh mint, chopped

1. Preheat the oven to 375ºF (190ºC). Line a rimmed baking sheet with parchment paper.
2. In a medium bowl, whisk together the vinegar, red pepper flakes, and ½ teaspoon of salt. Add the cucumbers and onion and toss to combine. Set aside.
3. In a large bowl, mix the lamb, coriander, cumin, garlic, mint, and remaining ½ teaspoon of salt. Form the mixture into 1-inch meatballs and place them on the prepared baking sheet.
4. Bake until the lamb reaches 140ºF (60ºC) internally, about 15 minutes.
5. Serve with the salad on the side.

Per Serving
calories: 346 | fat: 27.1g | protein: 20.1g
carbs: 6.9g | fiber: 1.1g | sugar: 5.0g
sodium: 363mg

Autumn Pork Chops

Prep time: 15 minutes | Cook time: 30 minutes | Serves 4

¼ cup apple cider vinegar
2 tablespoons granulated sweetener
4 (4-ounce / 113-g) pork chops, about 1 inch thick
Sea salt and freshly ground black pepper, to taste
1 tablespoon extra-virgin olive oil
½ red cabbage, finely shredded
1 sweet onion, thinly sliced
1 apple, peeled, cored, and sliced
1 teaspoon chopped fresh thyme

1. In a small bowl, whisk together the vinegar and sweetener. Set it aside.
2. Season the pork with salt and pepper.
3. Place a large skillet over medium-high heat and add the olive oil.
4. Cook the pork chops until no longer pink, turning once, about 8 minutes per side.
5. Transfer the chops to a plate and set aside.
6. Add the cabbage and onion to the skillet and sauté until the vegetables have softened, about 5 minutes.
7. Add the vinegar mixture and the apple slices to the skillet and bring the mixture to a boil.
8. Reduce the heat to low and simmer, covered, for 5 additional minutes.
9. Return the pork chops to the skillet, along with any accumulated juices and thyme, cover, and cook for 5 more minutes.

Per Serving
calories: 224 | fat: 8.1g | protein: 26.1g
carbs: 12.1g | fiber: 3.1g | sugar: 8.0g
sodium: 293mg

Roasted Pork Loin with Carrots

Prep time: 5 minutes | Cook time: 40 minutes | Serves 4

1 pound (454 g) pork loin
1 tablespoon extra-virgin olive oil, divided
2 teaspoons honey
¼ teaspoon freshly
ground black pepper
½ teaspoon dried rosemary
4 (6-inch) carrots, chopped into ½-inch rounds

1. Preheat the oven to 350ºF (180ºC).
2. Rub the pork loin with ½ tablespoon of oil and the honey. Season with the pepper and rosemary.
3. In a medium bowl, toss the carrots in the remaining ½ tablespoon of oil.
4. Place the pork and the carrots on a baking sheet in a single layer. Cook for 40 minutes.
5. Remove the baking sheet from the oven and let the pork rest for at least 10 minutes before slicing. Divide the pork and carrots into four equal portions.

Per Serving
calories: 344 | fat: 10.1g | protein: 26.1g
carbs: 25.9g | fiber: 3.9g | sugar: 6.0g
sodium: 110mg

Herbed Meatballs

Prep time: 10 minutes | Cook time: 15 minutes | Serves 4

½ pound (227 g) lean ground pork
½ pound (227 g) lean ground beef
1 sweet onion, finely chopped
¼ cup bread crumbs
2 tablespoons

chopped fresh basil
2 teaspoons minced garlic
1 egg
Pinch sea salt
Pinch freshly ground black pepper

1. Preheat the oven to 350ºF (180ºC).
2. Line a baking tray with parchment paper and set it aside.
3. In a large bowl, mix together the pork, beef, onion, bread crumbs, basil, garlic, egg, salt, and pepper until very well mixed.
4. Roll the meat mixture into 2-inch meatballs.
5. Transfer the meatballs to the baking sheet and bake until they are browned and cooked through, about 15 minutes.
6. Serve the meatballs with your favorite marinara sauce and some steamed green beans.

Per Serving
calories: 333 | fat: 19.1g | protein: 24.1g
carbs: 12.9g | fiber: 0.9g | sugar: 2.9g
sodium: 189mg

Beef Stroganoff

Prep time: 10 minutes | Cook time: 30 minutes | Serves 4

1 teaspoon extra-virgin olive oil
1 pound (454 g) top sirloin, cut into thin strips
1 cup sliced button mushrooms
½ sweet onion, finely chopped
1 teaspoon minced garlic
1 tablespoon whole-

wheat flour
½ cup low-sodium beef broth
¼ cup dry sherry
½ cup fat-free sour cream
1 tablespoon chopped fresh parsley
Sea salt and freshly ground black pepper, to taste

1. Place a large skillet over medium-high heat and add the oil.

2. Sauté the beef until browned, about 10 minutes, then remove the beef with a slotted spoon to a plate and set it aside.
3. Add the mushrooms, onion, and garlic to the skillet and sauté until lightly browned, about 5 minutes.
4. Whisk in the flour and then whisk in the beef broth and sherry.
5. Return the sirloin to the skillet and bring the mixture to a boil.
6. Reduce the heat to low and simmer until the beef is tender, about 10 minutes.
7. Stir in the sour cream and parsley. Season with salt and pepper.

Per Serving
calories: 258 | fat: 14.1g | protein: 26.1g
carbs: 6.1g | fiber: 1.1g | sugar: 1.0g
sodium: 142mg

Grilled Lamb Racks

Prep time: 15 minutes | Cook time: 20 minutes | Serves 4

1 tablespoon olive oil, plus more for brushing the grill grates
1 tablespoon garlic, minced
½ teaspoon salt
Freshly ground black pepper, to taste

2 (1-inch) sprig fresh rosemary
2 (1½-pounds / 680-g) French lamb racks, trimmed of fat, cut into four pieces with two bones, and leave one bone with an equal amount of meat

1. Combine all the ingredients in a large bowl. Toss to coat the lamb racks well.
2. Wrap the bowl in plastic and refrigerate to marinate for at least 2 hours.
3. Preheat the grill over medium heat. Brush the grill grates with olive oil.
4. Remove the bowl from the refrigerator, and arrange the lamb racks on the grill grates, bone side down.
5. Grill for 3 minutes until lightly browned, then flip the lamb racks, and cover and grill for 15 minutes or until it reaches your desired doneness.
6. Remove the lamb racks from the grill grates and serve hot.

Per Serving
calories: 192 | fat: 9.9g | protein: 22.2g
carbs: 1.0g | fiber: 0g | sugar: 0g
sodium: 347mg

Ritzy Beef Stew

Prep time: 20 minutes | Cook time: 2 hours | Serves 6

2 tablespoons all-purpose flour
1 tablespoon Italian seasoning
2 pounds (907 g) top round, cut into ¾-inch cubes
2 tablespoons olive oil
4 cups low-sodium chicken broth, divided
1½ pounds (680 g) cremini mushrooms, rinsed, stems removed, and quartered
1 large onion, coarsely chopped
3 cloves garlic, minced
3 medium carrots, peeled and cut into ½-inch pieces
1 cup frozen peas
1 tablespoon fresh thyme, minced
1 tablespoon red wine vinegar
½ teaspoon freshly ground black pepper

1. Combine the flour and Italian seasoning in a large bowl. Dredge the beef cubes in the bowl to coat well.
2. Heat the olive oil in a pot over medium heat until shimmering.
3. Add the beef to the single layer in the pot and cook for 2 to 4 minutes or until golden brown on all sides. Flip the beef cubes frequently.
4. Remove the beef from the pot and set aside, then add ¼ cup of chicken broth to the pot.
5. Add the mushrooms and sauté for 4 minutes or until soft. Remove the mushrooms from the pot and set aside.
6. Pour ¼ cup of chicken broth in the pot. Add the onions and garlic to the pot and sauté for 4 minutes or until translucent.
7. Put the beef back to the pot and pour in the remaining broth. Bring to a boil.
8. Reduce the heat to low and cover. Simmer for 45 minutes. Stir periodically.
9. Add the carrots, mushroom, peas, and thyme to the pot and simmer for 45 more minutes or until the vegetables are soft.
10. Open the lid, drizzle with red wine vinegar and season with black pepper. Stir and serve in a large bowl.

Per Serving
calories: 250 | fat: 7.0g | protein: 25.0g
carbs: 24.0g | fiber: 3.0g | sugar: 5.0g
sodium: 290mg

Roasted Pork Tenderloin with Mango Sauce

Prep time: 10 minutes | Cook time: 20 minutes | Serves 4

1 pound (454 g) boneless pork tenderloin, trimmed of fat
1 teaspoon fresh thyme, chopped
1 teaspoon fresh rosemary, chopped
¼ teaspoon salt, divided
¼ teaspoon freshly
ground black pepper, divided
1 teaspoon olive oil
2 tablespoons white wine vinegar
2 tablespoons dry cooking wine
1 tablespoon honey
1 tablespoon fresh ginger, minced
1 cup mango, diced

1. Preheat the oven to 400ºF (205ºC).
2. On a clean work surface, rub the pork tenderloin with thyme, rosemary, ⅛ teaspoon of salt, and ⅛ teaspoon of black pepper.
3. In an oven-safe skillet, heat the olive oil over medium-high heat.
4. Add the tenderloin to the skillet and sear for 5 minutes to brown on both sides. Flip the tenderloin halfway through the cooking time.
5. Move the skillet in the preheated oven and roast for 14 minutes or until an instant-read thermometer inserted in the thickest part of the tenderloin registers at least 145ºF (63ºC). Transfer to a plate and set aside.
6. Combine the vinegar, wine, honey, and ginger in a bowl. Stir to mix well.
7. Pour the mixture in the same skillet and simmer over medium-high heat for a minute, then pour the simmered mixture in a food processor.
8. Add the mango to the food processor, then pulse to purée until the mixture is smooth. Sprinkle with remaining salt and black pepper.
9. Top the pork tenderloin with the mango sauce and slice to serve.

Per Serving
calories: 183 | fat: 3.9g | protein: 24.2g
carbs: 11.9g | fiber: 1.2g | sugar: 9.8g
sodium: 237mg

Grilled Beef, Cucumber, and Lettuce Salad

Prep time: 15 minutes | Cook time: 15 minutes | Serves 4

Dressing:

¼ teaspoon red pepper flakes
¼ cup freshly squeezed lime juice
1 teaspoon honey
1 tablespoon tamari
1 garlic clove, minced
1 tablespoon extra-virgin olive oil

Salad:

1 pound (454 g) grass-fed flank steak
¼ teaspoon salt
Freshly ground black pepper, to taste
1 tablespoon olive oil
1 cucumber, halved lengthwise and thinly cut into half moons
1 carrot, cut into ribbons
6 cups leaf lettuce, chopped
¼ cup fresh cilantro, chopped
½ small red onion, sliced

1. Combine all the ingredients for the dressing in a bowl. Stir to mix well. Set aside.
2. On a clean work surface, rub the beef with salt and black pepper.
3. Heat the olive oil in a nonstick skillet over high heat until shimmering.
4. Add the steak to the skillet and grill for 10 minutes or until it reaches your desired doneness. Flip the steak halfway through the cooking time. Transfer to a large plate and cover with aluminum foil to keep it warm, if necessary.
5. Put the cucumber, carrot, lettuce, cilantro, and onion to a separate bowl. Toss to combine well.
6. Use two forks to slice the steak into strips, then put the strips into the bowl of vegetables. Pour the dressing over and toss to serve.

Per Serving

calories: 233 | fat: 9.8g | protein: 26.1g
carbs: 9.7g | fiber: 2.1g | sugar: 3.8g
sodium: 347mg

Easy Beef Roast with Green Peppercorn Sauce

Prep time: 10 minutes | Cook time: 1 hour 40 minutes | Serves 4

1½ pounds (680 g) top rump beef roast
Salt and freshly ground black pepper, to taste
3 teaspoons olive oil, divided
3 shallots, diced
1 tablespoon green peppercorns
2 teaspoons garlic, minced
2 tablespoons dry sherry
2 tablespoons all-purpose flour
1 cup low-sodium beef broth

1. Preheat the oven to 300ºF (150ºC).
2. On a clean work surface, rub the beef with salt and black pepper.
3. Heat 2 teaspoons olive oil in an oven-safe skillet over medium-high heat until shimmering.
4. Add the beef to the skillet and cook for 10 minutes until well browned on both sides. Flip the beef halfway through the cooking time.
5. Roast in the preheated oven for 1 hour and 30 minutes or until the beef reaches the desired doneness.
6. Meanwhile, heat the remaining olive oil in a saucepan over medium-high heat.
7. Add the shallots to the saucepan and sauté for 4 minutes or until translucent.
8. Add the peppercorns and garlic to the pan and sauté for 1 minutes until fragrant.
9. Pour the sherry into the pan for deglazing, then fold in the flour and stir until the mixture has a thick consistency. Cook for an additional minute. Keep stirring during the cooking.
10. Add the beef broth to the pan and stir until the sauce is thick and smooth, then sprinkle with salt and black pepper.
11. Remove the beef from the oven and serve with the peppercorn sauce on top.

Per Serving

calories: 332 | fat: 17.8g | protein: 36.1g
carbs: 3.9g | fiber: 0g | sugar: 1.1g
sodium: 205mg

Pulled Pork Sandwiches with Apricot Jelly

Prep time: 5 minutes | Cook time: 15 minutes | Serves 4

Avocado oil cooking spray
8 ounces (227 g) store-bought pulled pork
½ cup chopped green bell pepper
2 slices provolone cheese
4 whole-wheat sandwich thins
2½ tablespoons apricot jelly

1. Heat the pulled pork according to the package instructions.
2. Heat a medium skillet over medium-low heat. When hot, coat the cooking surface with cooking spray.
3. Put the bell pepper in the skillet and cook for 5 minutes. Transfer to a small bowl and set aside.
4. Meanwhile, tear each slice of cheese into 2 strips, and halve the sandwich thins so you have a top and bottom.
5. Reduce the heat to low, and place the sandwich thins in the skillet cut-side down to toast, about 2 minutes.
6. Remove the sandwich thins from the skillet. Spread one-quarter of the jelly on the bottom half of each sandwich thin, then place one-quarter of the cheese, pulled pork, and pepper on top. Cover with the top half of the sandwich thin.

Per Serving
calories: 250 | fat: 8.1g | protein: 16.1g
carbs: 34.1g | fiber: 6.1g | sugar: 8.0g
sodium: 510mg

Beef and Mushroom Cauliflower Wraps

Prep time: 5 minutes | Cook time: 20 minutes | Serves 4

Avocado oil cooking spray
½ cup chopped white onion
1 cup chopped portobello mushrooms
1 pound (454 g) 93% lean ground beef
½ teaspoon garlic
powder
Pinch salt
1 (10-ounce / 283-g) bag frozen cauliflower rice
12 iceberg lettuce leaves
¾ cup shredded Cheddar cheese

1. Heat a large skillet over medium heat. When hot, coat the cooking surface with cooking spray and add the onion and mushrooms. Cook for 5 minutes, stirring occasionally.
2. Add the beef, garlic powder, and salt, stirring and breaking apart the meat as needed. Cook for 5 minutes.
3. Stir in the frozen cauliflower rice and increase the heat to medium-high. Cook for 5 minutes more, or until the water evaporates.
4. For each portion, use three lettuce leaves. Spoon one-quarter of the filling onto the lettuce leaves, and top with one-quarter of the cheese. Then, working from the side closest to you, roll up the lettuce to close the wrap. Repeat with the remaining lettuce leaves and filling.

Per Serving
calories: 290 | fat: 15.1g | protein: 31.1g
carbs: 7.1g | fiber: 3.1g | sugar: 4.0g
sodium: 265mg

Parmesan Golden Pork Chops

Prep time: 10 minutes | Cook time: 25 minutes | Serves 4

Nonstick cooking spray
4 bone-in, thin-cut pork chops
2 tablespoons butter
½ cup grated Parmesan cheese
3 garlic cloves, minced
¼ teaspoon salt
¼ teaspoon dried thyme
Freshly ground black pepper, to taste

1. Preheat the oven to 400ºF (205ºC). Line a baking sheet with parchment paper and spray with nonstick cooking spray.
2. Arrange the pork chops on the prepared baking sheet so they do not overlap.
3. In a small bowl, combine the butter, cheese, garlic, salt, thyme, and pepper. Press 2 tablespoons of the cheese mixture onto the top of each pork chop.
4. Bake for 18 to 22 minutes until the pork is cooked through and its juices run clear. Set the broiler to high, then broil for 1 to 2 minutes to brown the tops.

Per Serving
calories: 333 | fat: 16.1g | protein: 44.1g
carbs: 1.1g | fiber: 0g | sugar: 0g
sodium: 441mg

Zucchini Carbonara

Prep time: 10 minutes | Cook time: 25 minutes | Serves 4

6 slices bacon, cut into pieces
1 red onion, finely chopped
3 zucchini, cut into noodles
1 cup peas
½ teaspoon sea salt
3 garlic cloves,

minced
3 large eggs, beaten
1 tablespoon heavy cream
Pinch red pepper flakes
½ cup grated Parmesan cheese (optional, for garnish)

1. In a large skillet over medium-high heat, cook the bacon until browned, about 5 minutes. With a slotted spoon, transfer the bacon to a plate.
2. Add the onion to the bacon fat in the pan and cook, stirring, until soft, 3 to 5 minutes. Add the zucchini, peas, and salt. Cook, stirring, until the zucchini softens, about 3 minutes. Add the garlic and cook, stirring constantly, for 5 minutes.
3. In a small bowl, whisk together the eggs, cream, and red pepper flakes. Add to the vegetables.
4. Remove the pan from the stove top and stir for 3 minutes, allowing the heat of the pan to cook the eggs without setting them.
5. Return the bacon to the pan and stir to mix.
6. Serve topped with Parmesan cheese, if desired.

Per Serving
calories: 327 | fat: 24.1g | protein: 14.1g
carbs: 14.9g | fiber: 3.9g | sugar: 11.0g
sodium: 556mg

Steak and Broccoli Bowls

Prep time: 10 minutes | Cook time: 15 minutes | Serves 4

2 tablespoons extra-virgin olive oil
1 pound (454 g) sirloin steak, cut into ¼-inch-thick strips
2 cups broccoli florets
1 garlic clove, minced
1 teaspoon peeled and grated fresh

ginger
2 tablespoons reduced-sodium soy sauce
¼ cup beef broth
½ teaspoon Chinese hot mustard
Pinch red pepper flakes

1. In a large skillet over medium-high heat, heat the olive oil until it shimmers. Add the beef. Cook, stirring, until it browns, 3 to 5 minutes. With a slotted spoon, remove the beef from the oil and set it aside on a plate.
2. Add the broccoli to the oil. Cook, stirring, until it is crisp-tender, about 4 minutes.
3. Add the garlic and ginger and cook, stirring constantly, for 30 seconds.
4. Return the beef to the pan, along with any juices that have collected.
5. In a small bowl, whisk together the soy sauce, broth, mustard, and red pepper flakes.
6. Add the soy sauce mixture to the skillet and cook, stirring, until everything warms through, about 3 minutes.

Per Serving
calories: 230 | fat: 11.1g | protein: 27.1g
carbs: 4.9g | fiber: 1.0g | sugar: 3.0g
sodium: 376mg

Beef Picadillo

Prep time: 10 minutes | Cook time: 3 to 4 hours | Serves 10

1½ pounds (680 g) lean ground beef
1 onion, diced fine
1 red bell pepper, diced
1 small tomato, diced
¼ cup cilantro, diced fine
1 cup tomato sauce
3 cloves garlic, diced

fine
¼ cup green olives, pitted
2 bay leaves
1½ teaspoons cumin
¼ teaspoon garlic powder
Salt and ground black pepper, to taste

1. In a large skillet, over medium heat, brown ground beef. Season with salt and pepper. Drain fat. Add onion, bell pepper, and garlic and cook for 3 to 4 minutes.
2. Transfer to crock pot and add remaining . Cover and cook on high 3 hours.
3. Discard bay leaves. Taste and adjust seasonings as desired. Serve.

Per Serving
calories: 256 | fat: 9.0g | protein: 35.1g
carbs: 6.1g | fiber: 1.0g | sugar: 3.0g
sodium: 227mg

Sumptuous Lamb and Pomegranate Salad Salad

Prep time: 8 hours 35 minutes | Cook time: 30 minutes | Serves 8

1½ cups pomegranate juice
4 tablespoons olive oil, divided
1 tablespoon ground cinnamon
1 teaspoon cumin
1 tablespoon ground ginger
3 cloves garlic, chopped
Salt and freshly ground black pepper, to taste
1 (4-pound / 1.8-kg) lamb leg, deboned, butterflied, and fat trimmed
2 tablespoons pomegranate balsamic vinegar
2 teaspoons Dijon mustard
½ cup pomegranate seeds
5 cups baby kale
4 cups fresh green beans, blanched
¼ cup toasted walnut halves
2 fennel bulbs, thinly sliced
2 tablespoons Gorgonzola cheese

1. Mix the pomegranate juice, 1 tablespoon of olive oil, cinnamon, cumin, ginger, garlic, salt, and black pepper in a large bowl. Stir to mix well.
2. Dunk the lamb leg in the mixture, press to coat well. Wrap the bowl in plastic and refrigerate to marinate for at least 8 hours.
3. Remove the bowl from the refrigerate and let sit for 20 minutes. Pat the lamb dry with paper towels.
4. Preheat the grill to high heat.
5. Brush the grill grates with 1 tablespoon of olive oil, then arrange the lamb on the grill grates.
6. Grill for 30 minutes or until the internal temperature of the lamb reaches at least 145ºF (63ºC). Flip the lamb halfway through the cooking time.
7. Remove the lamb from the grill and wrap with aluminum foil. Let stand for 15 minutes.
8. Meanwhile, Combine the vinegar, mustard, salt, black pepper, and remaining olive oil in a separate large bowl. Stir to mix well.
9. Add the remaining ingredients and lamb leg to the bowl and toss to combine well. Serve immediately.

Per Serving
calories: 380 | fat: 21.0g | protein: 32.0g
carbs: 16.0g | fiber: 5.0g | sugar: 6.0g
sodium: 240mg

Pork Souvlakia with Tzatziki Sauce

Prep time: 20 minutes | Cook time: 12 minutes | Serves 4

¼ cup lemon juice
1 tablespoon dried oregano
¼ teaspoon salt
¼ teaspoon ground black pepper
1 pound (454 g) pork tenderloin, cut into 1-inch cubes
1 tablespoon olive oil
Tzatziki Sauce:
½ cup plain Greek yogurt
1 large cucumber, peeled, deseeded and grated
1 tablespoon fresh lemon juice
4 cloves garlic, minced or grated
¼ teaspoon ground black pepper

Special Equipment:
8 bamboo skewers, soaked in water for at least 30 minutes

1. Combine the lemon juice, oregano, salt, and ground black pepper in a large bowl. Stir to mix well.
2. Dunk the pork cubes in the bowl of mixture, then toss to coat well. Wrap the bowl in plastic and refrigerate to marinate for 10 minutes or overnight.
3. Preheat the oven to 450ºF (235ºC) or broil. Grease a baking sheet with the olive oil.
4. Remove the bowl from the refrigerator. Run the bamboo skewers through the pork cubes. Set the skewers on the baking sheet, then brush with marinade.
5. Broil the skewers in the preheated oven for 12 minutes or until well browned. Flip skewers at least 3 times during the broiling.
6. Meanwhile, combine the ingredients for the tzatziki sauce in a small bowl.
7. Remove the skewers from the oven and baste with the tzatziki sauce and serve immediately.

Per Serving
calories: 260 | fat: 7.0g | protein: 28.0g
carbs: 21.0g | fiber: 3.0g | sugar: 3.0g
sodium: 360mg

Roasted Beef with Shallot Sauce

Prep time: 10 minutes | Cook time: 1 hour 40 minutes | Serves 4

1½ pounds (680 g) top rump beef roast
Sea salt and freshly ground black pepper, to taste
3 teaspoons extra-virgin olive oil, divided
3 shallots, minced
2 teaspoons minced garlic
1 tablespoon green peppercorns
2 tablespoons dry sherry
2 tablespoons all-purpose flour
1 cup sodium-free beef broth

1. Heat the oven to 300°F (150°C).
2. Season the roast with salt and pepper.
3. Place a large skillet over medium-high heat and add 2 teaspoons of olive oil.
4. Brown the beef on all sides, about 10 minutes in total, and transfer the roast to a baking dish.
5. Roast until desired doneness, about 1½ hours for medium. When the roast has been in the oven for 1 hour, start the sauce.
6. In a medium saucepan over medium-high heat, sauté the shallots in the remaining 1 teaspoon of olive oil until translucent, about 4 minutes.
7. Stir in the garlic and peppercorns, and cook for another minute. Whisk in the sherry to deglaze the pan.
8. Whisk in the flour to form a thick paste, cooking for 1 minute and stirring constantly.
9. Pour in the beef broth and whisk until the sauce is thick and glossy, about 4 minutes. Season the sauce with salt and pepper.
10. Serve the beef with a generous spoonful of sauce.

Per Serving
calories: 331 | fat: 18.1g | protein: 36.1g
carbs: 3.9g | fiber: 0g | sugar: 1.0g
sodium: 208mg

Mustard Pork Chops

Prep time: 5 minutes | Cook time: 25 minutes | Serves 4

¼ cup Dijon mustard
1 tablespoon pure maple syrup
2 tablespoons rice vinegar
4 bone-in, thin-cut pork chops

1. Preheat the oven to 400°F (205°C).
2. In a small saucepan, combine the mustard, maple syrup, and rice vinegar. Stir to mix and bring to a simmer over medium heat. Cook for about 2 minutes until just slightly thickened.
3. In a baking dish, place the pork chops and spoon the sauce over them, flipping to coat.
4. Bake, uncovered, for 18 to 22 minutes until the juices run clear.

Per Serving
calories: 258 | fat: 7.1g | protein: 39.1g
carbs: 6.9g | fiber: 0g | sugar: 4.0g
sodium: 465mg

Pork Diane

Prep time: 10 minutes | Cook time: 20 minutes | Serves 4

2 teaspoons Worcestershire sauce
1 tablespoon freshly squeezed lemon juice
¼ cup low-sodium chicken broth
2 teaspoons Dijon mustard
4 (5-ounce / 142-g) boneless pork top loin chops, about 1 inch thick
Sea salt and freshly ground black pepper, to taste
1 teaspoon extra-virgin olive oil
2 teaspoons chopped fresh chives
1 teaspoon lemon zest

1. Combine the Worcestershire sauce, lemon juice, broth, and Dijon mustard in a bowl. Stir to mix well.
2. On a clean work surface, rub the pork chops with salt and ground black pepper.
3. Heat the olive oil in a nonstick skillet over medium-high heat until shimmering.
4. Add the pork chops and sear for 16 minutes or until well browned. Flip the pork halfway through the cooking time. Transfer to a plate and set aside.
5. Pour the sauce mixture in the skillet and cook for 2 minutes or until warmed through and lightly thickened. Mix in the chives and lemon zest.
6. Baste the pork with the sauce mixture and serve immediately.

Per Serving
calories: 200 | fat: 8.0g | protein: 30.0g
carbs: 1.0g | fiber: 0g | sugar: 1.0g
sodium: 394mg

Beer Braised Brisket

Prep time: 10 minutes | Cook time: 8 hours | Serves 10

5 pounds (2.3 kg) beef brisket
1 bottle of lite beer
1 onion, sliced thin
1 (15-ounce / 425-g) can tomatoes, diced
3 cloves garlic, diced
fine
1 tablespoon plus 1 teaspoon oregano
1 tablespoon salt
1 tablespoon black pepper

1. Place the onion on the bottom of the crock pot. Add brisket, fat side up. Add the tomatoes, undrained and beer. Sprinkle the garlic and seasonings on the top.
2. Cover and cook on low heat 8 hours, or until beef is fork tender.

Per Serving
calories: 450 | fat: 14.0g | protein: 69.1g carbs: 4.1g | fiber: 1.0g | sugar: 2.0g sodium: 941mg

Steaks with Brandied Mushrooms

Prep time: 10 minutes | Cook time: 20 minutes | Serves 4

4 beef tenderloin steaks, about ¾ inch thick
3½ cups Portobello mushrooms, sliced
1 tablespoon margarine
½ cup brandy, divided
1 teaspoon balsamic
vinegar
½ teaspoon salt
½ teaspoon coarsely ground pepper
½ teaspoon instant coffee granules
Nonstick cooking spray

1. Heat oven to 200ºF (93ºC).
2. Salt and pepper both sides of the steaks and let sit 15 minutes.
3. In a small bowl, mix together coffee, vinegar, all but 1 tablespoon brandy, salt and pepper.
4. Spray a large skillet with cooking spray and place over medium-high heat.
5. Spray the mushrooms with cooking spray and add to the hot pan. Cook 5 minutes or until most of the liquid is absorbed. Transfer the mushrooms to a bowl.
6. Add the steaks to the skillet and cook 3 minutes per side. Reduce heat to medium-low and cook 2 more minutes or to desired doneness. Place on dinner plates, cover with foil and place in oven.
7. Add the brandy mixture to the skillet and bring to a boil. Boil 1 minute, or until reduced to about ¼ cup liquid. Stir in mushrooms and cook 1 to 2 minutes, or most of the liquid has evaporated.
8. Remove from heat and stir in remaining 1 tablespoon brandy and the margarine.
9. Spoon evenly over steaks and serve immediately.

Per Serving
calories: 352 | fat: 12.0g | protein: 44.1g carbs: 1.1g | fiber: 0g | sugar: 0g sodium: 374mg

Blue Cheese Crusted Beef Tenderloin

Prep time: 10 minutes | Cook time: 15 minutes | Serves 4

4 beef tenderloin steaks
2 tablespoons blue cheese, crumbled
4½ teaspoon fresh parsley, diced
4½ teaspoon chives, diced
1½ teaspoons butter
½ cup low sodium
beef broth
4½ teaspoon bread crumbs
1 tablespoon flour
1 tablespoon Madeira wine
¼ teaspoon pepper
Nonstick cooking spray

1. Heat oven to 350ºF (180ºC). Spray a large baking sheet with cooking spray.
2. In a small bowl, combine blue cheese, bread crumbs, parsley, chives, and pepper. Press onto one side of the steaks.
3. Spray a large skillet with cooking spray and place over medium-high heat.
4. Add steaks and sear 2 minutes per side. Transfer to prepared baking sheet and bake for 6 to 8 minutes, or steaks reach desired doneness.
5. Melt butter in a small saucepan over medium heat. Whisk in flour until smooth. Slowly whisk in broth and wine. Bring to a boil, cook, stirring, 2 minutes or until thickened.
6. Plate the steaks and top with gravy. Serve.

Per Serving
calories: 265 | fat: 10.0g | protein: 36.1g carbs: 4.1g | fiber: 0g | sugar: 0g sodium: 879mg

Sloppy Joes

Prep time: 10 minutes | Cook time: 15 minutes | Serves 4

1 tablespoon extra-virgin olive oil
1 pound (454 g) 93% lean ground beef
1 medium red bell pepper, chopped
½ medium yellow onion, chopped
2 tablespoons low-sodium Worcestershire sauce
1 (15-ounce / 425-g) can low-sodium tomato sauce
2 tablespoons low-sodium, sugar-free ketchup
4 whole-wheat sandwich thins, cut in half
1 cup cabbage, shredded

1. Heat the olive oil in a nonstick skillet over medium heat until shimmering.
2. Add the beef, bell pepper, and onion to the skillet and sauté for 8 minutes or until the beef is browned and the onion is translucent.
3. Pour the Worcestershire sauce, tomato sauce, and ketchup in the skillet. Turn up the heat to medium-high and simmer for 5 minutes.
4. Assemble the sandwich thin halves with beef mixture and cabbage to make the sloppy Joes, then serve warm.

Per Serving
calories: 329 | fat: 8.9g | protein: 31.2g
carbs: 35.9g | fiber: 7.9g | sugar: 10.9g
sodium: 271mg

Chipotle Chili Pork

Prep time: 4 hours 20 minutes | Cook time: 20 minutes | Serves 4

4 (5-ounce / 142-g) pork chops, about 1 inch thick
1 tablespoon chipotle chili powder
Juice and zest of 1 lime
2 teaspoons minced
garlic
1 teaspoon ground cinnamon
1 tablespoon extra-virgin olive oil
Pinch sea salt
Lime wedges, for garnish

1. Combine all the ingredients, except for the lemon wedges, in a large bowl. Toss to combine well.
2. Wrap the bowl in plastic and refrigerate to marinate for at least 4 hours.
3. Preheat the oven to 400ºF (205ºC). Set a rack on a baking sheet.
4. Remove the bowl from the refrigerator and let sit for 15 minutes. Discard the marinade and place the pork on the rack.
5. Roast in the preheated oven for 20 minutes or until well browned. Flip the pork halfway through the cooking time.
6. Serve immediately with lime wedges.

Per Serving
calories: 204 | fat: 9.0g | protein: 30.0g
carbs: 1.0g | fiber: 0g | sugar: 1.0g
sodium: 317mg

Mushroom, Beef, and Cauliflower Rice in Lettuce

Prep time: 5 minutes | Cook time: 20 minutes | Serves 4

1 tablespoon avocado oil
1 cup portobello mushrooms, chopped
½ cup white onion, chopped
1 pound (454 g) 93% lean ground beef
½ teaspoon garlic
powder
Salt, to taste
1 (10-ounce / 284-g) bag frozen cauliflower rice
¾ cup Cheddar cheese, shredded
12 iceberg lettuce leaves

1. Heath the avocado oil in a nonstick skillet over medium heat.
2. Add the mushrooms and onion to the skillet and sauté for 5 minutes until the mushrooms are soft and the onion starts to become translucent.
3. Add the beef, garlic powder, and salt to the skillet and sauté for another 5 minutes to brown the beef.
4. Increase the heat to medium-high, then add the cauliflower rice and sauté for an additional 5 minutes.
5. Divide the mixture and cheese on all lettuce leaves with a spoon, then roll up the lettuce to seal the wrap and serve warm.

Per Serving
calories: 289 | fat: 14.8g | protein: 31.2g
carbs: 6.9g | fiber: 3.1g | sugar: 3.8g
sodium: 262mg

Citrus Pork Tenderloin

Prep time: 10 minutes | Cook time: 30 minutes | Serves 4

¼ cup freshly squeezed orange juice
2 teaspoons orange zest
1 teaspoon low-sodium soy sauce
1 teaspoon honey
1 teaspoon grated

fresh ginger
2 teaspoons minced garlic
1½ pounds (680 g) pork tenderloin roast, fat trimmed
1 tablespoon extra-virgin olive oil

1. Combine the orange juice and zest, soy sauce, honey, ginger, and garlic in a large bowl. Stir to mix well. Dunk the pork in the bowl and press to coat well.
2. Wrap the bowl in plastic and refrigerate to marinate for at least 2 hours.
3. Preheat the oven to 400ºF (205ºC).
4. Remove the bowl from the refrigerator and discard the marinade.
5. Heat the olive oil in an oven-safe skillet over medium-high heat until shimmering.
6. Add the pork and sear for 5 minutes. Flip the pork halfway through the cooking time.
7. Arrange the skillet in the preheated oven and roast the pork for 25 minutes or until well browned. Flip the pork halfway through the cooking time.
8. Transfer the pork on a plate. Allow to cool before serving.

Per Serving
calories: 228 | fat: 9.0g | protein: 34.0g
carbs: 4.0g | fiber: 0g | sugar: 3.0g
sodium: 486mg

Beef, Tomato, and Pepper Tortillas

Prep time: 15 minutes | Cook time: 0 minutes | Serves 6

6 whole wheat flour tortillas (10-inch)
6 large romaine lettuce leaves
12 ounces (340 g) cooked deli roast beef, thinly sliced
1 cup diced red bell

peppers
1 cup diced tomatoes
1 tablespoon red wine vinegar
1 teaspoon cumin
¼ teaspoon freshly ground black pepper
1 tablespoon olive oil

1. Unfold the tortillas on a clean work surface, then top each tortilla with a lettuce leaf. Divide the roast beef over the leaf.
2. Combine the remaining ingredients in a bowl. Stir to mix well. Pour the mixture over the beef.
3. Fold the tortillas over the fillings, then roll them up. Serve immediately.

Per Serving
calories: 295 | fat: 6.0g | protein: 19.0g
carbs: 43.0g | fiber: 6.0g | sugar: 3.0g
sodium: 600mg

Easy Lime Lamb Cutlets

Prep time: 4 hours 20 minutes | Cook time: 8 minutes | Serves 4

¼ cup freshly squeezed lime juice
2 tablespoons lime zest
2 tablespoons chopped fresh parsley
Sea salt and freshly

ground black pepper, to taste
1 tablespoon extra-virgin olive oil
12 lamb cutlets (about 1½ pounds / 680 g in total)

1. Combine the lime juice and zest, parsley, salt, black pepper, and olive oil in a large bowl. Stir to mix well.
2. Dunk the lamb cutlets in the bowl of the lime mixture, then toss to coat well. Wrap the bowl in plastic and refrigerate to marinate for at least 4 hours.
3. Preheat the oven to 450ºF (235ºC) or broil. Line a baking sheet with aluminum foil.
4. Remove the bowl from the refrigerator and let sit for 10 minutes, then discard the marinade. Arrange the lamb cutlets on the baking sheet.
5. Broil the lamb in the preheated oven for 8 minutes or until it reaches your desired doneness. Flip the cutlets with tongs to make sure they are cooked evenly.
6. Serve immediately.

Per Serving
calories: 297 | fat: 18.8g | protein: 31.0g
carbs: 1.0g | fiber: 0g | sugar: 0g
sodium: 100mg

Slow Cooked Beef and Vegetables Roast

Prep time: 15 minutes | Cook time: 4 hours | Serves 4

1 tablespoon olive oil
2 medium celery stalks, halved lengthwise and cut into 3-inch pieces
4 medium carrots, scrubbed, halved lengthwise, and cut into 3-inch pieces
1 medium onion, cut in eighths
1¼ pounds (567 g)
lean chuck roast, boneless, trimmed of fat
2 teaspoons Worcestershire sauce
1 tablespoon balsamic vinegar
2 tablespoons water
1 tablespoon onion soup mix
½ teaspoon ground black pepper

1. Grease a slow cooker with olive oil.
2. Put the celery, carrots, and onion in the slow cooker, then add the beef.
3. Top them with Worcestershire sauce, balsamic vinegar, and water, then sprinkle with onion soup mix and black pepper.
4. Cover and cook on high for 4 hours.
5. Allow to cool for 20 minutes, then serve them on a large plate.

Per Serving
calories: 250 | fat: 6.0g | protein: 33.0g
carbs: 15.0g | fiber: 3.0g | sugar: 6.0g
sodium: 510mg

Asian Beef Bowls

Prep time: 15 minutes | Cook time: 15 minutes | Serves 4

1 pound (454 g) lean ground beef
1 bunch green onions, sliced
¼ cup fresh ginger, grated
1 cup riced cauliflower
¼ cup toasted sesame
oil
5 cloves garlic, diced fine
2 tablespoons light soy sauce
2 teaspoons sesame seeds

1. Heat oil in a large, cast iron skillet over high heat. Add all but 2 tablespoons, of the onions and cook until soft and starting to brown, about 5 minutes.
2. Add beef, and cook, breaking up with a spatula, until no longer pink. About 8 minutes.

3. Add remaining and simmer for 2 to 3 minutes, stirring frequently. Serve over hot cauliflower rice garnished with sesame seeds and reserved green onions.

Per Serving
calories: 385 | fat: 21.0g | protein: 40.1g
carbs: 24.1g | fiber: 2.0g | sugar: 11.0g
sodium: 209mg

Beef and Veggie Quesadillas

Prep time: 15 minutes | Cook time: 10 minutes | Serves 4

¾ pound (340 g) lean ground beef
2 tomatoes, seeded and diced
1 onion, diced
1 zucchini, grated
1 carrot, grated
¾ cup mushrooms, diced
½ cup Mozzarella cheese, grated
¼ cup cilantro, diced
4 (8-inch) whole wheat tortillas, warmed
2 cloves garlic, diced
2 teaspoons chili powder
¼ teaspoon salt
¼ teaspoon hot pepper sauce
Nonstick cooking spray

1. Heat oven to 400ºF (205ºC). Spray a large baking sheet with cooking spray.
2. Cook beef and onions in a large nonstick skillet over medium heat, until beef is no longer pink, drain fat. Transfer to a bowl and keep warm.
3. Add the mushrooms, zucchini, carrot, garlic, chili powder, salt and pepper sauce to the skillet and cook until vegetables are tender.
4. Stir in the tomatoes, cilantro and beef.
5. Lay the tortillas on the prepared pan. Cover half of each with beef mixture, and top with cheese. Fold other half over filling. Bake 5 minutes. Flip over and bake 5 to 6 minute more or until cheese has melted. Cut into wedges and serve.

Per Serving
calories: 320 | fat: 7.0g | protein: 33.1g
carbs: 31.1g | fiber: 5.0g | sugar: 5.0g
sodium: 575mg

Bacon and Cauliflower Casserole

Prep time: 15 minutes | Cook time: 20 minutes | Serves 6

6 slices bacon, cooked and crumbled, divided
3 scallions, sliced thin, divided
5 cup cauliflower
2 cup cheddar cheese, grated and divided
1 cup fat free sour cream
½ teaspoon salt
¼ teaspoon fresh cracked pepper
Nonstick cooking spray

1. Heat oven to 350ºF (180ºC). Spray casserole dish with cooking spray.
2. Steam cauliflower until just tender.
3. In a large bowl, combine cauliflower, sour cream, half the bacon, half the scallions and half the cheese. Stir in salt and pepper. Place in prepared baking dish and sprinkle remaining cheese over top.
4. Bake 18 to 20 minutes until heated through. Sprinkle remaining scallions and bacon over top and serve.

Per Serving
calories: 333 | fat: 20.0g | protein: 21.1g
carbs: 15.1g | fiber: 4.0g | sugar: 6.0g
sodium: 681mg

BBQ Pork Tacos

Prep time: 20 minutes | Cook time: 6 hours | Serves 16

2 pounds (907 g) pork shoulder, trim off excess fat
2 onions, diced fine
2 cups cabbages, shredded
16 (6-inch) low carb whole wheat tortillas
4 chipotle peppers in adobo sauce, puréed
1 cup light barbecue sauce
2 cloves garlic, diced fine
1½ teaspoons paprika

1. In a medium bowl, whisk together garlic, barbecue sauce and chipotles, cover and chill.
2. Place pork in the crock pot. Cover and cook on low 8 to 10 hours, or on high 4 to 6 hours.
3. Transfer pork to a cutting board. Use two forks and shred the pork, discarding the fat. Place pork back in the crock pot. Sprinkle with paprika then pour the barbecue sauce over mixture.
4. Stir to combine, cover and cook 1 hour. Skim off excess fat.
5. To assemble the tacos: place about ¼ cup of pork on warmed tortilla. Top with cabbage and onions and serve. Refrigerate any leftover pork up to 3 days.

Per Serving
calories: 266 | fat: 14.0g | protein: 17.1g
carbs: 14.1g | fiber: 9.0g | sugar: 3.0g
sodium: 434mg

Ham and Brie Turnovers

Prep time: 15 minutes | Cook time: 25 minutes | Serves 8

8 slices ham, diced
3 ounces (85 g) brie cheese
1 egg
2 (9-inch) pie crusts, unbaked
2 tablespoons sugar
free fig preserves
2 tablespoons stone ground mustard
1 tablespoon water
⅛ teaspoon salt
⅛ teaspoon pepper

1. Heat oven to 400ºF (205ºC). Line two cookie sheets with parchment paper.
2. On a lightly floured surface unroll one pie crust and cut 4 4-inch circles and place on prepared pan.
3. Gather up remaining dough, roll out and cut 4 more 4-inch circles and set aside
4. In a small bowl, combine fig preserves, mustard, salt, and pepper. Place a heaping teaspoon of fig mustard mixture in the center of dough on the pan and shape into a half dollar size
5. Use your hands to make a smaller circle of the brie and place on top of fig mixture. Place ham on top of the cheese, leaving ¼-inch edge.
6. In another small bowl, beat egg and water together. Brush around edge and top with 4-inch circle of dough. Repeat. Use a fork to seal the edges and cut a small X in the top. Brush with remaining egg wash.
7. Bake 25 minutes, or until golden brown. Remove from oven and cool on wire rack at least 5 minutes before serving. Repeat these steps with the second pie crust.

Per Serving
calories: 340 | fat: 21.0g | protein: 10.1g
carbs: 25.1g | fiber: 1.0g | sugar: 2.0g
sodium: 700mg

Beef Goulash

Prep time: 15 minutes | Cook time: 1 hour | Serves 6

2 pounds (907 g) chuck steak, trim fat and cut into bite-sized pieces
3 onions, quartered
1 green pepper, chopped
1 red pepper, chopped
1 orange pepper, chopped
3 cups water
1 can tomatoes, chopped

1 cup low sodium beef broth
3 cloves garlic, diced fine
2 tablespoons tomato paste
1 tablespoon olive oil
1 tablespoon paprika
2 teaspoons hot smoked paprika
2 bay leaves
Salt and ground black pepper, to taste

1. Heat oil in a large soup pot over medium-high. Add steak and cook until browned, stirring frequently. Add onions and cook 5 minutes, or until soft. Add garlic and cook another minute, stirring frequently.
2. Add remaining . Stir well and bring to a boil. Reduce heat to medium-low and simmer 45 to 50 minutes, stirring occasionally. Goulash is done when steak is tender. Stir well before serving.

Per Serving
calories: 412 | fat: 15.0g | protein: 53.1g carbs: 14.1g | fiber: 3.0g | sugar: 8.0g sodium: 159mg

Cajun Beef and Rice Skillet

Prep time: 10 minutes | Cook time: 25 minutes | Serves 4

¾ pound (340 g) lean ground beef
2 cup cauliflower rice, cooked
1 red bell pepper, sliced thin
½ yellow onion, diced
1 stalk celery, sliced thin

1 jalapeño pepper, seeds removed and diced fine
¼ cup fresh parsley, diced
½ cup low sodium beef broth
4 teaspoons Cajun seasoning

1. Place beef and 1½ teaspoons Cajun seasoning in a large skillet over medium-high heat. Cook, breaking apart with wooden spoon, until no longer pink, about 10 minutes.

2. Add vegetables, except cauliflower, and remaining Cajun seasoning. Cook, stirring occasionally, 6 to 8 minutes, or until vegetables are tender.
3. Add broth and stir, scraping brown bits from the bottom of the pan. Cook 2 to 3 minutes until mixture has thickened. Stir in cauliflower and cook just until heated through. Remove from heat, stir in parsley and serve.

Per Serving
calories: 200 | fat: 6.0g | protein: 28.1g carbs: 8.1g | fiber: 2.0g | sugar: 4.0g sodium: 291mg

Alfredo Sausage and Vegetables

Prep time: 10 minutes | Cook time: 15 minutes | Serves 6

1 package smoked sausage, cut in ¼-inch slices
1 cup half-and-half
½ cup zucchini, cut in matchsticks
½ cup carrots, cut in matchsticks
½ cup red bell pepper, cut in matchsticks
½ cup peas, frozen
¼ cup margarine

¼ cup onion, diced
2 tablespoons fresh parsley, diced
1 cup whole-wheat pasta, cooked and drained
¹⁄₃ cup reduced fat Parmesan cheese
1 clove garlic, diced fine
Salt and ground black pepper, to taste

1. Melt margarine in a large skillet over medium heat. Add onion and garlic and cook, stirring occasionally, 3 to 4 minutes or until onion is soft.
2. Increase heat to medium-high. Add sausage, zucchini, carrots, and red pepper. Cook, stirring frequently, 5 to 6 minutes, or until carrots are tender crisp.
3. Stir in peas and half-and-half, cook for 1 to 2 minutes until heated through. Stir in cheese, parsley, salt, and pepper. Add pasta and toss to mix. Serve.

Per Serving
calories: 285 | fat: 15.0g | protein: 21.1g carbs: 18.1g | fiber: 4.0g | sugar: 8.0g sodium: 807mg

Classic Stroganoff

Prep time: 15 minutes | Cook time: 20 minutes | Serves 5

5 ounces (142 g) cooked egg noodles
2 teaspoons olive oil
1 pound (454 g) beef tenderloin tips, boneless, sliced into 2-inch strips
1½ cups white button mushrooms, sliced
½ cup onion, minced
1 tablespoon all-purpose flour
½ cup dry white wine
1 (14.5-ounce / 411-g) can fat-free, low-sodium beef broth
1 teaspoon Dijon mustard
½ cup fat-free sour cream
¼ teaspoon salt
¼ teaspoon black pepper

1. Put the cooked egg noodles on a large plate.
2. Heat the olive oil in a nonstick skillet over high heat until shimmering.
3. Add the beef and sauté for 3 minutes or until lightly browned. Remove the beef from the skillet and set on the plate with noodles.
4. Add the mushrooms and onion to the skillet and sauté for 5 minutes or until tender and the onion browns.
5. Add the flour and cook for a minute. Add the white wine and cook for 2 more minutes.
6. Add the beef broth and Dijon mustard. Bring to a boil. Keep stirring. Reduce the heat to low and simmer for another 5 minutes.
7. Add the beef back to the skillet and simmer for an additional 3 minutes. Add the remaining ingredients and simmer for 1 minute.
8. Pour them over the egg noodles and beef, and serve immediately.

Per Serving
calories: 275 | fat: 7.0g | protein: 23.0g
carbs: 29.0g | fiber: 4.0g | sugar: 3.0g
sodium: 250mg

Cajun Smothered Pork Chops

Prep time: 5 minutes | Cook time: 25 minutes | Serves 4

4 pork chops, thick-cut
1 small onion, diced fine
1 cup mushrooms, sliced
1 cup fat free sour cream
2 tablespoons margarine
1 cup low sodium chicken broth
3 cloves garlic, diced fine
1 tablespoon Cajun seasoning
2 bay leaves
1 teaspoon smoked paprika
Salt and ground black pepper, to taste to taste

1. Melt margarine in a large skillet over medium heat. Sprinkle chops with salt and pepper and cook until nicely browned, about 5 minutes per side. Transfer to a plate.
2. Add onions and mushrooms and cook until soft, about 5 minutes. Add garlic and cook one minute more.
3. Add broth and stir to incorporate brown bits on bottom of the pan. Add a dash of salt and the bay leaves. Add pork chops back to sauce. Bring to a simmer, cover, and reduce heat. Cook 5 to 8 minutes, or until chops are cooked through.
4. Transfer chops to a plate and keep warm. Bring sauce to a boil and cook until it has reduced by half, stirring occasionally.
5. Reduce heat to low and whisk in sour cream, Cajun seasoning, and paprika. Cook, stirring frequently, 3 minutes. Add chops back to the sauce and heat through. Serve.

Per Serving
calories: 325 | fat: 18.0g | protein: 24.1g
carbs: 13.1g | fiber: 1.0g | sugar: 5.0g
sodium: 383mg

Steak Sandwich

Prep time: 10 minutes | Cook time: 10 minutes | Serves 4

2 tablespoons balsamic vinegar
2 teaspoons freshly squeezed lemon juice
1 teaspoon fresh parsley, chopped
2 teaspoons fresh oregano, chopped
2 teaspoons garlic, minced
2 tablespoons olive oil
1 pound (454 g) flank steak, trimmed of fat
4 whole-wheat pitas
1 tomato, chopped
1 ounce (28 g) low-sodium feta cheese
2 cups lettuce, shredded
1 red onion, thinly sliced

1. Combine the balsamic vinegar, lemon juice, parsley, oregano, garlic, and olive oil in a bowl.
2. Dunk the steak in the bowl to coat well, then wrap the bowl in plastic and refrigerate for at least 1 hour.
3. Preheat the oven to 450°F (235°C).
4. Remove the bowl from the refrigerator. Discard the marinade and arrange the steak on a baking sheet lined with aluminum foil.
5. Broil in the preheated oven for 10 minutes for medium. Flip the steak halfway through the cooking time.
6. Remove the steak from the oven and allow to cool for 10 minutes. Slice the steak into strips.
7. Assemble the pitas with steak, tomato, feta cheese, lettuce, and onion to make the sandwich, and serve warm.

Per Serving
calories: 345 | fat: 15.8g | protein: 28.1g
carbs: 21.9g | fiber: 3.1g | carbs: 18.8g
sodium: 295mg

Coffeed and Herbed Steak

Prep time: 10 minutes | Cook time: 10 minutes | Serves 4

¼ cup whole coffee beans
2 teaspoons fresh rosemary, chopped
2 teaspoons fresh thyme, chopped
2 teaspoons garlic, minced
1 teaspoon freshly ground black pepper
2 tablespoons apple cider vinegar
2 tablespoons olive oil
1 pound (454 g) flank steak, trimmed of fat

1. Put the coffee beans, rosemary, thyme, garlic, and black pepper in a food processor. Pulse until well ground and combined.
2. Pour the mixture in a large bowl, then pour the vinegar and olive oil in the bowl. Stir to mix well.
3. Dunk the steak in the mixture, then wrap the bowl in plastic and refrigerate to marinate for 2 hours.
4. Preheat the broiler to MEDIUM.
5. Remove the bowl from the refrigerator, and discard the marinade.
6. Place the marinated steak on a baking sheet lined with aluminum foil.
7. Broil in the preheated broiler for 10 minutes or until the steak reaches your desired doneness. Flip the steak halfway through the cooking time.
8. Remove the steak from the broiler. Allow to cool for a few minutes and slice to serve.

Per Serving
calories: 316 | fat: 19.8g | protein: 31.1g
carbs: 0g | fiber: 0g | sugar: 0g
sodium: 78mg

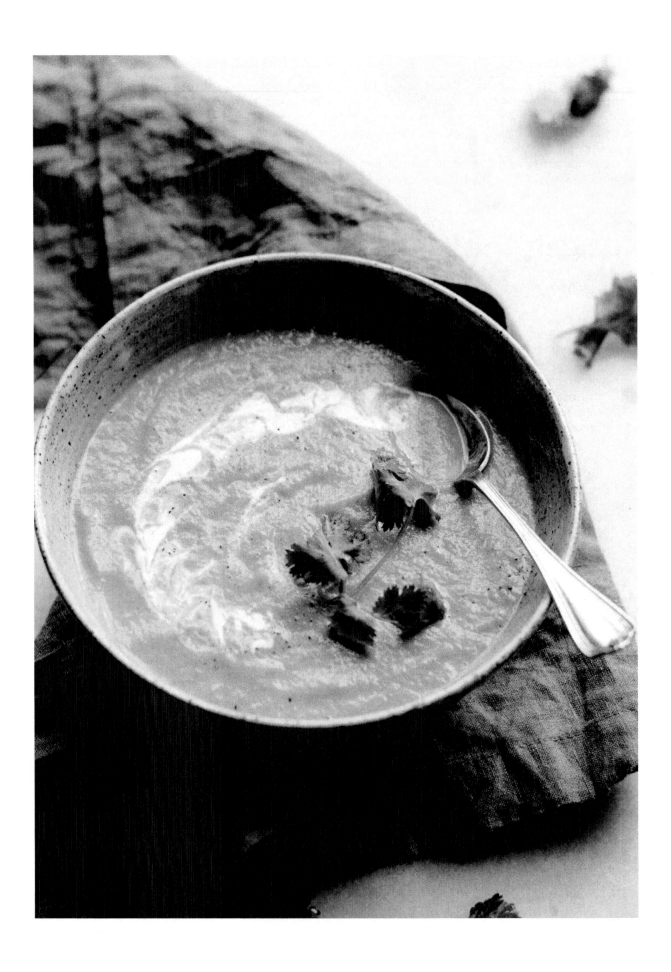

Chapter 10: Soups and Stews

North Carolina Stew

Prep time: 20 minutes | Cook time: 20 minutes | Serves 8

½ cup seafood broth
2 large white onions, chopped
4 garlic cloves, minced
¼ cup tomato paste
1 teaspoon red pepper flakes
2 teaspoons smoked

paprika
3 bay leaves
3 cups water
2 pounds (907 g) fish fillets, such as rockfish, striped bass, or cod, cut into ½- to 1-inch dice
8 medium eggs

1. Select the Sauté setting on an electric pressure cooker, and combine the broth, onions, garlic, tomato paste, red pepper flakes, paprika, and bay leaves. Cook for 2 minutes, or until the onions and garlic are translucent.
2. Add 1 cup of water.
3. Close and lock the lid, and set the pressure valve to sealing.
4. Change to the Manual/Pressure Cook setting, and cook for 3 minutes.
5. Once cooking is complete, quick-release the pressure. Carefully remove the lid.
6. Add the fish and enough of the water just to cover the fish.
7. Close and lock the lid, and set the pressure valve to sealing.
8. Select the Manual/Pressure Cook setting, and cook for 3 more minutes.
9. Once cooking is complete, quick-release the pressure. Carefully remove the lid.
10. Carefully crack the eggs one by one into the stew, keeping the yolks intact.
11. Close and lock the lid, and set the pressure valve to sealing.
12. Select the Manual/Pressure Cook setting, and cook for 1 minute.
13. Once cooking is complete, quick-release the pressure. Carefully remove the lid, discard the bay leaves, and serve in bowls.

Per Serving
calories: 220 | fat: 6.1g | protein: 28.1g
carbs: 14.9g | fiber: 3.1g | sugar: 4.0g
sodium: 146mg

Beef, Mushroom, and Pearl Barley Soup

Prep time: 10 minutes | Cook time: 1 hour 20 minutes | Serves 6

1 pound (454 g) beef stew meat, cubed
¼ teaspoon salt
¼ teaspoon freshly ground black pepper
1 tablespoon extra-virgin olive oil
8 ounces (227 g) sliced mushrooms
1 onion, chopped
2 carrots, chopped

3 celery stalks, chopped
6 garlic cloves, minced
½ teaspoon dried thyme
4 cups low-sodium beef broth
1 cup water
½ cup pearl barley

1. Season the meat with the salt and pepper.
2. In an Instant Pot, heat the oil over high heat. Add the meat and brown on all sides. Remove the meat from the pot and set aside.
3. Add the mushrooms to the pot and cook for 1 to 2 minutes, until they begin to soften. Remove the mushrooms and set aside with the meat.
4. Add the onion, carrots, and celery to the pot. Sauté for 3 to 4 minutes until the vegetables begin to soften. Add the garlic and continue to cook until fragrant, about 30 seconds longer.
5. Return the meat and mushrooms to the pot, then add the thyme, beef broth, and water. Set the pressure to high and cook for 15 minutes. Let the pressure release naturally.
6. Open the Instant Pot and add the barley. Use the slow cooker function on the Instant Pot, affix the lid (vent open), and continue to cook for 1 hour until the barley is cooked through and tender. Serve.

Per Serving
calories: 250 | fat: 9.1g | protein: 21.1g
carbs: 18.9g | fiber: 4.1g | sugar: 3.0g
sodium: 515mg

Classic Gazpacho

Prep time: 15 minutes | Cook time: 0 minutes | Serves 4

3 pounds (1.4 kg) ripe tomatoes, chopped
1 cup low-sodium tomato juice
½ red onion, chopped
1 cucumber, peeled, seeded, and chopped
1 red bell pepper, seeded and chopped
2 celery stalks, chopped
2 tablespoons

chopped fresh parsley
2 garlic cloves, chopped
2 tablespoons extra-virgin olive oil
2 tablespoons red wine vinegar
1 teaspoon honey
½ teaspoon salt
¼ teaspoon freshly ground black pepper

1. In a blender jar, combine the tomatoes, tomato juice, onion, cucumber, bell pepper, celery, parsley, garlic, olive oil, vinegar, honey, salt, and pepper. Pulse until blended but still slightly chunky.
2. Adjust the seasonings as needed and serve.
3. To store, transfer to a nonreactive, airtight container and refrigerate for up to 3 days.

Per Serving
calories: 172 | fat: 8.1g | protein: 5.1g
carbs: 23.9g | fiber: 6.1g | sugar: 16.0g
sodium: 333mg

Italian Minestrone

Prep time: 10 minutes | Cook time: 20 minutes | Serves 4

2 tablespoons extra-virgin olive oil
1 onion, chopped
1 red bell pepper, seeded and chopped
2 garlic cloves, minced
2 cups green beans (fresh or frozen; halved if fresh)
6 cups low-sodium

vegetable broth
1 (14-ounce / 397-g) can crushed tomatoes
1 tablespoon Italian seasoning
½ cup dried whole-wheat elbow macaroni
½ teaspoon sea salt
Pinch red pepper flakes (or to taste)

1. In a large pot over medium-high heat, heat the olive oil until it shimmers. Add the onion and bell pepper and cook, stirring occasionally, until they soften, about 3 minutes. Add the garlic and cook,

stirring constantly, for 30 seconds. Add the green beans, vegetable broth, tomatoes, and Italian seasoning and bring to a boil.
2. Add the elbow macaroni, salt, and red pepper flakes. Cook, stirring occasionally, until the macaroni is soft, about 8 minutes.

Per Serving
calories: 200 | fat: 7.1g | protein: 5.1g
carbs: 28.9g | fiber: 7.1g | sugar: 12.8g
sodium: 478mg

Carrot Curry Soup

Prep time: 10 minutes | Cook time: 5 minutes | Serves 6

1 tablespoon extra-virgin olive oil
1 small onion, coarsely chopped
2 celery stalks, coarsely chopped
1½ teaspoons curry powder
1 teaspoon ground cumin
1 teaspoon minced fresh ginger

6 medium carrots, roughly chopped
4 cups low-sodium vegetable broth
¼ teaspoon salt
1 cup canned coconut milk
¼ teaspoon freshly ground black pepper
1 tablespoon chopped fresh cilantro

1. Heat an Instant Pot to high and add the olive oil.
2. Sauté the onion and celery for 2 to 3 minutes. Add the curry powder, cumin, and ginger to the pot and cook until fragrant, about 30 seconds.
3. Add the carrots, vegetable broth, and salt to the pot. Close and seal, and set for 5 minutes on high. Allow the pressure to release naturally.
4. In a blender jar, carefully purée the soup in batches and transfer back to the pot.
5. Stir in the coconut milk and pepper, and heat through. Top with the cilantro and serve.

Per Serving
calories: 146 | fat: 11.1g | protein: 2.1g
carbs: 12.9g | fiber: 3.1g | sugar: 4.0g
sodium: 240mg

Kale and Tomato Soup

Prep time: 10 minutes | Cook time: 15 minutes | Serves 4

1 tablespoon extra-virgin olive oil
1 medium onion, chopped
2 carrots, finely chopped
3 garlic cloves, minced
4 cups low-sodium vegetable broth
1 (28-ounce / 794-g) can crushed tomatoes
½ teaspoon dried oregano
¼ teaspoon dried basil
4 cups chopped baby kale leaves
¼ teaspoon salt

1. In a large pot, heat the oil over medium heat. Add the onion and carrots to the pan. Sauté for 3 to 5 minutes until they begin to soften. Add the garlic and sauté for 30 seconds more, until fragrant.
2. Add the vegetable broth, tomatoes, oregano, and basil to the pot and bring to a boil. Reduce the heat to low and simmer for 5 minutes.
3. Using an immersion blender, purée the soup.
4. Add the kale and simmer for 3 more minutes. Season with the salt. Serve immediately.

Per Serving
calories: 172 | fat: 5.1g | protein: 6.1g
carbs: 30.9g | fiber: 9.1g | sugar: 13.0g
sodium: 583mg

Thai Shrimp and Peanut Soup

Prep time: 10 minutes | Cook time: 10 minutes | Serves 4

1 tablespoon coconut oil
1 tablespoon Thai red curry paste
½ onion, sliced
3 garlic cloves, minced
2 cups chopped carrots
½ cup whole unsalted peanuts
4 cups low-sodium vegetable broth
½ cup unsweetened plain almond milk
½ pound (227 g) shrimp, peeled and deveined
Minced fresh cilantro, for garnish

1. In a large pan, heat the oil over medium-high heat until shimmering.
2. Add the curry paste and cook, stirring constantly, for 1 minute. Add the onion, garlic, carrots, and peanuts to the pan, and continue to cook for 2 to 3 minutes until the onion begins to soften.
3. Add the broth and bring to a boil. Reduce the heat to low and simmer for 5 to 6 minutes until the carrots are tender.
4. Using an immersion blender or in a blender, purée the soup until smooth and return it to the pot. With the heat still on low, add the almond milk and stir to combine. Add the shrimp to the pot and cook for 2 to 3 minutes until cooked through.
5. Garnish with cilantro and serve.

Per Serving
calories: 240 | fat: 14.1g | protein: 14.1g
carbs: 16.9g | fiber: 5.1g | sugar: 6.0g
sodium: 620mg

Leek and Cauliflower Soup

Prep time: 10 minutes | Cook time: 20 minutes | Serves 2

Avocado oil cooking spray
2½ cups chopped leeks (2 to 3 leeks)
2½ cups cauliflower florets
1 garlic clove, peeled
⅓ cup low-sodium vegetable broth
½ cup half-and-half
¼ teaspoon salt
¼ teaspoon freshly ground black pepper

1. Heat a large stockpot over medium-low heat. When hot, coat the cooking surface with cooking spray. Put the leeks and cauliflower into the pot.
2. Increase the heat to medium and cover the pan. Cook for 10 minutes, stirring halfway through.
3. Add the garlic and cook for 5 minutes.
4. Add the broth and deglaze the pan, stirring to scrape up the browned bits from the bottom.
5. Transfer the broth and vegetables to a food processor or blender and add the half-and-half, salt, and pepper. Blend well.

Per Serving
calories: 174 | fat: 7.1g | protein: 6.1g
carbs: 23.9g | fiber: 5.1g | sugar: 8.0g
sodium: 490mg

Mushroom and Beef Cheeseburger Soup

Prep time: 5 minutes | Cook time: 25 minutes | Serves 4

Avocado oil cooking spray
½ cup diced white onion
½ cup diced celery
½ cup sliced portobello mushrooms
1 pound (454 g) 93% lean ground beef
1 (15-ounce / 425-g) can no-salt-added diced tomatoes
2 cups low-sodium beef broth
⅓ cup half-and-half
¾ cup shredded sharp Cheddar cheese

1. Heat a large stockpot over medium-low heat. When hot, coat the cooking surface with cooking spray. Put the onion, celery, and mushrooms into the pot. Cook for 7 minutes, stirring occasionally.
2. Add the ground beef and cook for 5 minutes, stirring and breaking apart as needed.
3. Add the diced tomatoes with their juices and the broth. Increase the heat to medium-high and simmer for 10 minutes.
4. Remove the pot from the heat and stir in the half-and-half.
5. Serve topped with the cheese.

Per Serving
calories: 332 | fat: 18.1g | protein: 33.1g carbs: 8.9g | fiber: 2.1g | sugar: 5.0g sodium: 320mg

Traditional Pot Liquor Soup

Prep time: 15 minutes | Cook time: 20 minutes | Serves 6

3 cups low-sodium chicken broth, divided
1 medium onion, chopped
3 garlic cloves, minced
1 bunch collard greens or mustard greens including stems,
roughly chopped
1 fresh ham bone
5 carrots, peeled and cut into 1-inch rounds
2 fresh thyme sprigs
3 bay leaves
Freshly ground black pepper, to taste

1. Select the Sauté setting on an electric pressure cooker, and combine ½ cup of chicken broth, the onion, and garlic and cook for 3 to 5 minutes, or until the onion and garlic are translucent.
2. Add the collard greens, ham bone, carrots, remaining 2½ cups of broth, the thyme, and bay leaves.
3. Close and lock the lid and set the pressure valve to sealing.
4. Change to the Manual/Pressure Cook setting, and cook for 15 minutes.
5. Once cooking is complete, quick-release the pressure. Carefully remove the lid. Discard the bay leaves.
6. Serve with Skillet Bivalves.

Per Serving
calories: 100 | fat: 4.1g | protein: 6.1g carbs: 9.9g | fiber: 3.1g | sugar: 4.0g sodium: 200mg

Beef Taco Soup

Prep time: 5 minutes | Cook time: 20 minutes | Serves 4

Avocado oil cooking spray
1 medium red bell pepper, chopped
½ cup chopped yellow onion
1 pound (454 g) 93% lean ground beef
1 teaspoon ground cumin
½ teaspoon salt
½ teaspoon chili powder
½ teaspoon garlic powder
2 cups low-sodium beef broth
1 (15-ounce / 425-g) can no-salt-added diced tomatoes
1½ cups frozen corn
⅓ cup half-and-half

1. Heat a large stockpot over medium-low heat. When hot, coat the cooking surface with cooking spray. Put the pepper and onion in the pan and cook for 5 minutes.
2. Add the ground beef, cumin, salt, chili powder, and garlic powder. Cook for 5 to 7 minutes, stirring and breaking apart the beef as needed.
3. Add the broth, diced tomatoes with their juices, and corn. Increase the heat to medium-high and simmer for 10 minutes.
4. Remove from the heat and stir in the half-and-half.

Per Serving
calories: 321 | fat: 12.1g | protein: 30.1g carbs: 22.9g | fiber: 4.1g | sugar: 7.0g sodium: 457mg

Clam Chowder

Prep time: 10 minutes | Cook time: 15 minutes | Serves 4

2 tablespoons extra-virgin olive oil
3 slices pepper bacon, chopped
1 onion, chopped
1 red bell pepper, seeded and chopped
1 fennel bulb, chopped

3 tablespoons flour
5 cups low-sodium or unsalted chicken broth
6 ounces (170 g) chopped canned clams, undrained
½ teaspoon sea salt
½ cup milk

1. In a large pot over medium-high heat, heat the olive oil until it shimmers. Add the bacon and cook, stirring, until browned, about 4 minutes. Remove the bacon from the fat with a slotted spoon, and set it aside on a plate.
2. Add the onion, bell pepper, and fennel to the fat in the pot. Cook, stirring occasionally, until the vegetables are soft, about 5 minutes. Add the flour and cook, stirring constantly, for 1 minute. Add the broth, clams, and salt. Bring to a simmer. Cook, stirring, until the soup thickens, about 5 minutes more.
3. Stir in the milk and return the bacon to the pot. Cook, stirring, 1 minute more.

Per Serving
calories: 336 | fat: 20.1g | protein: 20.1g
carbs: 20.9g | fiber: 3.1g | sugar: 11.4g
sodium: 495mg

Spicy Beef and Vegetable Soup

Prep time: 20 minutes | Cook time: 30 minutes | Serves 4

2 teaspoons olive oil
1 tablespoon garlic, minced
1 sweet onion, chopped
2 carrots, peeled, diced
1 sweet potato, peeled, diced
4 celery stalks, with greens, chopped
2 cups cooked beef, diced

1 cup cooked pearl barley
8 cups low-sodium beef broth
2 teaspoons hot sauce
2 bay leaves
1 cup kale, shredded
2 teaspoons fresh thyme, chopped
Salt and freshly ground black pepper, to taste

1. Heat the olive oil in a stockpot over medium-high heat.
2. Add the garlic and onion to the pot and sauté for 3 minutes or until the onion is translucent and the garlic is fragrant.
3. Add the carrot, sweet potato, and celery to the pot and sauté for 5 minutes more.
4. Add the beef, barley, beef broth, hot sauce, and bay leaves to the pot. Bring to a boil, then reduce the heat to low and simmer for 15 minutes until the beef is browned and the vegetables are tender.
5. Discard the bay leaves, then add the kale and thyme to the pot. Sprinkle with salt and black pepper, and simmer for an additional 5 minutes.
6. Pour the soup in a large bowl, then serve warm.

Per Serving
calories: 697 | fat: 23.9g | protein: 54.6g
carbs: 76.6g | fiber: 5.7g | sugar: 11.9g
sodium: 282mg

Beef and Vegetable Soup

Prep time: 10 minutes | Cook time: 15 minutes | Serves 4

1 pound (454 g) ground beef
1 onion, chopped
2 celery stalks, chopped
1 carrot, chopped
1 teaspoon dried

rosemary
6 cups low-sodium beef or chicken broth
½ teaspoon sea salt
⅛ teaspoon freshly ground black pepper
2 cups peas

1. In a large pot over medium-high heat, cook the ground beef, crumbling with the side of a spoon, until browned, about 5 minutes.
2. Add the onion, celery, carrot, and rosemary. Cook, stirring occasionally, until the vegetables start to soften, about 5 minutes.
3. Add the broth, salt, pepper, and peas. Bring to a simmer. Reduce the heat and simmer, stirring, until warmed through, about 5 minutes more.

Per Serving
calories: 356 | fat: 17.1g | protein: 34.1g
carbs: 17.9g | fiber: 5.1g | sugar: 12.6g
sodium: 363mg

Ritzy Calabaza Squash Soup

Prep time: 15 minutes | Cook time: 45 minutes | Serves 8

2 pounds (907 g) calabaza squash, peeled and chopped	8 scallions, chopped
	3 sprigs fresh thyme
1 large tomato, chopped	1 tablespoon minced ginger root
1 medium onion, chopped	8 cups low-sodium vegetable broth
1 medium green bell pepper, chopped	Juice of 1 lime
	¼ cup chopped cilantro
1 scotch bonnet chili, deseeded and minced	Salt, to taste
	¼ cup toasted pepitas

1. Put the calabaza squash, tomato, onion, bell pepper, scotch bonnet, scallions, thyme, and ginger roots in a saucepan, then pour in the vegetable broth.
2. Bring to a boil over medium-high heat. Reduce the heat to low, then simmer for 45 minutes or until the vegetables are soft. Stir constantly.
3. Add the lime juice, cilantro, and salt. Pour the soup in a large bowl, then discard the thyme sprigs and garnish with pepitas before serving.

Per Serving
calories: 50 | fat: 0g | protein: 2.0g
carbs: 12.0g | fiber: 4.0g | sugar: 5.0g
sodium: 20mg

Simple Buttercup Squash Soup

Prep time: 15 minutes | Cook time: 33 minutes | Serves 6

2 tablespoons extra-virgin olive oil	4 cups vegetable broth
1 medium onion, chopped	½ teaspoon kosher salt
1½ pounds (680 g) buttercup squash, peeled, deseeded, and cut into 1-inch chunks	¼ teaspoon ground white pepper
	Ground nutmeg, to taste

1. Heat the olive oil in a pot over medium-high heat until shimmering.
2. Add the onion and sauté for 3 minutes or until translucent.
3. Add the buttercup squash, vegetable broth, salt, and pepper. Stir to mix well. Bring to a boil.
4. Reduce the heat to low and simmer for 30 minutes or until the buttercup squash is soft.
5. Pour the soup in a food processor, then pulse to purée until creamy and smooth.
6. Pour the soup in a large serving bowl, then sprinkle with ground nutmeg and serve.

Per Serving (1¹/₃ Cups)
calories: 110 | fat: 5.0g | protein: 1.0g
carbs: 18.0g | fiber: 4.0g | sugar: 4.0g
sodium: 166mg

Turkey, Barley and Vegetable Stock

Prep time: 25 minutes | Cook time: 3 hours 7 minutes | Serves 8

2 tablespoons avocado oil	peppers and onions (about 2½ cups)
1 pound (454 g) ground turkey	1 (15-ounce / 425-g) package frozen chopped carrots (about 2½ cups)
28 ounces (1.3 kg) tomatoes, diced	
2 tablespoons sugar-free tomato paste	¹/₃ cup dry barley
4 cups low-sodium chicken broth	2 bay leaves
	1 teaspoon kosher salt
1 (15-ounce / 425-g) package frozen	¼ teaspoon freshly ground black pepper

1. Heat the avocado oil in a pot over medium-high heat.
2. Add the turkey and sauté for 7 minutes or until lightly browned.
3. Add the tomatoes, tomato paste, and chicken broth. Stir to mix well.
4. Add the peppers and onions, carrots, barley, bay leaves, salt, and pepper. Stir to mix well.
5. Bring to a boil. Reduce the heat to low, then cover the pot and simmer for 3 hours.
6. Once the simmering is finished, allow to cool for 20 minutes, then discard the bay leaves and pour the soup in a large bowl to serve.

Per Serving (1¼ Cups)
calories: 253 | fat: 12.0g | protein: 19.0g
carbs: 21.0g | fiber: 7.0g | sugar: 7.0g
sodium: 560mg

African Christmas Stew

Prep time: 15 minutes | Cook time: 1 hour 40 minutes | Serves 6

3½ pounds (1.6 kg) chicken, whole pieces with bones in
6 Roma tomatoes
2 scallions, diced white and green parts
1 onion, sliced thin
1 cup carrots, sliced
2 cups water
⅛ cup vegetable oil
3 tablespoons parsley
2 cloves garlic, diced fine
1 tablespoon paprika
1½ teaspoons thyme
¼ teaspoon curry powder
1 bay leaf
Salt and ground black pepper, to taste

1. Season chicken with salt and pepper on both sides.
2. Place the tomatoes, onion, and scallions in a food processor and pulse until puréed.
3. In a large soup pot, heat the oil over medium heat. Add chicken and brown on both sides.
4. Pour the tomato mixture over the chicken and add the remaining . Bring to a low boil.
5. Reduce heat to low, cover, and simmer 60 to 90 minutes until the chicken is cooked through and the carrots are tender. Discard bay leaf before serving. Serve as is or over cauliflower rice.

Per Serving
calories: 481 | fat: 13.0g | protein: 78.0g
carbs: 9.1g | fiber: 2.0g | sugar: 5.1g
sodium: 235mg

Asian Meatball Soup

Prep time: 15 minutes | Cook time: 5 hours | Serves 4

½ pound (227 g) ground pork
4 cup mustard greens, torn
4 scallions, sliced thin
2 teaspoons fresh ginger, peeled and grated fine
4 cup low sodium chicken broth
2 tablespoons soy sauce
1 tablespoon
vegetable oil
2 cloves garlic, diced fine
1 teaspoon peppercorns, crushed
1 teaspoon fish sauce
¾ teaspoon red pepper flakes,
½ teaspoon cumin seeds, chopped coarse
Sea salt and black pepper, to taste

1. In a large bowl, combine pork, garlic, ginger, and spices. Season with salt and pepper. Use your hands to combine all thoroughly.
2. Heat oil in a large skillet over medium heat. Form pork into 1-inch balls and cook in oil till brown on all sides. Use a slotted spoon to transfer the meatballs to a crock pot.
3. Add remaining and stir. Cover and cook on low for 4 to 5 hours or until meatballs are cooked through. Serve.

Per Serving
calories: 157 | fat: 6.0g | protein: 19.0g
carbs: 7.1g | fiber: 2.0g | sugar: 2.1g
sodium: 571mg

Lentil, Carrot, and Celery Soup

Prep time: 10 minutes | Cook time: 55 minutes | Serves 8

1 teaspoon olive oil
1 tablespoon garlic, minced
1 sweet onion, chopped
3 carrots, peeled and diced
4 celery stalks, with the greens, chopped
2 bay leaves
3 cups red lentils,
picked over, washed, and drained
4 cups low-sodium vegetable soup
3 cups water
2 teaspoons fresh thyme, chopped
Salt and freshly ground black pepper, to taste

1. Heat the olive oil in a stockpot over medium-high heat.
2. Add the garlic and onion to the pot and sauté for 3 minutes until the onion is translucent.
3. Add the carrots and celery to the pot and sauté for 5 minutes.
4. Add the bay leaves, lentils, vegetables soup, and water to the pot. Bring to a boil.
5. Turn down the heat to low and simmer for 45 minutes until lentils are tender and soup starts to have a thick consistency.
6. Pour the soup in a large bowl. Discard the bay leaves, and top with thyme, salt, and black pepper before serving.

Per Serving
calories: 285 | fat: 1.9g | protein: 20.1g
carbs: 46.8g | fiber: 24.2g | sugar: 3.8g
sodium: 417mg

Bacon and Cabbage Soup

Prep time: 15 minutes | Cook time: 6 hours | Serves 6

6 bacon strips, cut into 1-inch pieces
3 cup cauliflower, separated into florets
2 cup cabbage, sliced thin
2 celery stalks, peeled and diced
1 onion, diced
1 carrot, peeled and diced
5 cup low sodium chicken broth
2 cloves garlic, diced fine
¼ teaspoon thyme

1. Cook bacon in a large skillet over medium-high heat until almost crisp. Remove from skillet and place on paper towels to drain.
2. Add the celery, garlic, and onion to the skillet and cook, stirring frequently, about 5 minutes. Use a slotted spoon to transfer to the crock pot.
3. Add the bacon, broth, cabbage, carrot, and thyme to the crock pot. Cover and cook on low for 4 to 5 hours or until the carrots are tender.
4. Add the cauliflower and cook until tender, about 1 to 2 hours. Serve.

Per Serving
calories: 150 | fat: 8.0g | protein: 10.0g
carbs: 8.1g | fiber: 3.0g | sugar: 3.1g
sodium: 216mg

Beef and Sweet Potato Stew

Prep time: 20 minutes | Cook time: 1 hour 10 minutes | Serves 6

2 pounds (907 g) top sirloin steak, diced
1½ pounds (680 g) sweet potato, peeled and cut in ½-inch cubes
½ pound (227 g) cremini mushrooms, quartered
2 stalks celery, diced
1 red onion, diced
1 carrot, peeled and diced
2 tablespoons fresh
parsley, chopped
4 sprigs fresh thyme
4 cup low sodium beef broth
½ cup dry red wine
¼ cup flour
3 cloves garlic, diced
2 tablespoons tomato paste
2 tablespoons olive oil
2 bay leaves
Salt and ground black pepper, to taste

1. Heat oil in a large stockpot over medium heat. Season steak with salt and pepper

and add to pot. Cook, stirring occasionally, until brown on all sides. Remove from pot and set aside.
2. Add onion, carrot, and celery. Cook, stirring occasionally, 3 to 4 minutes or until tender.
3. Add garlic and mushrooms and cook another 3 to 4 minutes. Whisk in flour and tomato paste and cook until lightly browned, about 1 minute.
4. Stir in wine, scraping up any browned bits from the bottom of the pot. Add the broth, thyme, bay leaves and steak. Bring to a boil, reduce heat and simmer about 30 minutes, or until steak is tender.
5. Add sweet potato and cook 20 minutes or until potatoes are tender and stew has thickened. Discard bay leaves and thyme sprigs. Stir in parsley and serve.

Per Serving
calories: 420 | fat: 15.0g | protein: 51.0g
carbs: 14.1g | fiber: 2.0g | sugar: 4.1g
sodium: 175mg

Beef Burgundy and Mushroom Stew

Prep time: 15 minutes | Cook time: 8 hours | Serves 4

1 pound (454 g) sirloin steak, cut into bite size pieces
2 carrots, peeled and cut into 1-inch pieces
1 cup mushrooms, sliced
¾ cup pearl onions, thawed if frozen
1 cup Burgundy wine
½ cup low sodium beef broth
3 cloves garlic, diced
2 tablespoons olive oil
1 bay leaf
1 teaspoon marjoram
½ teaspoon salt
½ teaspoon thyme
¼ teaspoon pepper

1. Heat the oil in a large skillet over medium-high heat. Add steak and brown on all sides. Transfer to a crock pot.
2. Add remaining and stir to combine. Cover and cook on low 7 to 8 hours or until steak is tender and vegetables are cooked through. Discard the bay leaf before serving.

Per Serving
calories: 352 | fat: 14.0g | protein: 36.0g
carbs: 8.1g | fiber: 1.0g | sugar: 3.1g
sodium: 470mg

Chicken and Pepper Stew

Prep time: 15 minutes | Cook time: 4 hours | Serves 4

2 small onions, quartered
1½ cup chicken, cut into 1-inch pieces
1 cup broccoli florets
½ cup green bell pepper, diced
½ cup yellow pepper, diced
½ cup red pepper, diced
½ cup mushrooms, diced
2 tablespoons margarine
4 cup low sodium chicken broth
⅛ cup water
4 cloves garlic, diced fine
1 teaspoon rosemary
1 teaspoon corn starch
½ teaspoon thyme
Salt and ground black pepper, to taste

1. Heat 1 tablespoon margarine in large skillet over medium heat. Add chicken and cook till no longer pink. Remove from skillet and add to crock pot.
2. Add remaining tablespoon of margarine to skillet along with onions and garlic. Sauté until onions begin to soften. Add to chicken.
3. Add the broth, vegetables and seasonings to the crock pot. Cover and cook on high 2 to 3 hours till chicken is cooked through and vegetables are tender.
4. Stir the corn starch into the ⅛ cup of water and stir into the stew. Cook another 60 minutes, or until thickened.

Per Serving
calories: 208 | fat: 8.0g | protein: 20.0g
carbs: 15.1g | fiber: 3.1g | sugar: 6.1g
sodium: 389mg

Chipotle Bacon and Chicken Chowder

Prep time: 5 minutes | Cook time: 30 minutes | Serves 6

1½ pounds (680 g) chicken breast, boneless, skinless and cut in 1-inch pieces
½ pound (227 g) bacon, chopped
3 cup half-and-half
4 chipotle peppers in adobo sauce, diced fine
2 tablespoons cilantro, diced
6 cup low sodium chicken broth
1 teaspoon salt
½ teaspoon onion powder
½ teaspoon garlic powder
½ teaspoon pepper

1. Place a large saucepan over medium-high heat. Add bacon and cook until crisp. Transfer to a paper towel lined plate.
2. Add the chicken and cook until browned on all sides.
3. Add the broth and seasonings and simmer for 10 to 15 minutes, or until the chicken is cooked through. Stir in the half-and-half and chipotles and simmer 5 minutes more. Serve topped with the bacon and cilantro.

Per Serving
calories: 500 | fat: 32.0g | protein: 46.0g
carbs: 7.1g | fiber: 1.1g | sugar: 0g
sodium: 827mg

Pork Posole

Prep time: 5 minutes | Cook time: 25 minutes | Serves 6

1 yellow onion, diced fine
1½ cup pork, cook and shred
1 fresh lime, cut in wedges
½ bunch cilantro, chopped
1 (15-ounce / 425-g) can hominy, drain
1 (4-ounce / 113-g) can green chilies, diced
3 ounces (85 g) tomato paste
3 cup low sodium chicken broth
2 cup water
2 tablespoons vegetable oil
2 tablespoons flour
2 tablespoons chili powder
¾ teaspoon salt
½ teaspoon cumin
½ teaspoon garlic powder
¼ teaspoon cayenne pepper

1. Heat oil in a large pot over medium heat. Add onion and cook 3 to 5 minutes, or until it softens.
2. Add the flour and chili powder and cook 2 minutes more, stirring continuously.
3. Add water, tomato paste, and seasonings. Whisk mixture until tomato paste dissolves. Bring to a simmer and let thicken, about 2 to 3 minutes.
4. Stir in broth, pork, chilies, and hominy and cook until heated through, about 10 minutes.
5. Ladle into bowls and garnish with a lime wedge and chopped cilantro.

Per Serving
calories: 235 | fat: 8.0g | protein: 11.2g
carbs: 33.1g | fiber: 9.2g | sugar: 12.1g
sodium: 913mg

Fast Split Pea Soup

Prep time: 8 minutes | Cook time: 15 minutes | Serves 4

1½ cups dried green split peas, rinsed and drained
4 cups vegetable broth or water
2 celery stalks, chopped
1 medium onion, chopped
2 carrots, chopped
3 garlic cloves,
minced
1 teaspoon herbes de Provence
1 teaspoon liquid smoke
Kosher salt and freshly ground black pepper, to taste
Shredded carrot, for garnish (optional)

1. In the electric pressure cooker, combine the peas, broth, celery, onion, carrots, garlic, herbes de Provence, and liquid smoke.
2. Close and lock the lid of the pressure cooker. Set the valve to sealing.
3. Cook on high pressure for 15 minutes.
4. When the cooking is complete, hit Cancel and allow the pressure to release naturally for 10 minutes, then quick release any remaining pressure.
5. Once the pin drops, unlock and remove the lid.
6. Stir the soup and season with salt and pepper.
7. Spoon into serving bowls and sprinkle shredded carrots on top (if using).

Per Serving
calories: 285 | fat: 1.1g | protein: 19.1g
carbs: 51.9g | fiber: 21.1g | sugar: 9.0g
sodium: 61mg

Hearty Bell Pepper Stew

Prep time: 20 minutes | Cook time: 4 hours | Serves 8

1 pound (454 g) hot Italian sausage
1 pound (454 g) lean ground sirloin
3½ cup tomatoes, diced
3 cup green pepper, diced
3 cup onion, diced
1 cup cauliflower,
grated
4 cup low sodium beef broth
1 cup tomato sauce
2 tablespoons olive oil
4 cloves garlic, diced fine
1 teaspoon basil
½ teaspoon oregano

1. Heat the oil in a large skillet over medium-high heat. Add in both kinds of meat and cook, breaking it up with a spoon, until no longer pink on the outside. Remove the meat with a slotted spoon and place in crock pot.
2. Add the green pepper, onion and garlic to the skillet. Cook, stirring frequently, about 5 minutes. Remove the vegetables with a slotted spoon and add to the meat mixture.
3. Add in the broth, tomatoes, tomato sauce and seasonings. Cover and cook on high 2 to 3 hours.
4. Add the cauliflower and cook another 60 minutes or until cauliflower is tender.

Per Serving
calories: 313 | fat: 20.0g | protein: 19.2g
carbs: 14.1g | fiber: 2.9g | sugar: 8.1g
sodium: 952mg

Tangy Asparagus Bisque

Prep time: 10 minutes | Cook time: 20 minutes | Serves 4

2 pounds (907 g) fresh asparagus, remove the bottom and cut into small pieces
1 yellow onion, diced
1 small lemon, zest and juice
1 teaspoon fresh
thyme, diced fine
4 cup low sodium vegetable broth
3 tablespoons olive oil
3 cloves garlic, diced fine
Salt and ground black pepper, to taste

1. Heat oil in a large saucepan over medium-high heat. Add asparagus and onion and cook, stirring occasionally, until nicely browned, about 5 minutes. Add garlic and cook 1 minute more.
2. Stir in remaining and bring to a boil. Reduce heat, and simmer 12 to 15 minutes or until asparagus is soft.
3. Use an immersion blender and process until smooth. Salt and ground black pepper, to taste and serve.

Per Serving
calories: 170 | fat: 11.0g | protein: 6.2g
carbs: 17.1g | fiber: 6.2g | sugar: 7.1g
sodium: 185mg

Summer Squash and Crispy Chickpeas Soup

Prep time: 10 minutes | Cook time: 20 minutes | Serves 4

1 (15-ounce / 425-g) can low-sodium chickpeas, drained and rinsed
1 teaspoon extra-virgin olive oil, plus 1 tablespoon
¼ teaspoon smoked paprika
Pinch salt, plus ½ teaspoon
3 medium zucchini, coarsely chopped
3 cups low-sodium vegetable broth
½ onion, diced
3 garlic cloves, minced
2 tablespoons plain low-fat Greek yogurt
Freshly ground black pepper, to taste

1. Preheat the oven to 425ºF (220ºC). Line a baking sheet with parchment paper.
2. In a medium mixing bowl, toss the chickpeas with 1 teaspoon of olive oil, the smoked paprika, and a pinch salt. Transfer to the prepared baking sheet and roast until crispy, about 20 minutes, stirring once. Set aside.
3. Meanwhile, in a medium pot, heat the remaining 1 tablespoon of oil over medium heat.
4. Add the zucchini, broth, onion, and garlic to the pot, and bring to a boil. Reduce the heat to a simmer, and cook until the zucchini and onion are tender, about 20 minutes.
5. In a blender jar, or using an immersion blender, purée the soup. Return to the pot.
6. Add the yogurt, remaining ½ teaspoon of salt, and pepper, and stir well. Serve topped with the roasted chickpeas.

Per Serving
calories: 190 | fat: 7.1g | protein: 8.1g
carbs: 23.9g | fiber: 7.1g | sugar: 7.0g
sodium: 529mg

Cheesy Chicken Tortilla Soup

Prep time: 10 minutes | Cook time: 35 minutes | Serves 4

1 tablespoon extra-virgin olive oil
1 onion, thinly sliced
1 garlic clove, minced
1 jalapeño pepper, diced
2 boneless, skinless chicken breasts
4 cups low-sodium chicken broth
1 Roma tomato, diced
½ teaspoon salt
2 (6-inch) corn tortillas, cut into thin strips
Nonstick cooking spray
Juice of 1 lime
Minced fresh cilantro, for garnish
¼ cup shredded Cheddar cheese, for garnish

1. In a medium pot, heat the oil over medium-high heat. Add the onion and cook for 3 to 5 minutes until it begins to soften. Add the garlic and jalapeño, and cook until fragrant, about 1 minute more.
2. Add the chicken, chicken broth, tomato, and salt to the pot and bring to a boil. Reduce the heat to medium and simmer gently for 20 to 25 minutes until the chicken breasts are cooked through. Remove the chicken from the pot and set aside.
3. Preheat a broiler to high.
4. Spray the tortilla strips with nonstick cooking spray and toss to coat. Spread in a single layer on a baking sheet and broil for 3 to 5 minutes, flipping once, until crisp.
5. When the chicken is cool enough to handle, shred it with two forks and return to the pot.
6. Season the soup with the lime juice. Serve hot, garnished with cilantro, cheese, and tortilla strips.

Per Serving
calories: 192 | fat: 8.1g | protein: 19.1g
carbs: 12.9g | fiber: 2.1g | sugar: 2.0g
sodium: 483mg

Lamb and Vegetable Stew

Prep time: 10 minutes | Cook time: 3 to 6 hours | Serves 6

1 pound (454 g) boneless lamb stew meat
1 pound (454 g) turnips, peeled and chopped
1 fennel bulb, trimmed and thinly sliced
10 ounces (283 g) mushrooms, sliced
1 onion, diced
3 garlic cloves, minced
2 cups low-sodium chicken broth
2 tablespoons tomato paste
¼ cup dry red wine (optional)
1 teaspoon chopped fresh thyme
½ teaspoon salt
¼ teaspoon freshly ground black pepper
Chopped fresh parsley, for garnish

1. In a slow cooker, combine the lamb, turnips, fennel, mushrooms, onion, garlic, chicken broth, tomato paste, red wine (if using), thyme, salt, and pepper.
2. Cover and cook on high for 3 hours or on low for 6 hours. When the meat is tender and falling apart, garnish with parsley and serve.
3. If you don't have a slow cooker, in a large pot, heat 2 teaspoons of olive oil over medium heat, and sear the lamb on all sides. Remove from the pot and set aside. Add the turnips, fennel, mushrooms, onion, and garlic to the pot, and cook for 3 to 4 minutes until the vegetables begin to soften. Add the chicken broth, tomato paste, red wine (if using), thyme, salt, pepper, and browned lamb. Bring to a boil, then reduce the heat to low. Simmer for 1½ to 2 hours until the meat is tender. Garnish with parsley and serve.

Per Serving
calories: 305 | fat: 7.1g | protein: 32.1g
carbs: 26.9g | fiber: 4.1g | sugar: 7.0g
sodium: 312mg

Thai Peanut and Shrimp Soup with Carrots

Prep time: 10 minutes | Cook time: 15 minutes | Serves 4

1 tablespoon coconut oil
1 tablespoon Thai red curry paste
3 garlic cloves, minced
½ onion, sliced
2 cups carrots, chopped
½ cup whole unsalted peanuts
4 cups low-sodium chicken broth
½ cup unsweetened almond milk
½ pound (227 g) shrimp, peeled and deveined
Minced fresh cilantro, for garnish

Special Equipment:
An immersion blender

1. Melt the coconut oil in a large skillet over medium-high heat until shimmering.
2. Add the red curry paste and cook for 1 minutes, stirring continuously.
3. Add the garlic, onion, carrots, and peanuts to the skillet, and sauté for 2 to 3 minutes until the garlic is fragrant.
4. Pour in the chicken broth and whisk to combine, then bring to a boil.
5. Reduce the heat to low and allow to simmer until the carrots are tender when pierced with a fork, about 5 to 6 minutes.
6. Purée the soup with an immersion blender until smooth.
7. Add the almond milk and mix well. Stir in the shrimp and cook for an additional 3 minutes , or until the flesh is totally pink and opaque.
8. Remove from the heat and ladle the soup into four bowls. Sprinkle the cilantro on top for garnish before serving.

Per Serving
calories: 240 | fat: 14.3g | protein: 14.2g
carbs: 17.3g | fiber: 5.2g | sugar: 6.2g
sodium: 618mg

Chicken and Egg Noodle Soup

Prep time: 15 minutes | Cook time: 30 minutes | Serves 12

2 tablespoons avocado oil
1 medium onion, chopped
3 celery stalks, chopped
1 teaspoon kosher salt
¼ teaspoon freshly ground black pepper
2 teaspoons minced garlic
5 large carrots, peeled and cut into ¼-inch-thick rounds
3 pounds (1.4 kg) bone-in chicken breasts (about 3)
4 cups low-sodium chicken broth
4 cups water
2 tablespoons soy sauce
6 ounces (170 g) whole grain wide egg noodles

1. Set the electric pressure cooker to the Sauté setting. When the pot is hot, pour in the avocado oil.
2. Sauté the onion, celery, salt, and pepper for 3 to 5 minutes or until the vegetables begin to soften.
3. Add the garlic and carrots, and stir to mix well. Hit Cancel.
4. Add the chicken to the pot, meat-side down. Add the broth, water, and soy sauce. Close and lock the lid of the pressure cooker. Set the valve to sealing.
5. Cook on high pressure for 20 minutes.
6. When the cooking is complete, hit Cancel and quick release the pressure. Unlock and remove the lid.
7. Using tongs, remove the chicken breasts to a cutting board. Hit Sauté/More and bring the soup to a boil.
8. Add the noodles and cook for 4 to 5 minutes or until the noodles are al dente.
9. While the noodles are cooking, use two forks to shred the chicken. Add the meat back to the pot and save the bones to make more bone broth.
10. Season with additional pepper, if desired, and serve.

Per Serving
calories: 331 | fat: 15.1g | protein: 32.1g
carbs: 16.9g | fiber: 4.1g | sugar: 3.0g
sodium: 450mg

Eggplant Stew

Prep time: 20 minutes | Cook time: 8 minutes | Serves 4

2 tablespoons avocado oil
1 large onion, minced
2 garlic cloves, minced
1 teaspoon ras el hanout spice blend or curry powder
¼ teaspoon cayenne pepper
1 teaspoon kosher salt
1 cup vegetable broth or water
1 tablespoon tomato paste
2 cups chopped eggplant
2 medium gold potatoes, peeled and chopped
4 ounces (113 g) tomatillos, husks removed, chopped
1 (14-ounce / 397-g) can diced tomatoes

1. Set the electric pressure cooker to the Sauté setting. When the pot is hot, pour in the avocado oil.
2. Sauté the onion for 3 to 5 minutes, until it begins to soften. Add the garlic, ras el hanout, cayenne, and salt. Cook and stir for about 30 seconds. Hit Cancel.
3. Stir in the broth and tomato paste. Add the eggplant, potatoes, tomatillos, and tomatoes with their juices.
4. Close and lock the lid of the pressure cooker. Set the valve to sealing.
5. Cook on high pressure for 3 minutes.
6. When the cooking is complete, hit Cancel and allow the pressure to release naturally.
7. Once the pin drops, unlock and remove the lid.
8. Stir well and spoon into serving bowls.

Per Serving
calories: 215 | fat: 8.1g | protein: 4.1g
carbs: 27.9g | fiber: 8.1g | sugar: 9.0g
sodium: 736mg

Roasted Tomato and Bell Pepper Soup

Prep time: 20 minutes | Cook time: 35 minutes | Serves 6

2 tablespoons extra-virgin olive oil, plus more for coating the baking dish
16 plum tomatoes, cored and halved
4 celery stalks, coarsely chopped
4 red bell peppers, seeded, halved
4 garlic cloves, lightly crushed
1 sweet onion, cut into eighths
Sea salt and freshly ground black pepper, to taste
6 cups low-sodium chicken broth
2 tablespoons chopped fresh basil
2 ounces (57 g) goat cheese, grated

1. Preheat the oven to 400ºF (205ºC). Coat a large baking dish lightly with olive oil.
2. Put the tomatoes in the oiled dish, cut-side down. Scatter the celery, bell peppers, garlic, and onion on top of the tomatoes. Drizzle with 2 tablespoons of olive oil and season with salt and pepper.
3. Roast in the preheated oven for about 30 minutes, or until the vegetables are fork-tender and slightly charred.
4. Remove the vegetables from the oven. Let them rest for a few minutes until cooled slightly.
5. Transfer to a food processor, along with the chicken broth, and purée until fully mixed and smooth.
6. Pour the purée soup into a medium saucepan and bring it to a simmer over medium-high heat.
7. Sprinkle the basil and grated cheese on top before serving.

Per Serving
calories: 187 | fat: 9.7g | protein: 7.8g
carbs: 21.3g | fiber: 6.1g | sugar: 14.0g
sodium: 825mg

Black Bean and Zucchini Pepper Stew

Prep time: 15 minutes | Cook time: 15 minutes | Serves 6

1 tablespoon extra-virgin olive oil
½ onion, chopped
½ red bell pepper, deseeded and chopped
½ green bell pepper, deseeded and chopped
2 small zucchini, chopped
3 garlic cloves, minced
1 (15-ounce / 425-g) can low-sodium black beans, drained and rinsed
1 (10-ounce / 284-g) can low-sodium enchilada sauce
1 teaspoon ground cumin
¼ teaspoon salt
¼ teaspoon freshly ground black pepper
½ cup shredded Cheddar cheese, divided
2 (6-inch / 15-cm) corn tortillas, cut into strips
Chopped fresh cilantro, for garnish
Plain yogurt, for serving

1. Preheat the broiler to high.
2. In a large skillet, heat the oil over medium-high heat until it shimmers.
3. Add the onion, red bell pepper, green bell pepper, zucchini, and garlic to the skillet, and cook for 3 to 5 minutes until the onion softens.
4. Add the black beans, enchilada sauce, cumin, salt, pepper, ¼ cup of cheese, and tortilla strips, and mix together. Top with the remaining ¼ cup of cheese.
5. Put the skillet under the broiler and broil for 5 to 8 minutes until the cheese is melted and bubbly.
6. Garnish with cilantro and serve with yogurt on the side.

Per Serving
calories: 172 | fat: 7.2g | protein: 8.3g
carbs: 21.2g | fiber: 7.2g | sugar: 3.2g
sodium: 563mg

Beef Zoodle Stew

Prep time: 15 minutes | Cook time: 1 hour 25 minutes | Serves 6

1 pound (454 g) beef stew meat
4 large zucchinis, spiralize
3 celery stalks, diced
3 carrots, peeled and diced
½ red onion, diced
1 (14-ounce / 397-g) can tomatoes, diced
4 cup low-sodium beef broth
2 cloves garlic, diced fine
1 to 2 bay leaves
3 tablespoons Worcestershire sauce
2 tablespoons olive oil
1 teaspoon thyme
½ teaspoon cayenne pepper
¼ teaspoon red pepper flakes
Salt and ground black pepper, to taste
Freshly chopped parsley, to garnish

1. Heat oil in a large saucepan over medium heat. Add beef and cook until brown on all sides. Remove from pan and set aside.
2. Add the garlic to the pan and cook 30 seconds. Then stir in onion and red pepper flakes. Cook 1 minute and add the celery and carrots. Sweat the vegetables for 2 minutes, stirring occasionally.
3. Add the beef back to the pan with the Worcestershire, thyme, and cayenne pepper and stir. Season with salt and pepper to taste. Add the broth, tomatoes, and bay leaves and bring to a boil.
4. Reduce heat, cover and let simmer 40 minutes. Remove the cover and cook 35 minutes more or until stew thickens.
5. Divide the zucchini noodles evenly among four bowls. Ladle stew evenly over zucchini and let set for a few minutes to cook the zucchini. Top with fresh parsley and serve.

Per Serving
calories: 226 | fat: 6.0g | protein: 29.0g
carbs: 13.1g | fiber: 3.1g | sugar: 8.1g
sodium: 320mg

Cajun Seafood Stew

Prep time: 20 minutes | Cook time: 40 minutes | Serves 8

6 live blue crabs
2 pounds (907 g) medium shrimp, peeled, deveined and tails removed
1 pound (454 g) jumbo lump crabmeat
5 scallions, diced
4 stalks celery, diced
1½ large yellow onions, diced
1 green bell pepper, diced
⅓ cup parsley, diced fine
¼ cup fresh lemon juice
8 cup low sodium vegetable broth
6 cloves garlic, diced fine
½ cup olive oil
½ cup flour
1 tablespoon Worcestershire sauce
2 bay leaves
½ teaspoon cayenne
Salt and ground black pepper, to taste to taste

1. Prepare crabs, working with one at a time. Remove and discard legs. Remove and save the claws. Discard the underside, the triangular section, and pull the body away from the shell. Remove gills and organs and rinse thoroughly. Place clean crabs in a bowl, cover and refrigerate till ready to use.
2. Heat oil in a large stock pot over medium-high heat. Whisk in flour and cook, stirring constantly, until you have a dark roux. Add vegetables and cook, stirring frequently, until vegetables are soft, about 10 to 12 minutes.
3. Add the cleaned crabs, broth, Worcestershire and spices and bring to a boil. Reduce heat, cover and simmer 15 to 20 minutes.
4. Add remaining seafood and cook until shrimp turn pink, 3 to 5 minutes. Stir in parsley, lemon juice and scallions. Serve.

Per Serving
calories: 441 | fat: 19.0g | protein: 54.0g
carbs: 17.1g | fiber: 1.1g | sugar: 3.1g
sodium: 1371mg

Guinness Beef Stew with Cauliflower Mash

Prep time: 10 minutes | Cook time: 8 hours | Serves 4

2 pounds (907 g) beef round steak, cut into 1-inch cubes
1 large head cauliflower, separated into florets
5 sprigs fresh thyme
1 medium carrot, cut into ½-inch pieces
1 stick of celery, cut into ½-inch pieces
1 cup yellow onion, cut into large pieces
²/₃ cup Guinness
1 tablespoon margarine
2 cups low sodium beef broth
2 tablespoons arrowroot starch
1 tablespoon plus 1 teaspoon garlic, diced fine
2 teaspoons olive oil
Sea salt and pepper to taste

1. Add oil to a large nonstick skillet and heat over medium-high heat. Add beef and sear on all sides. Transfer to crock pot.
2. Add thyme, Guinness, carrot, onion, celery, garlic, and broth. Set to low and cook 6 to 8 hours, or 4 to 5 on high.
3. One hour before the stew is ready, mix arrowroot with 1½ tablespoons water and stir into stew.
4. For the mash: bring 2 cups water to a boil in a large pot and add cauliflower. Cover and cook 10 to 12 minutes, or until cauliflower is soft.
5. Drain. Add salt, pepper, 1 teaspoon garlic, and margarine. Use an immersion blender and process until it resembles mashed potatoes.
6. To serve: ladle stew in a bowl and spoon about ¼ cup of the mash on top. Garnish with fresh thyme, parsley, and cracked pepper if desired.

Per Serving
calories: 564 | fat: 28.0g | protein: 75.2g
carbs: 17.1g | fiber: 5.9g | sugar: 7.1g
sodium: 248mg

Mexican Beef Stew

Prep time: 15 minutes | Cook time: 1 hour 30 minutes | Serves 6

1½ pound (680 g) beef round steak, cut into ½-inch pieces
1¾ cup tomatoes, diced
1 cup carrots, sliced
1 cup onion, diced
¼ cup sweet red pepper, diced
1 jalapeno, seeded and diced
2 tablespoons cilantro, diced
1¾ cup low sodium beef broth
1 clove garlic, diced
2 tablespoons flour
2 tablespoons water
1 tablespoon vegetable oil
1½ teaspoons chili powder
½ teaspoon salt

1. Heat the oil in a large pot over medium-high heat. Add the steak and cook until brown on all sides.
2. Add the broth, carrots, onion, red pepper, jalapeno, garlic, and seasonings and bring to a low boil. Reduce heat to low, cover and simmer 45 minutes, stirring occasionally.
3. Add the tomatoes and continue cooking 15 minutes.
4. Stir the flour and water together in a measuring up until smooth. Add to stew with the cilantro and continue cooking another 20 to 30 minutes or until stew has thickened. Serve.

Per Serving
calories: 313 | fat: 13.0g | protein: 39.2g
carbs: 9.1g | fiber: 2.2g | sugar: 4.1g
sodium: 306mg

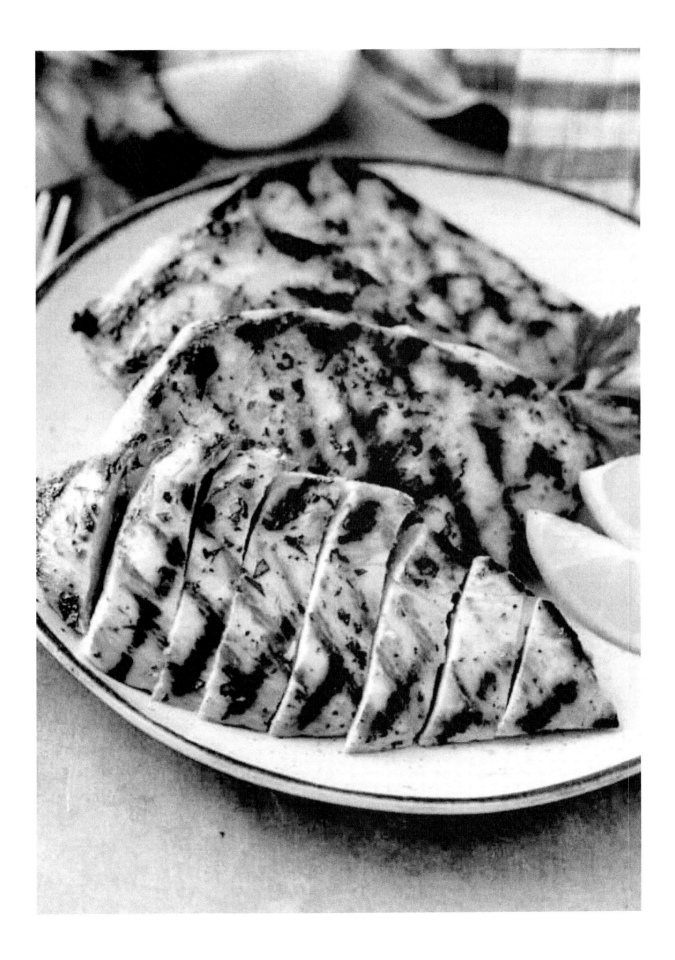

Chapter 11: Poultry

Peach Chicken Thighs with Dandelion Greens

Prep time: 10 minutes | Cook time: 30 minutes | Serves 4

4 boneless, skinless chicken thighs
Juice of 1 lime
½ cup white vinegar
2 garlic cloves, smashed
1 cup frozen peaches
½ cup water
Pinch ground cinnamon
Pinch ground cloves
Pinch ground nutmeg
⅛ teaspoon vanilla extract
½ cup low-sodium chicken broth
1 bunch dandelion greens, cut into ribbons
1 medium onion, thinly sliced

1. Set oven to broil. In a bowl, combine the chicken, lime juice, vinegar, and garlic, coating the chicken thoroughly.
2. Meanwhile, to make the peach glaze, in a small pot, combine the peaches, water, cinnamon, cloves, nutmeg, and vanilla. Cook over medium heat, stirring often, for 10 minutes, or until the peaches have softened.
3. In a large cast iron skillet, bring the broth to a simmer over medium heat.
4. Add the greens, and sauté for 5 minutes, or until the greens are wilted.
5. Add the onion and cook, stirring occasionally, for 3 minutes, or until slightly reduced.
6. Add the chicken and cover with the peach glaze.
7. Transfer the pan to the oven, and broil for 10 to 12 minutes, or until the chicken is golden brown.

Per Serving
calories: 201 | fat: 4.9g | protein: 24.1g
carbs: 13.9g | fiber: 4.1g | sugar: 6.0g
sodium: 156mg

Turkey Stuffed Red Bell Peppers

Prep time: 15 minutes | Cook time: 50 minutes | Serves 4

1 teaspoon extra-virgin olive oil, plus more for greasing the baking dish
1 pound (454 g) ground turkey breast
½ sweet onion, chopped
1 teaspoon minced garlic
1 tomato, diced
½ teaspoon chopped fresh basil
Sea salt and freshly ground black pepper, to taste
4 red bell peppers, tops cut off, seeded
2 ounces (57 g) low-sodium feta cheese

1. Preheat the oven to 350ºF (180ºC).
2. Lightly grease a baking dish with olive oil and set it aside.
3. Place a large skillet over medium heat and add 1 teaspoon of olive oil.
4. Add the turkey to the skillet and cook until it is no longer pink, stirring occasionally to break up the meat and brown it evenly, about 6 minutes.
5. Add the onion and garlic and sauté until softened and translucent, about 3 minutes.
6. Stir in the tomato and basil. Season with salt and pepper.
7. Place the peppers cut-side up in the baking dish. Divide the filling into four equal portions and spoon it into the peppers.
8. Sprinkle the feta cheese on top of the filling.
9. Add ¼ cup of water to the dish and cover with aluminum foil.
10. Bake the peppers until they are soft and heated through, about 40 minutes.

Per Serving
calories: 282 | fat: 14.1g | protein: 24.1g
carbs: 14.0g | fiber: 4.1g | sugar: 9.0g
sodium: 270mg

Strawberry and Peach Chicken

Prep time: 20 minutes | Cook time: 40 minutes | Serves 4

For the Barbecue Sauce:
1 cup frozen peaches	paprika
1 cup frozen strawberries	1 teaspoon garlic powder
¼ cup tomato purée	½ teaspoon cayenne pepper
½ cup white vinegar	
1 tablespoon yellow mustard	½ teaspoon onion powder
1 teaspoon mustard seeds	½ teaspoon freshly ground black pepper
1 teaspoon turmeric	1 teaspoon celery seeds
1 teaspoon sweet	

For the Chicken:
4 boneless, skinless chicken thighs

To Make the Barbecue Sauce
1. In a stockpot, combine the peaches, strawberries, tomato purée, vinegar, mustard, mustard seeds, turmeric, paprika, garlic powder, cayenne, onion powder, black pepper, and celery seeds. Cook over low heat for 15 minutes, or until the flavors come together.
2. Remove the sauce from the heat, and let cool for 5 minutes.
3. Transfer the sauce to a blender, and purée until smooth.

To Make the Chicken
1. Preheat the oven to 350ºF (180ºC).
2. Put the chicken in a medium bowl. Coat well with ½ cup of barbecue sauce.
3. Place the chicken on a rimmed baking sheet.
4. Place the baking sheet on the middle rack of the oven, and bake for about 20 minutes (depending on the thickness of thighs), or until the juices run clear.
5. Brush the chicken with additional sauce, return to the oven, and broil on high for 3 to 5 minutes, or until a light crust forms.
6. Serve immediately.

Per Serving
calories: 190 | fat: 5.1g | protein: 23.1g
carbs: 11.1g | fiber: 3.1g | sugar: 7.0g
sodium: 150mg

Rosemary Turkey Scaloppini

Prep time: 10 minutes | Cook time: 20 minutes | Serves 4

½ cup whole-wheat flour	1 garlic clove, minced
½ teaspoon sea salt	½ cup dry white wine
¼ teaspoon freshly ground black pepper	2 tablespoons chopped fresh rosemary
3 tablespoons extra-virgin olive oil	1 cup low-sodium chicken broth
12 ounces (340 g) turkey breast, cut into ½-inch-thick cutlets and pounded flat	2 tablespoons salted butter, cold, cut into small pieces

1. Preheat the oven to 200ºF (93ºC). Line a baking sheet with parchment paper.
2. In a medium bowl, whisk together the flour, salt, and pepper.
3. In a large skillet over medium-high heat, heat the olive oil until it shimmers.
4. Working in batches with one or two pieces of turkey at a time (depending on how much room you have in the pan), dredge the turkey cutlets in the flour and pat off any excess. Cook in the hot oil until the turkey is cooked through, about 3 minutes per side. Add more oil if needed.
5. Place the cooked cutlets on the lined baking sheet and keep them warm in the oven while you cook the remaining turkey and make the pan sauce.
6. Once all the turkey is cooked and warming in the oven, add the garlic to the pan and cook, stirring constantly, for 30 seconds. Add the wine and use the side of a spoon to scrape any browned bits off the bottom of the pan. Simmer, stirring, for 1 minute. Add the rosemary and chicken broth. Simmer, stirring, until it thickens, 1 to 2 minutes more.
7. Whisk in the cold butter, one piece at a time, until incorporated. Return the turkey cutlets to the sauce and turn once to coat. Serve with any remaining sauce spooned over the top.

Per Serving
calories: 346 | fat: 20.1g | protein: 24.1g
carbs: 14.9g | fiber: 2.1g | sugar: 7.4g
sodium: 267mg

Turkey Taco

Prep time: 10 minutes | Cook time: 20 minutes | Serves 4

3 tablespoons extra-virgin olive oil
1 pound (454 g) ground turkey
1 onion, chopped
1 green bell pepper, seeded and chopped
½ teaspoon sea salt
1 small head cauliflower, grated
1 cup corn kernels
½ cup prepared salsa
1 cup shredded pepper Jack cheese

1. In a large nonstick skillet over medium-high heat, heat the olive oil until it shimmers.
2. Add the turkey. Cook, crumbling with a spoon, until browned, about 5 minutes.
3. Add the onion, bell pepper, and salt. Cook, stirring occasionally, until the vegetables soften, 4 to 5 minutes.
4. Add the cauliflower, corn, and salsa. Cook, stirring, until the cauliflower rice softens, about 3 minutes more.
5. Sprinkle with the cheese. Reduce heat to low, cover, and allow the cheese to melt, 2 or 3 minutes.

Per Serving
calories: 449 | fat: 30.1g | protein: 30.1g
carbs: 17.9g | fiber: 4.1g | sugar: 8.7g
sodium: 650mg

Wochestershire Turkey Meatballs

Prep time: 10 minutes | Cook time: 20 minutes | Serves 4

¼ cup tomato paste
1 tablespoon honey
1 tablespoon Worcestershire sauce
½ cup milk
½ cup whole-wheat bread crumbs
1 pound (454 g)
ground turkey
1 onion, grated
1 tablespoon Dijon mustard
1 teaspoon dried thyme
½ teaspoon sea salt

1. Preheat the oven to 375ºF (190ºC). Line a rimmed baking sheet with parchment paper.
2. In a small saucepan on medium-low heat, whisk together the tomato paste, honey, and Worcestershire sauce. Bring to a simmer and then remove from the heat.
3. In a large bowl, combine the milk and bread crumbs. Let rest for 5 minutes.

4. Add the ground turkey, onion, mustard, thyme, and salt. Using your hands, mix well without overmixing.
5. Form into 1-inch meatballs and place on the prepared baking sheet. Brush the tops with the tomato paste mixture.
6. Bake until the meatballs reach 165ºF (74ºC) internally, about 15 minutes.

Per Serving
calories: 286 | fat: 11.1g | protein: 24.1g
carbs: 21.9g | fiber: 2.1g | sugar: 13.6g
sodium: 464mg

Golden Chicken Tenders

Prep time: 10 minutes | Cook time: 15 minutes | Serves 4

1 cup whole-wheat bread crumbs
1 tablespoon dried thyme
1 teaspoon garlic powder
1 teaspoon paprika
½ teaspoon sea salt
3 large eggs, beaten
1 tablespoon Dijon mustard
1 pound (454 g) chicken, cut into ½-inch-thick pieces and pounded to even thickness

1. Preheat the oven to 375ºF (190ºC). Line a rimmed baking sheet with parchment paper.
2. In a medium bowl, whisk together the bread crumbs, thyme, garlic powder, paprika, and salt.
3. In another bowl, whisk together the eggs and mustard.
4. Dip each piece of chicken in the egg mixture and then in the bread crumb mixture. Place on the prepared baking sheet.
5. Bake until the chicken reaches an internal temperature of 165ºF (74ºC) and the bread crumbs are golden, about 15 minutes.

Per Serving
calories: 277 | fat: 6.1g | protein: 34.1g
carbs: 16.9g | fiber: 3.1g | sugar: 8.8g
sodium: 488mg

Chicken with Lemony Caper Sauce

Prep time: 10 minutes | Cook time: 15 minutes | Serves 4

3 tablespoons extra-virgin olive oil
4 chicken breast halves or thighs, pounded slightly to even thickness
½ teaspoon sea salt
⅛ teaspoon freshly ground black pepper
¼ cup freshly squeezed lemon juice
¼ cup dry white wine
2 tablespoons capers, rinsed
2 tablespoons salted butter, cold, cut into pieces

1. In a large skillet over medium-high heat, heat the olive oil until it shimmers.
2. Season the chicken with the salt and pepper. Add it to the hot oil and cook until opaque with an internal temperature of 165ºF (74ºC), about 5 minutes per side. Transfer the chicken to a plate and tent loosely with foil to keep warm. Keep the pan on the heat.
3. Add the lemon juice and wine to the pan, using the side of a spoon to scrape any browned bits from the bottom of the pan. Add the capers. Simmer until the liquid is reduced by half, about 3 minutes. Reduce the heat to low.
4. Whisk in the butter, one piece at a time, until incorporated.
5. Return the chicken to the pan, turning once to coat with the sauce. Serve with additional sauce spooned over the top.

Per Serving

calories: 282 | fat: 17.1g | protein: 26.1g
carbs: 1.9g | fiber: 1.0g | sugar: 0.9g
sodium: 388mg

Asian Chicken and Edamame Stir-Fry

Prep time: 10 minutes | Cook time: 10 minutes | Serves 4

3 tablespoons extra-virgin olive oil
1 pound (454 g) chicken breasts or thighs, cut into ¾-inch pieces
2 cups edamame or pea pods
3 garlic cloves, chopped
1 tablespoon peeled
and grated fresh ginger
2 tablespoons reduced-sodium soy sauce
Juice of 2 limes
1 teaspoon sesame oil
2 teaspoons toasted sesame seeds
1 tablespoon chopped fresh cilantro

1. In a large skillet over medium-high heat, heat the olive oil until it shimmers. Add the chicken to the oil and cook, stirring occasionally, until opaque, about 5 minutes. Add the edamame and cook, stirring occasionally, until crisp-tender, 3 to 5 minutes. Add the garlic and ginger and cook, stirring constantly, for 30 seconds.
2. In a small bowl, whisk together the soy sauce, lime juice, and sesame oil. Add the sauce mixture to the pan. Bring to a simmer, stirring, and cook for 2 minutes.
3. Remove from heat and garnish with the sesame seeds and cilantro.

Per Serving

calories: 332 | fat: 17.1g | protein: 31.1g
carbs: 10.9g | fiber: 5.1g | sugar: 5.0g
sodium: 341mg

Citrus Chicken

Prep time: 10 minutes | Cook time: 10 minutes | Serves 4

3 tablespoons extra-virgin olive oil
1 pound (454 g) chicken breasts or thighs, cut into ¾-inch pieces
1 teaspoon peeled and grated fresh ginger
2 garlic cloves, minced
1 tablespoon honey
Juice and zest of 1 orange
1 teaspoon cornstarch
½ teaspoon sriracha (or to taste)
Sesame seeds (optional, for garnish)
Thinly sliced scallion (optional, for garnish)

1. In a large skillet over medium-high heat, heat the olive oil until it shimmers. Add the chicken to the oil and cook, stirring occasionally, until opaque, about 5 minutes. Add the ginger and garlic and cook, stirring constantly, for 30 seconds.
2. In a small bowl, whisk together the honey, orange juice and zest, cornstarch, and sriracha. Add the sauce mixture to the chicken and cook, stirring, until the sauce thickens, about 2 minutes.
3. Serve garnished with sesame seeds and sliced scallions, if desired.

Per Serving

calories: 246 | fat: 12.1g | protein: 26.1g
carbs: 8.9g | fiber: 1.1g | sugar: 6.7g
sodium: 76mg

Thai Chicken Roll-Ups with Sauce

Prep time: 15 minutes | Cook time: 0 minutes | Serves 4

Filling:

1½ cups cooked chicken breast, shredded
1 cup shredded green cabbage
1 cup bean sprouts
½ cup carrots,

shredded
¼ cup chopped fresh cilantro
¼ cup chopped scallions, both white and green parts

Sauce:

2 tablespoons water
2 tablespoons natural peanut butter
1 garlic clove, minced

1 tablespoon rice wine vinegar
¼ teaspoon salt

4 (8-inch) low-carb whole-wheat tortillas

1. Make the filling: Put the chicken breast, cabbage, bean sprouts, carrots, cilantro, and scallion in a large bowl. Gently toss to combine well and set aside.
2. Make the sauce: Mix the water, peanut butter, garlic, rice vinegar, and salt together in a separate bowl. Stir well with a fork until blended.
3. Arrange each tortilla on a clean work surface. Evenly divide the chicken and vegetable mixture among the tortillas, then spread 1 tablespoon of the sauce over the filling.
4. Fold each tortilla in half to enclose filling and roll up. Serve immediately.

Per Serving
calories: 212 | fat: 8.2g | protein: 21.2g carbs: 17.1g | fiber: 10.2g | sugar: 3.1g sodium: 358mg

Greek Chicken Sandwiches

Prep time: 10 minutes | Cook time: 0 minutes | Serves 3

3 slices 100% whole-wheat bread, toasted
3 tablespoons red pepper hummus
3 cups arugula
¾ cup cucumber slices

1 cup rotisserie chicken, shredded
¼ cup sliced red onion
Oregano, for garnish (optional)

1. Place the toasted bread slices on a clean work surface, and spoon 1 tablespoon of red pepper hummus on each slice of bread.
2. Top each bread slice evenly with arugula, cucumber slices, chicken, and red onion.
3. Serve garnished with the oregano, if desired.

Per Serving
calories: 227 | fat: 6.1g | protein: 23.1g carbs: 24.8g | fiber: 4.1g | sugar: 4.1g sodium: 330mg

Chicken Sandwiches with Caesar Dressing

Prep time: 5 minutes | Cook time: 0 minutes | Serves 4

For the Dressing:

4 tablespoons plain low-fat Greek yogurt
4 teaspoons Dijon mustard
4 teaspoons freshly squeezed lemon juice

4 teaspoons shredded Parmesan cheese
¼ teaspoon freshly ground black pepper
⅛ teaspoon garlic powder

For the Sandwiches:

2 cups shredded rotisserie chicken
1½ cups chopped romaine lettuce
12 cherry tomatoes,

halved
4 whole-wheat sandwich thins
¼ cup thinly sliced red onion (optional)

To Make the Dressing
1. In a small bowl, whisk together the yogurt, mustard, lemon juice, Parmesan cheese, black pepper, and garlic powder.

To Make the Sandwiches
1. In a large bowl, combine the chicken, lettuce, and tomatoes. Add the dressing and stir until evenly coated. Divide the filling into four equal portions.
2. Slice the sandwich thins so there is a top and bottom half for each. Put one portion of filling on each of the bottom halves and cover with the top halves.

Per Serving
calories: 243 | fat: 5.1g | protein: 28.1g carbs: 24.9g | fiber: 8.1g | sugar: 4.0g sodium: 360mg

Coconut-Encrusted Chicken

Prep time: 10 minutes | Cook time: 20 minutes | Serves 6

4 chicken breasts, each cut lengthwise into 3 strips
½ teaspoon salt
¼ teaspoon freshly ground black pepper
2 eggs

2 tablespoons unsweetened plain almond milk
½ cup coconut flour
1 cup unsweetened coconut flakes

1. Preheat the oven to 400ºF (205ºC).
2. On a clean work surface, rub the chicken with salt and black pepper.
3. Whisk together the eggs and almond milk in a bowl. Put the coconut flour in another bowl. Put the coconut flakes in a third bowl.
4. Dunk the chicken in the bowl of flour to coat, then dredge in the egg mixture, and then dip in coconut flakes. Shake the excess off.
5. Arrange the well coated chicken in a baking pan lined with parchment paper. Bake in the preheated oven for 16 minutes. Flip the chicken halfway through the cooking time or until well browned.
6. Remove the chicken from the oven and serve in a plate.

Per Serving
calories: 218 | fat: 12.8g | protein: 20.1g
carbs: 8.8g | fiber: 6.1g | sugar: 1.8g
sodium: 345mg

Easy Chicken Leg Roast

Prep time: 10 minutes | Cook time: 35 minutes | Serves 6

1 teaspoon ground paprika
1 teaspoon garlic powder
½ teaspoon ground coriander
½ teaspoon ground

cumin
½ teaspoon salt
¼ teaspoon ground cayenne pepper
6 chicken legs
1 teaspoon extra-virgin olive oil

1. Preheat the oven to 400ºF (205ºC).
2. Combine the coriander, cumin, paprika, garlic powder, salt, and cayenne pepper in a bowl. Dunk the chicken legs in the mixture to coat well.
3. Heat the olive oil in an oven-safe skillet over medium heat.
4. Add the chicken legs and sear for 9 minutes or until browned and crisp. Flip the legs halfway through the cooking time.
5. Place the skillet in the oven and roast for 14 minutes or until the internal temperature of the chicken legs reaches at least 165ºF (74ºC).
6. Remove the chicken legs from the oven and serve warm.

Per Serving
calories: 278 | fat: 15.8g | protein: 30.1g
carbs: 0.8g | fiber: 0g | sugar: 0g
sodium: 254mg

Teriyaki Turkey Balls

Prep time: 20 minutes | Cook time: 20 minutes | Serves 6

1 pound (454 g) lean ground turkey
1 egg, beaten
2 tablespoons tamari
2 teaspoons mirin
¼ cup scallions, both white and green parts, finely chopped

1 teaspoon fresh ginger, grated
2 garlic cloves, minced
1 tablespoon honey
1 teaspoon toasted sesame oil

1. Preheat the oven to 400ºF (205ºC).
2. Combine the ground turkey, beaten egg, tamari, mirin, scallions, ginger, garlic, honey, and sesame oil in a bowl. Stir to mix well.
3. Use a tablespoon to shape the turkey mixture into balls, then arrange the balls on a baking sheet lined with parchment paper.
4. Bake the balls in the preheated oven for 20 minutes until the balls are well browned. Flip the balls with a spatula halfway through the cooking time.
5. Remove the balls from the oven and serve hot.

Per Serving
calories: 156 | fat: 7.8g | protein: 16.1g
carbs: 4.8g | fiber: 0g | sugar: 3.9g
sodium: 267mg

Goat Cheese Stuffed Chicken Breasts

Prep time: 15 minutes | Cook time: 30 minutes | Serves 4

1 cup chopped roasted red pepper
2 ounces (57 g) goat cheese
4 Kalamata olives, pitted, finely chopped
1 tablespoon chopped

fresh basil
4 (5-ounce / 142-g) boneless, skinless chicken breasts
1 tablespoon extra-virgin olive oil

1. Preheat the oven to 400ºF (205ºC).
2. In a small bowl, stir together the red pepper, goat cheese, olives, and basil until well mixed.
3. Place the filling in the refrigerator for about 15 minutes to firm it up.
4. Cut a slit horizontally in each chicken breast to create a pocket in the middle.
5. Evenly divide the filling between the chicken breast pockets and secure them closed with wooden toothpicks.
6. Place a large skillet over medium-high heat and add the olive oil.
7. Brown the chicken breasts on both sides, about 10 minutes in total.
8. Transfer to the oven. Bake the chicken breasts until the chicken is cooked through, about 20 minutes.
9. Let the chicken breasts rest for 10 minutes, remove the toothpicks, and serve.

Per Serving
calories: 246 | fat: 9.1g | protein: 35.1g
carbs: 3.0g | fiber: 1.1g | sugar: 2.0g
sodium: 280mg

Turkey Burgers

Prep time: 10 minutes | Cook time: 20 minutes | Serves 4

1½ pounds (680 g) lean ground turkey
½ cup bread crumbs
½ sweet onion, chopped
1 carrot, peeled, grated
1 teaspoon minced

garlic
1 teaspoon chopped fresh thyme
Sea salt and freshly ground black pepper, to taste
Nonstick cooking spray

1. In a large bowl, mix together the turkey, bread crumbs, onion, carrot, garlic, and thyme until very well mixed.
2. Season the mixture lightly with salt and pepper.
3. Shape the turkey mixture into 4 equal patties.
4. Place a large skillet over medium-high heat and coat it lightly with cooking spray.
5. Cook the turkey patties until golden and completely cooked through, about 10 minutes per side.
6. Serve the burgers plain or with your favorite toppings on a whole-wheat bun.

Per Serving
calories: 320 | fat: 15.1g | protein: 32.1g
carbs: 11.9g | fiber: 1.1g | sugar: 2.0g
sodium: 271mg

Chicken with Balsamic Kale

Prep time: 5 minutes | Cook time: 15 minutes | Serves 4

4 (4-ounce / 113-g) boneless, skinless chicken breasts
¼ teaspoon salt
1 tablespoon freshly ground black pepper
2 tablespoons unsalted butter
1 tablespoon extra-

virgin olive oil
8 cups stemmed and roughly chopped kale, loosely packed (about 2 bunches)
½ cup balsamic vinegar
20 cherry tomatoes, halved

1. Season both sides of the chicken breasts with the salt and pepper.
2. Heat a large skillet over medium heat. When hot, heat the butter and oil. Add the chicken and cook for 8 to 10 minutes, flipping halfway through. When cooked all the way through, remove the chicken from the skillet and set aside.
3. Increase the heat to medium-high. Put the kale in the skillet and cook for 3 minutes, stirring every minute.
4. Add the vinegar and the tomatoes and cook for another 3 to 5 minutes.
5. Divide the kale and tomato mixture into four equal portions, and top each portion with 1 chicken breast.

Per Serving
calories: 294 | fat: 11.1g | protein: 31.1g
carbs: 17.9g | fiber: 3.1g | sugar: 4.0g
sodium: 330mg

Yogurt Chicken Salad Sandwiches

Prep time: 10 minutes | Cook time: 10 minutes | Serves 4

2 (4-ounce / 113-g) boneless, skinless chicken breasts
⅛ teaspoon freshly ground black pepper
1½ tablespoons plain low-fat Greek yogurt
¼ cup halved purple seedless grapes
¼ cup chopped pecans
2 tablespoons chopped celery
4 whole-wheat sandwich thins
Avocado oil cooking spray

1. Heat a small skillet over medium-low heat. When hot, coat the cooking surface with cooking spray.
2. Season the chicken with the pepper. Place the chicken in the skillet and cook for 6 minutes. Flip and cook for 3 to 5 minutes more, or until cooked through.
3. Remove the chicken from the skillet and let cool for 5 minutes.
4. Chop or shred the chicken.
5. Combine the chicken, yogurt, grapes, pecans, and celery.
6. Cut the sandwich thins in half, so there is a top and bottom.
7. Divide the chicken salad into four equal portions, spoon one portion on each of the bottom halves of the sandwich thins, and cover with the top halves.

Per Serving
calories: 251 | fat: 8.1g | protein: 23.1g
carbs: 23.9g | fiber: 6.1g | sugar: 4.0g
sodium: 210mg

Indian Flavor Milky Curry Chicken

Prep time: 15 minutes | Cook time: 35 minutes | Serves 4

2 teaspoons olive oil
3 (5-ounce / 142-g) boneless, skinless chicken breasts, cut into 1-inch chunks
1 tablespoon garlic, minced
2 tablespoons curry powder
1 tablespoon fresh
ginger, grated
1 cup coconut milk
2 cups low-sodium chicken broth
1 sweet potato, diced
1 carrot, peeled and diced
2 tablespoons fresh cilantro, chopped

1. Heat the olive oil in a saucepan over medium-high heat until shimmering.
2. Add the chicken to the saucepan and sauté for 10 minutes until browned on all sides.
3. Add the garlic, curry powder, and ginger to the saucepan and sauté for 3 minutes until fragrant.
4. Pour the coconut milk and chicken broth in the saucepan, then add the sweet potato and carrot to the saucepan. Stir to mix well. Bring to a boil.
5. Turn down the heat to low, then simmer for 20 minutes until tender. Stir periodically.
6. Pour them in a large bowl and spread the cilantro on top before serving.

Per Serving
calories: 328 | fat: 16.9g | protein: 29.1g
carbs: 14.8g | fiber: 1.1g | sugar: 3.9g
sodium: 274mg

Blackened Spatchcock with Lime Aioli

Prep time: 15 minutes | Cook time: 45 minutes | Serves 6

4 pounds (1.8 kg) chicken, spatchcocked
3 tablespoons
blackened seasoning
2 tablespoons olive oil
Lime Aioli:
½ cup mayonnaise
Juice and zest of 1 lime
¼ teaspoon kosher
salt
¼ teaspoon ground black pepper

1. Preheat the grill to medium high heat.
2. On a clean work surface, rub the chicken with blackened seasoning and olive oil.
3. Place the chicken on the preheated grill, skin side up, and grill for 45 minutes or until the internal temperature of the chicken reaches at least 165ºF (74ºC).
4. Meanwhile, combine the ingredients for the aioli in a small bowl and stir to mix well.
5. Once the chicken is fully grilled, transfer it to a large plate and baste with the lime aioli. Allow to cool and serve.

Per Serving
calories: 436 | fat: 16.3g | protein: 61.8g
carbs: 6.8g | fiber: 0.7g | sugar: 1.5g
sodium: 653mg

Turkey Burger with Homemade Barbecue Sauce

Prep time: 15 minutes | Cook time: 15 minutes | Serves 4

Barbecue Sauce:

½ cup low-carb ketchup
½ teaspoon onion powder
½ teaspoon Worcestershire sauce
½ teaspoon freshly ground black pepper

1 tablespoon pure maple syrup
2 tablespoons apple cider vinegar
Juice of ½ lemon
Freshly ground white pepper, to taste

Burgers:

8 ounces (227 g) lean ground turkey
1 scallion, both white and green parts, finely chopped
1 celery stalk, finely chopped

1 tablespoon olive oil, plus more for greasing your hands
4 whole-wheat dinner rolls, split
4 tomato slices
4 lettuce leaves

1. Combine all the ingredients for the barbecue sauce in a saucepan. Bring to a boil over medium heat.
2. Reduce the heat to low, then simmer for 5 minutes or until the sauce has a thick consistency. Set aside until ready to use.
3. Combine the turkey, scallion, and celery in a large bowl. Stir to mix well.
4. Grease your hands with olive oil, then shape the turkey mixture into 4 patties with your hands.
5. Heat the olive oil in a grill pan over medium-high heat until shimmering.
6. Arrange the patties in the grill pan, then cook for 6 minutes or until well browned. Flip the patties halfway through the cooking time.
7. Brush the patties with barbecue sauce on both sides, then keep cooking until the juices run clear.
8. Remove the turkey patties from the grill pan. Assemble the patties with dinner rolls, tomato, and lettuce, then serve warm.

Per Serving

calories: 216 | fat: 6.8g | protein: 15.2g
carbs: 25.9g | fiber: 4.1g | sugar: 10.8g
sodium: 270mg

Chicken, Avocado, and Tomato in Lettuce

Prep time: 10 minutes | Cook time: 0 minutes | Serves 4

8 romaine lettuce leaves
1½ cups shredded rotisserie chicken
1 avocado, sliced
2 hard-boiled eggs,

sliced
1 medium tomato, sliced
4 teaspoons honey mustard

1. Divide the rotisserie chicken, sliced avocado, sliced tomato, and eggs among the lettuce leaves.
2. Drizzle with honey mustard, then roll the lettuce up before serving.

Per Serving

calories: 229 | fat: 10.8g | protein: 24.2g
carbs: 7.8g | fiber: 4.2g | sugar: 2.8g
sodium: 158mg

Creole Chicken

Prep time: 15 minutes | Cook time: 25 minutes | Serves 2

2 chicken breast halves, boneless and skinless
1 cup cauliflower rice, cooked
1/3 cup green bell pepper, julienned
¼ cup celery, diced
¼ cup onion, diced

14½ ounces (411 g) stewed tomatoes, diced
1 teaspoon sunflower oil
1 teaspoon chili powder
½ teaspoon thyme
⅛ teaspoon pepper

1. Heat oil in a small skillet over medium heat. Add chicken and cook 5 to 6 minutes per side or cooked through. Transfer to plate and keep warm.
2. Add the pepper, celery, onion, tomatoes, and seasonings. Bring to a boil. Reduce heat, cover, and simmer 10 minutes or until vegetables start to soften.
3. Add chicken back to pan to heat through. Serve over cauliflower rice.

Per Serving

calories: 361 | fat: 14.0g | protein: 45.2g
carbs: 14.1g | fiber: 4.0g | sugar: 8.0g
sodium: 335mg

Arroz Con Pollo

Prep time: 10 minutes | Cook time: 25 minutes | Serves 4

1 onion, diced
1 red pepper, diced
2 cup chicken breast, cooked and cubed
1 cup cauliflower, grated
1 cup peas, thaw
2 tablespoons cilantro, diced
½ teaspoon lemon zest
14½ ounces (411 g) low sodium chicken broth
¼ cup black olives, sliced
¼ cup sherry
1 clove garlic, diced
2 teaspoons olive oil
¼ teaspoon salt
¼ teaspoon cayenne pepper

1. Heat oil in a large skillet over medium-high heat. Add pepper, onion and garlic and cook 1 minute. Add the cauliflower and cook, stirring frequently, until light brown, 4 to 5 minutes.
2. Stir in broth, sherry, zest and seasonings. Bring to a boil. Reduce heat, cover and simmer 15 minutes.
3. Stir in the chicken, peas and olives. Cover and simmer another 3 to 6 minutes or until heated through. Serve garnished with cilantro.

Per Serving
calories: 162 | fat: 5.0g | protein: 14.2g
carbs: 13.1g | fiber: 4.2g | sugar: 5.1g
sodium: 307mg

Sesame Chicken and Cucumber Soba

Prep time: 10 minutes | Cook time: 15 minutes | Serves 6

8 ounces (227 g) soba noodles
2 boneless, skinless chicken breasts, halved lengthwise
¼ cup tahini
1 tablespoon tamari
1 (1-inch) piece fresh ginger, finely grated
2 tablespoons rice vinegar
1 teaspoon toasted sesame oil
1/3 cup water
1 large cucumber, deseeded and diced
1 scallions bunch, green parts only, cut into 1-inch segments
1 tablespoon sesame seeds

1. Preheat the broiler to high.
2. Add the soba noodles in a pot of salted boiling water and cook for 5 minutes or until al dente. Transfer to a plate and pat dry with paper towels.
3. Place the chicken in a single layer on a baking sheet. Broil in the preheated broiler for 6 to 7 minutes or until the chicken is fork-tender. Transfer the chicken to a bowl and shred with forks.
4. Combine the tahini, tamari, ginger, rice vinegar, sesame oil, and water in a small bowl. Stir to combine well.
5. Put the soba noddles, chicken, cucumber, and scallions in a large bowl. Top them with the tahini sauce, then toss to combine well. Serve with sesame seeds on top.

Per Serving
calories: 253 | fat: 7.8g | protein: 16.1g
carbs: 34.8g | fiber: 2.2g | sugar: 1.8g
sodium: 479mg

Roasted Vegetable and Chicken Tortillas

Prep time: 10 minutes | Cook time: 20 minutes | Serves 4

1 red bell pepper, seeded and cut into 1-inch-wide strips
½ small eggplant, cut into ¼-inch-thick slices
½ small red onion, sliced
1 medium zucchini, cut lengthwise into strips
1 tablespoon extra-virgin olive oil
Salt and freshly ground black pepper, to taste
4 whole-wheat tortilla wraps
2 (8-ounce / 227-g) cooked chicken breasts, sliced

1. Preheat the oven to 400ºF (205ºC). Line a baking sheet with aluminum foil.
2. Combine the bell pepper, eggplant, red onion, zucchini, and olive oil in a large bowl. Toss to coat well.
3. Pour the vegetables into the baking sheet, then sprinkle with salt and pepper.
4. Roast in the preheated oven for 20 minutes or until tender and charred.
5. Unfold the tortillas on a clean work surface, then divide the vegetables and chicken slices on the tortillas.
6. Wrap and serve immediately.

Per Serving
calories: 483 | fat: 25.0g | protein: 20.0g
carbs: 45.0g | fiber: 3.0g | sugar: 4.0g
sodium: 730mg

Turkey Zoodles with Spaghetti Sauce

Prep time: 5 minutes | Cook time: 20 minutes | Serves 4

1 (10-ounce / 284-g) package zucchini noodles, rinsed and patted dry
2 tablespoons olive oil, divided
1 pound (454 g) 93%
lean ground turkey
½ teaspoon dried oregano
2 cups low-sodium spaghetti sauce
½ cup Cheddar cheese, shredded

1. Preheat the broiler to high.
2. Warm 1 tablespoon olive oil over in an oven-safe skillet over medium heat.
3. Add the zucchini noodles to the skillet and cook for 3 minutes until soft. Stir the zucchini noodles frequently.
4. Drizzle the remaining olive oil over, then add the ground turkey and oregano to the skillet. Cook for 8 minutes until the turkey is well browned.
5. Pour the spaghetti sauce over the turkey and stir to coat well.
6. Spread the Cheddar on top, then broil in the preheated broiler for 5 minutes until the cheese is melted and frothy.
7. Remove them from the broiler and serve warm.

Per Serving
calories: 337 | fat: 20.8g | protein: 28.2g carbs: 20.7g | fiber: 3.2g | sugar: 3.8g sodium: 214mg

Chicken Marsala

Prep time: 10 minutes | Cook time: 25 minutes | Serves 4

4 boneless chicken breasts
½ pound (227 g) mushrooms, sliced
1 tablespoon margarine
1 cup Marsala wine
¼ cup flour
1 tablespoon oil
Pinch of white pepper
Pinch of oregano
Pinch of basil

1. On a shallow plate, combine flour and seasonings.
2. Dredge the chicken in the flour mixture to coat both sides.
3. In a large skillet, over medium heat, heat oil until hot. Add chicken and cook until brown on both sides, about 15 minutes. Transfer chicken to a plate.

4. Reduce heat to low and add mushrooms and ¼ cup of the wine. Cook about 5 minutes. Scrape bottom of pan to loosen any flour. Stir in reserved flour mixture and the remaining wine.
5. Simmer until mixture starts to thicken, stirring constantly. Add the chicken back to the pan and cook an additional 5 minutes. Serve.

Per Serving
calories: 328 | fat: 14.0g | protein: 21.2g carbs: 9.1g | fiber: 1.0g | sugar: 1.0g sodium: 190mg

Citrus Chicken Thighs

Prep time: 15 minutes | Cook time: 30 minutes | Serves 4

1 tablespoon grated fresh ginger
Sea salt, to taste
4 chicken thighs, bone-in, skinless
1 tablespoon extra-virgin olive oil
Juice and zest of ½ orange
Juice and zest of ½ lemon
1 tablespoon low-sodium soy sauce
Pinch red pepper flakes, to taste
2 tablespoons honey
1 tablespoon chopped fresh cilantro

1. In a large bowl, combine the ginger and salt. Dunk the chicken thighs and toss to coat well.
2. Heat the olive oil in a nonstick skillet over medium-high heat until shimmering.
3. Add the chicken thighs and cook for 10 minutes or until well browned. Flip halfway through the cooking time.
4. Meanwhile, combine the orange juice and zest, lemon juice and zest, soy sauce, red pepper flakes, and honey. Stir to mix well.
5. Pour the mixture in the skillet. Reduce the heat to low, then cover and braise for 20 minutes. Add tablespoons of water if too dry.
6. Serve the chicken thighs garnished with cilantro.

Per Serving
calories: 114 | fat: 5.0g | protein: 9.0g carbs: 9.0g | fiber: 0g | sugar: 9.0g sodium: 287mg

Mexican Turkey Sliders

Prep time: 15 minutes | Cook time: 6 minutes | Serves 7

1 pound (454 g) lean ground turkey
1 tablespoon chili powder
½ teaspoon garlic powder
¼ teaspoon ground black pepper

7 mini whole-wheat hamburger buns
7 tomato slices
3½ slices reduced-fat pepper Jack cheese, cut in half
½ mashed avocado

1. Preheat the grill to high heat.
2. Combine the ground turkey, chili powder, garlic powder, and black pepper in a large bow. Stir to mix well.
3. Divide and shape the mixture into 7 patties, then arrange the patties on the preheated grill grates.
4. Grill for 6 minutes or until well browned. Flip the patties halfway through.
5. Assemble the patties with buns, tomato slices, cheese slices, and mashed avocado to make the sliders, then serve immediately.

Per Serving
calories: 225 | fat: 9.0g | protein: 17.0g
carbs: 21.0g | fiber: 4.0g | sugar: 6.0g
sodium: 230mg

Asian Roasted Duck Legs

Prep time: 10 minutes | Cook time: 1 hour 30 minutes | Serves 4

4 duck legs
3 plum tomatoes, diced
1 red chili, deseeded and sliced
½ small Savoy cabbage, quartered
2 teaspoons fresh

ginger, grated
3 cloves garlic, sliced
2 tablespoons soy sauce
2 tablespoons honey
1 teaspoon five-spice powder

1. Heat oven to 350ºF (180ºC).
2. Place the duck in a large skillet over low heat and cook until brown on all sides and most of the fat is rendered, about 10 minutes. Transfer duck to a deep baking dish. Drain off all but 2 tablespoons of the fat.
3. Add ginger, garlic, and chili to the skillet and cook 2 minutes until soft. Add soy sauce, tomatoes and 2 tablespoons water and bring to a boil.
4. Rub the duck with the five spice seasoning. Pour the sauce over the duck and drizzle with the honey. Cover with foil and bake 1 hour. Add the cabbage for the last 10 minutes.

Per Serving
calories: 212 | fat: 5.0g | protein: 25.2g
carbs: 19.1g | fiber: 3.2g | sugar: 14.1g
sodium: 365mg

Chicken Zucchini Patties with Salsa

Prep time: 10 minutes | Cook time: 10 minutes | Serves 8

2 cup chicken breast, cooked, divided
1 zucchini, cut in ¾-inch pieces
¼ cup cilantro, diced
1/3 cup bread crumbs
1/3 cup lite mayonnaise
2 teaspoons olive oil
½ teaspoon salt
¼ teaspoon pepper

Roasted Tomato Salsa:
6 plum tomatoes
1¼ cups cilantro
2 teaspoons olive oil
1 teaspoon adobo sauce
½ teaspoon salt, divided
Nonstick cooking spray

1. Place 1½ cups chicken and zucchini into a food processor. Cover and process until coarsely chopped. Add bread crumbs, mayonnaise, pepper, cilantro, remaining chicken, and salt. Cover and pulse until chunky.
2. Heat oil in a large skillet over medium-high heat. Shape chicken mixture into 8 patties and cook 4 minutes per side, or until golden brown.
3. Meanwhile, combine the ingredients for the salsa in a small bowl.
4. Serve the patties topped with salsa.

Per Serving
calories: 147 | fat: 7.0g | protein: 12.2g
carbs: 10.1g | fiber: 2.0g | sugar: 5.0g
sodium: 461mg

Cheesy Chicken and Spinach

Prep time: 10 minutes | Cook time: 45 minutes | Serves 6

3 chicken breasts, boneless, skinless and halved lengthwise
6 ounces (170 g) low fat cream cheese, soft
2 cup baby spinach
1 cup Mozzarella cheese, grated
2 tablespoons olive oil, divided
3 cloves garlic, diced fine
1 teaspoon Italian seasoning
Nonstick cooking spray

1. Heat oven to 350ºF (180ºC). Spray a glass baking dish with cooking spray.
2. Lay chicken breast cutlets in baking dish. Drizzle 1 tablespoon oil over chicken. Sprinkle evenly with garlic and Italian seasoning. Spread cream cheese over the top of chicken.
3. Heat remaining tablespoon of oil in a small skillet over medium heat. Add spinach and cook until spinach wilts, about 3 minutes. Place evenly over cream cheese layer. Sprinkle Mozzarella over top.
4. Bake for 35 to 40 minutes, or until chicken is cooked through. Serve.

Per Serving
calories: 362 | fat: 25.0g | protein: 31.2g
carbs: 3.1g | fiber: 0g | sugar: 0g
sodium: 376mg

Pecan Chicken Enchiladas

Prep time: 20 minutes | Cook time: 45 minutes | Serves 12

1 onion, diced
4 cup chicken breast, cooked and cubed
1 cup fat free sour cream
1 cup skim milk
4 ounces (113 g) low fat cream cheese
½ cup reduced fat cheddar cheese, grated
2 tablespoons cilantro, diced
12 (6-inch) flour
tortillas, warm
1 can low fat condensed cream of chicken soup
¼ cup pecans, toasted
2 tablespoons green chilies, diced
1 tablespoon water
1 teaspoon cumin
¼ teaspoon pepper
⅛ teaspoon salt
Nonstick cooking spray

1. Heat oven to 350ºF (180ºC). Spray a baking dish with cooking spray.
2. Spray a nonstick skillet with cooking spray and place over medium heat. Add onion and cook until tender.
3. In a large bowl, beat cream cheese, water, cumin, salt, and pepper until smooth. Stir in the onion, chicken, and pecans.
4. Spoon ⅓ cup chicken mixture down the middle of each tortilla. Roll up and place, seam side down, in prepared baking dish.
5. In a medium bowl, combine soup, sour cream, milk, and chilies and pour over enchiladas.
6. Cover with foil and bake 40 minutes. Uncover and sprinkle cheese over top and bake another 5 minutes until cheese is melted. Sprinkle with cilantro and serve.

Per Serving
calories: 321 | fat: 13.0g | protein: 21.2g
carbs: 27.1g | fiber: 2.0g | sugar: 4.0g
sodium: 684mg

Chicken Tuscany

Prep time: 10 minutes | Cook time: 15 minutes | Serves 4

1½ pounds (680 g) chicken breasts, boneless, skinless and sliced thin
1 cup spinach, chopped
1 cup half-and-half
½ cup reduced fat Parmesan cheese
½ cup low sodium chicken broth
½ cup sun dried tomatoes
2 tablespoons olive oil
1 teaspoon Italian seasoning
1 teaspoon garlic powder

1. Heat oil in a large skillet over medium-high heat. Add chicken and cook 3 to 5 minutes per side, or until browned and cooked through. Transfer to a plate.
2. Add half-and-half, broth, cheese and seasonings to the pan. Whisk constantly until sauce starts to thicken. Add spinach and tomatoes and cook, stirring frequently, until spinach starts to wilt, about 2 to 3 minutes.
3. Add chicken back to the pan and cook just long enough to heat through.

Per Serving
calories: 463 | fat: 23.0g | protein: 55.2g
carbs: 6.1g | fiber: 1.0g | sugar: 0g
sodium: 441mg

Cheesy Chicken and "Potato" Casserole

Prep time: 10 minutes | Cook time: 40 minutes | Serves 6

4 slices bacon, cooked and crumbled
3 cups cauliflower
3 cups chicken, cooked and chopped
3 cups broccoli florets
2 cups reduced fat cheddar cheese, grated
1 cup fat free sour cream
4 tablespoons margarine, soft
1 teaspoon salt
½ teaspoon black pepper
½ teaspoon garlic powder
½ teaspoon paprika
Nonstick cooking spray

1. In a large saucepan add 4 to 5 cups of water and bring to a boil. Add the cauliflower and cook about 4 to 5 minutes, or until it is tender drain well. Repeat with broccoli.
2. Heat oven to 350°F (180°C). Spray a baking dish with cooking spray.
3. In a medium bowl, mash the cauliflower with the margarine, sour cream and seasonings. Add remaining , saving ½ the cheese, and mix well.
4. Spread mixture in prepared baking dish and sprinkle remaining cheese on top. Bake 20 to 25 minutes, or until heated through and cheese has melted. Serve.

Per Serving
calories: 345 | fat: 15.0g | protein: 28.2g
carbs: 10.1g | fiber: 2.2g | sugar: 4.1g
sodium: 990mg

Korean Chicken

Prep time: 15 minutes | Cook time: 3 to 4 hours | Serves 6

2 pounds (907 g) chicken thighs, boneless and skinless
2 tablespoons fresh ginger, grated
4 cloves garlic, diced fine
¼ cup lite soy sauce
¼ cup honey
2 tablespoons Korean chili paste
2 tablespoons toasted sesame oil
2 teaspoons cornstarch
Pinch of red pepper flakes

1. Add the soy sauce, honey, chili paste, sesame oil, ginger, garlic and pepper flakes to the crock pot, stir to combine. Add the chicken and turn to coat in the sauce.
2. Cover and cook on low 3–4 hours or till chicken is cooked through.
3. When the chicken is cooked, transfer it to a plate.
4. Pour the sauce into a medium saucepan. Whisk the cornstarch and ¼ cup cold water until smooth. Add it to the sauce. Cook over medium heat, stirring constantly, about 5 minutes, or until sauce is thick and glossy.
5. Use 2 forks and shred the chicken. Add it to the sauce and stir to coat. Serve.

Per Serving
calories: 400 | fat: 16.0g | protein: 44.2g
carbs: 18.1g | fiber: 0g | sugar: 13.0g
sodium: 583mg

Curried Chicken and Apples

Prep time: 15 minutes | Cook time: 30 minutes | Serves 4

1 pound (454 g) chicken breasts, boneless, skinless, cut in 1-inch cubes
2 tart apples, peel and slice
1 sweet onion, cut in half and slice
1 jalapeno, seeded and diced
2 tablespoons cilantro, diced
½ teaspoon ginger, grated
14½ ounces (411 g) tomatoes, diced and drained
½ cup water
3 cloves garlic, diced
2 tablespoons sunflower oil
1 teaspoon salt
1 teaspoon coriander
½ teaspoon turmeric
¼ teaspoon cayenne pepper

1. Heat oil in a large skillet over medium-high heat. Add chicken and onion, and cook until onion is tender. Add garlic and cook 1 more minute.
2. Add apples, water and seasonings and stir to combine. Bring to a boil. Reduce heat and simmer 12 to 15 minutes, or until chicken is cooked through, stirring occasionally.
3. Stir in tomatoes, jalapeno, and cilantro and serve.

Per Serving
calories: 372 | fat: 16.0g | protein: 34.2g
carbs: 23.1g | fiber: 5.0g | sugar: 15.0g
sodium: 705mg

Chicken, Cabbage, and Sweet Potato Roast

Prep time: 10 minutes | Cook time: 40 minutes | Serves 6

¼ cup olive oil, divided
½ head cabbage, cut into 2-inch chunks
1 sweet potato, peeled and cut into 1-inch chunks
1 onion, peeled and cut into eighths
4 garlic cloves, peeled and lightly crushed
2 teaspoons fresh thyme, minced
Salt and freshly ground black pepper, to taste
2½ pounds (1.1 kg) bone-in chicken thighs and drumsticks

1. Preheat the oven to 450ºF (235ºC). Coat a baking pan with 1 tablespoon of olive oil.
2. Place the cabbage, sweet potato, onion, and garlic in the baking pan. Sprinkle with thyme, salt, and black pepper, and drizzle 1 tablespoon of olive oil on top. Set aside.
3. On a clean work surface, rub the chicken with salt and black pepper.
4. Heat 2 tablespoons olive oil in a large skillet over medium-high heat.
5. Add the chicken to the skillet and cook for 10 minutes or until lightly browned on both sides. Flip the chicken halfway through the cooking time.
6. Put the chicken over the vegetables in the baking pan, then roast in the preheated oven for 30 minutes until an instant-read thermometer inserted in the thickest part of the chicken registers at least 165ºF (74ºC).
7. Remove them from the oven and serve hot on a large platter.

Per Serving
calories: 542 | fat: 33.8g | protein: 43.1g
carbs: 13.8g | fiber: 4.1g | sugar: 4.9g
sodium: 210mg

Turkey and Cabbage Broth

Prep time: 15 minutes | Cook time: 30 minutes | Serves 4

1 tablespoon olive oil
2 celery stalks, chopped
2 teaspoons fresh garlic, minced
1 sweet onion, chopped
1 sweet potato, peeled, diced
4 cups green cabbage, finely shredded
8 cups low-sodium chicken broth
2 bay leaves
1 cup cooked turkey, chopped
2 teaspoons fresh thyme, chopped
Salt and freshly ground black pepper, to taste

1. Heat the olive oil in a large saucepan over medium-high heat until shimmering.
2. Add the celery, garlic, and onion to the saucepan and sauté for 3 minutes until the onion is translucent.
3. Add the sweet potato and cabbage to the saucepan and sauté for 3 minutes to soft the vegetables a little.
4. Pour the chicken broth in the saucepan and add the bay leaves. Bring to a boil.
5. Turn down the heat to low, then simmer for 20 minutes or until the vegetables are tender.
6. Add the turkey and thyme to the pan and simmer for 4 minutes until the turkey is heated through.
7. Pour the turkey broth in a large bowl, and discard the bay leaves. Sprinkle with salt and black pepper to taste before serving warm.

Per Serving
calories: 328 | fat: 10.8g | protein: 24.1g
carbs: 29.8g | fiber: 4.3g | sugar: 12.7g
sodium: 710mg

Herbed Turkey and Vegetable Chunk Roast

Prep time: 20 minutes | Cook time: 2 hours | Serves 6

1 tablespoon fresh parsley, chopped
1 teaspoon fresh rosemary, chopped
1 teaspoon fresh thyme, chopped
2 teaspoons garlic, minced
Salt and freshly ground black pepper, to taste
2 pounds (907 g) boneless, skinless
whole turkey breast
3 teaspoons extra-virgin olive oil, divided
2 carrots, peeled and cut into 2-inch chunks
1 sweet onion, peeled and cut into eighths
2 parsnips, peeled and cut into 2-inch chunks
2 sweet potatoes, peeled and cut into 2-inch chunks

1. Preheat the oven to 350°F (180°C).
2. Combine the parsley, rosemary, thyme, garlic, salt, and black pepper in a bowl.
3. Arrange the turkey breast in the baking pan lined with aluminum foil. Brush 1 teaspoon of olive oil on all sides. Rub the with parsley mixture.
4. Roast in the preheated oven for 30 minuets.
5. Meanwhile, put the remaining olive oil in a large bowl. Add the carrots, onion, parsnips, and sweet potatoes to the bowl. Toss to coat well.
6. Set the vegetables around the turkey and move the pan back to the oven and keep roasting for an additional one and a half hours or until the internal temperature of the turkey reaches at least 165°F (74°C).
7. Remove the

Per Serving
calories: 274 | fat: 2.8g | protein: 38.1g
carbs: 19.7g | fiber: 4.2g | sugar: 5.8g
sodium: 114mg

Creamy Chicken with Quinoa and Broccoli

Prep time: 5 minutes | Cook time: 15 minutes | Serves 4

½ cup uncooked quinoa
4 (4-ounce / 113-g) boneless, skinless chicken breasts
1 teaspoon garlic powder, divided
¼ teaspoon salt
¼ teaspoon freshly ground black pepper
1 tablespoon avocado oil
3 cups fresh or frozen broccoli, cut into florets
1 cup half-and-half

1. Put the quinoa in a pot of salted water. Bring to a boil. Reduce the heat to low and simmer for 15 minutes or until the quinoa is soft and has a white "tail". Cover and turn off the heat. Let sit for 5 minutes.
2. On a clean work surface, rub the chicken breasts with ½ teaspoon of garlic powder, salt, and pepper.
3. Heat the avocado oil in a nonstick skillet over medium-low heat.
4. Add the chicken and broccoli in the skillet and cook for 9 minutes or until the chicken is browned and the broccoli is tender. Flip the chicken and shake the skillet halfway through the cooking time.
5. Pour the half-and-half in the skillet, and sprinkle with remaining garlic powder. Turn up the heat to high and simmer for 2 minutes until creamy.
6. Divide the rice, chicken breasts, broccoli florets, and the sauce remains in the skillet in four bowls and serve warm.

Per Serving
calories: 305 | fat: 9.8g | protein: 33.1g
carbs: 21.8g | fiber: 3.1g | sugar: 3.9g
sodium: 270mg

Teriyaki Chicken with Vegetables

Prep time: 5 minutes | Cook time: 20 minutes | Serves 4

Teriyaki Sauce:

¼ teaspoon garlic powder
½ cup water
1 tablespoon cornstarch
1 tablespoon rice vinegar
2 tablespoons honey
2 tablespoons tamari
Pinch ground ginger
1 tablespoon sesame

oil
4 (4-ounce / 113-g) boneless, skinless chicken breasts, cut into bite-size cubes
1 (12-ounce / 340-g) bag frozen cauliflower rice
1 (12-ounce / 340-g) bag frozen broccoli

1. Put all the ingredients for the teriyaki sauce in a saucepan, then whisk to combine well.
2. Bring to a boil over medium heat, then let boil for 1 minute until thickened. Transfer the sauce in a bowl and set aside until ready to use.
3. Heat the sesame oil in a nonstick skillet over medium-low heat.
4. Add the chicken to the skillet and cook for 6 minutes until browned on all sides. Remove the chicken from the skillet and set aside.
5. Put the cauliflower rice and broccoli in a microwave-safe bowl, then add 1 tablespoon of water and sprinkle with salt. Microwave for 2 minutes or until they are soft.
6. Divide the chicken, cauliflower rice, and broccoli among four bowls, then serve with teriyaki sauce on top.

Per Serving

calories: 250 | fat: 6.7g | protein: 29.1g
carbs: 19.9g | fiber: 5.2g | sugar: 11.8g
sodium: 416mg

Creamy and Aromatic Chicken

Prep time: 15 minutes | Cook time: 30 minutes | Serves 4

4 (4-ounce / 113-g) boneless, skinless chicken breasts
Salt and freshly ground black pepper, to taste
1 tablespoon extra-virgin olive oil
½ sweet onion,

chopped
2 teaspoons chopped fresh thyme
1 cup low-sodium chicken broth
¼ cup heavy whipping cream
1 scallion, white and green parts, chopped

1. Preheat the oven to 375°F (190°C).
2. On a clean work surface, rub the chicken with salt and pepper.
3. Heat the olive oil in an oven-safe skillet over medium-high heat until shimmering.
4. Put the chicken in the skillet and cook for 10 minutes or until well browned. Flip halfway through. Transfer onto a platter and set aside.
5. Add the onion to the skillet and sauté for 3 minutes or until translucent.
6. Add the thyme and broth and simmer for 6 minutes or until the liquid reduces in half.
7. Mix in the cream, then put the chicken back to the skillet.
8. Arrange the skillet in the oven and bake for 10 minutes.
9. Remove the skillet from the oven and serve them with scallion.

Per Serving

calories: 287 | fat: 14.0g | protein: 34.0g
carbs: 4.0g | fiber: 1.0g | sugar: 1.0g
sodium: 184mg

Creamy and Cheesy Chicken Chile Casserole

Prep time: 25 minutes | Cook time: 32 minutes | Serves 4

1 tablespoon olive oil
4 eggs, beaten
3 tablespoons softened cream cheese
¾ cup heavy whipping cream
1 teaspoon cumin
½ garlic powder
½ teaspoon salt
½ teaspoon ground black pepper
2 (6- to 8-ounce / 170- to 227-g) chicken breast, cooked and shredded
4 large whole green chiles, rinsed and patted dry, flattened
1 cup shredded Jack cheese
1 cup shredded Cheddar cheese
¼ teaspoon red pepper flakes, optional

1. Preheat the oven to 350ºF (180ºC). Grease a casserole dish with olive oil.
2. Combine the eggs, cream cheese, cream, cumin, garlic powder, salt, and black pepper in a large bowl. Stir to mix well.
3. Dunk the chicken in the mixture. Press to coat well. Set aside.
4. Lay two chiles on the casserole dish, then flatten to cover the bottom. Pour half of the cream chicken mixture over the chiles.
5. Scatter ½ cup of Jack cheese and ½ cup of Cheddar cheese on the cream chicken, then top them with remaining two flattened chiles.
6. Pour the remaining cream chicken mixture over, then scatter the remaining cheeses and sprinkle them with red pepper flakes.
7. Arrange the casserole dish in the preheated oven and bake for 30 minutes, then turn the oven to broil for 2 minutes until the top of the casserole is well browned.
8. Remove the casserole from the oven. Allow to cool for 15 minutes, then serve warm.

Per Serving
calories: 412 | fat: 30.0g | protein: 30.0g
carbs: 4.0g | fiber: 1.0g | sugar: 1.0g
sodium: 727mg

Herbed Chicken and Artichoke Hearts

Prep time: 10 minutes | Cook time: 20 minutes | Serves 4

2 tablespoons olive oil, divided
4 (6-ounce / 170-g) boneless, skinless chicken breast halves
½ teaspoon dried thyme, divided
1 teaspoon crushed dried rosemary, divided
½ teaspoon ground black pepper, divided
2 (14-ounce / 397-g) cans water-packed, low-sodium artichoke hearts, drained and quartered
½ cup low-sodium chicken broth
2 garlic cloves, chopped
1 medium onion, coarsely chopped
¼ cup shredded Parmesan cheese
1 lemon, cut into 8 slices
2 green onions, thinly sliced

1. Preheat the oven to 375ºF (190ºC). Grease a baking sheet with 1 teaspoon of olive oil.
2. Place the chicken breasts on the baking sheet and rub with ¼ teaspoon of thyme, ½ teaspoon of rosemary, ¼ teaspoon of black pepper, and 1 tablespoon of olive oil.
3. Combine the artichoke hearts, chicken broth, garlic, onion, and remaining thyme, rosemary, black pepper, and olive oil. Toss to coat well.
4. Spread the artichoke around the chicken breasts, then scatter with Parmesan and lemon slices.
5. Place the baking sheet in the preheated oven and roast for 20 minutes or until the internal temperature of the chicken breasts reaches at least 165ºF (74ºC).
6. Remove the sheet from the oven. Allow to cool for 10 minutes, then serve with green onions on top.

Per Serving
calories: 339 | fat: 9.0g | protein: 42.0g
carbs: 18.0g | fiber: 1.0g | sugar: 2.0g
sodium: 667mg

Ritzy Jerked Chicken Breasts

Prep time: 4 hours 10 minutes | Cook time: 15 minutes | Serves 4

2 habanero chile peppers, halved lengthwise, seeded
½ sweet onion, cut into chunks
1 tablespoon minced garlic
1 tablespoon ground allspice
2 teaspoons chopped fresh thyme
¼ cup freshly squeezed lime juice
½ teaspoon ground nutmeg
¼ teaspoon ground cinnamon
1 teaspoon freshly ground black pepper
2 tablespoons extra-virgin olive oil
4 (5-ounce / 142-g) boneless, skinless chicken breasts
2 cups fresh arugula
1 cup halved cherry tomatoes

1. Combine the habaneros, onion, garlic, allspice, thyme, lime juice, nutmeg, cinnamon, black pepper, and olive oil in a blender. Pulse to blender well.
2. Transfer the mixture into a large bowl or two medium bowls, then dunk the chicken in the bowl and press to coat well.
3. Put the bowl in the refrigerator and marinate for at least 4 hours.
4. Preheat the oven to 400ºF (205ºC).
5. Remove the bowl from the refrigerator, then discard the marinade.
6. Arrange the chicken on a baking sheet, then roast in the preheated oven for 15 minutes or until golden brown and lightly charred. Flip the chicken halfway through the cooking time.
7. Remove the baking sheet from the oven and let sit for 5 minutes. Transfer the chicken on a large plate and serve with arugula and cherry tomatoes.

Per Serving
calories: 226 | fat: 9.0g | protein: 33.0g
carbs: 3.0g | fiber: 0g | sugar: 1.0g
sodium: 92mg

Roasted Chicken with Root Vegetables

Prep time: 20 minutes | Cook time: 41 minutes | Serves 6

1 teaspoon minced fresh rosemary
1 teaspoon minced fresh thyme
1 teaspoon salt
1 teaspoon ground black pepper
2 tablespoons olive oil, divided
6 (6-ounce / 170-g) boneless, skinless chicken breast halves
2 medium fennel bulbs, chopped
4 medium peeled carrots, chopped
3 peeled medium radishes, chopped
3 tablespoons honey
½ cup white wine
2 cups chicken stock
3 bay leaves

1. Preheat the oven to 375ºF (190ºC).
2. Mix the rosemary, thyme, salt, and black pepper in a small bowl.
3. Heat 1 tablespoon of olive oil in a nonstick skillet over medium-high heat until shimmering.
4. On a clean work surface, rub the chicken breasts with half of the seasoning mixture.
5. Place the chicken in the skillet and cook for 6 minutes or until lightly browned on both sides. Remove the chicken from the skillet and set aside.
6. Mix the fennel bulbs, carrots, and radishes in a microwave-safe bowl, then sprinkle with remaining seasoning mixture and drizzle with honey, white wine, and remaining olive oil. Toss to combine well.
7. Cover the bowl and microwave the root vegetables for 10 minutes or until soft.
8. Arrange the root vegetables and chicken in a baking sheet, then pour in the chicken stock and honey mixture remains in the bowl. Top them with bay leaves.
9. Place the sheet in the preheated oven and roast for 25 minutes or until the internal temperature of the chicken reaches at least 165ºF (74ºC).
10. Remove the sheet from the oven and transfer the chicken and vegetables on a large plate. Discard the bay leaves, then allow to cool for a few minutes before serving.

Per Serving
calories: 364 | fat: 10.2g | protein: 41.8g
carbs: 22.2g | fiber: 3.8g | sugar: 15.1g
sodium: 650mg

Chicken with Couscous and Kale

Prep time: 15 minutes | Cook time: 27 minutes | Serves 2

½ cup couscous
1 cup water, divided
⅓ cup basil pesto
3 teaspoons olive oil, divided
3 (2-ounce / 57-g) whole carrots, rinsed, thinly sliced
Salt and ground black pepper, to taste
1 (about 6-ounce / 170-g) bunch kale, rinsed, stems removed, chopped
2 cloves garlic, minced
2 tablespoons dried currants
1 tablespoon red wine vinegar
2 (6-ounce / 170-g) boneless, skinless chicken breasts, rinsed
1 tablespoon Italian seasoning

1. Pour the couscous and ¾ cup of water in a pot. Bring to a boil on high heat. Reduce the heat to low. Simmer for 7 minutes or until most of the water has been absorbed. Fluffy with a fork and mix in the basil pesto.
2. Heat 1 teaspoon of olive oil in a nonstick skillet over medium-high heat until shimmering.
3. Add the carrots, then sprinkle with salt and pepper. Sauté for 3 minutes or until tender.
4. Add the kale and garlic and sauté for 2 minutes or until the kale is lightly wilted.
5. Add the currents and remaining water and sauté for 3 minutes or until most of the water is cooked off.
6. Turn off the heat, then mix in the red wine vinegar. Transfer them in a large bowl and cover to keep warm.
7. On a clean work surface, rub the chicken with Italian seasoning, salt, and pepper.
8. Clean the skillet and heat 2 teaspoons of olive oil over medium-high heat until shimmering.
9. Add the chicken and sear for 12 minutes or until well browned. Flip the chicken halfway through the cooking time.
10. Transfer the chicken to a large plate, then spread with vegetables and couscous. Slice to serve.

Per Serving
calories: 461 | fat: 14.2g | protein: 57.0g
carbs: 26.1g | fiber: 6.5g | sugar: 5.0g
sodium: 1210mg

Turkey Meatball and Vegetable Kabobs

Prep time: 50 minutes | Cook time: 20 minutes | Serves 6

20 ounces (567 g) lean ground turkey (93% fat-free)
2 egg whites
2 tablespoons grated Parmesan cheese
2 cloves garlic, minced
½ teaspoon salt, or to taste
¼ teaspoon ground black pepper
1 tablespoon olive oil
8 ounces (227 g) fresh cremini mushrooms, cut in half to make 12 pieces
24 cherry tomatoes
1 medium onion, cut into 12 pieces
¼ cup balsamic vinegar

Special Equipment:
12 bamboo skewers, soaked in water for at least 30 minutes

1. Mix the ground turkey, egg whites, Parmesan, garlic, salt, and pepper in a large bowl. Stir to combine well.
2. Shape the mixture into 12 meatballs and place on a baking sheet. Refrigerate for at least 30 minutes.
3. Preheat the oven to 375ºF (190ºC). Grease another baking sheet with 1 tablespoon of olive oil.
4. Remove the meatballs from the refrigerator. Run the bamboo skewers through 2 meatballs, 1 mushroom, 2 cherry tomatoes, and 1 onion piece alternatively.
5. Arrange the kabobs on the greased baking sheet and brush with balsamic vinegar.
6. Grill in the preheated oven for 20 minutes or until an instant-read thermometer inserted in the middle of the meatballs reads at least 165ºF (74ºC). Flip the kabobs halfway through the cooking time.
7. Allow the kabobs to cool for 10 minutes, then serve warm.

Per Serving
calories: 200 | fat: 8.0g | protein: 22.0g
carbs: 7.0g | fiber: 1.0g | sugar: 4.0g
sodium: 120mg

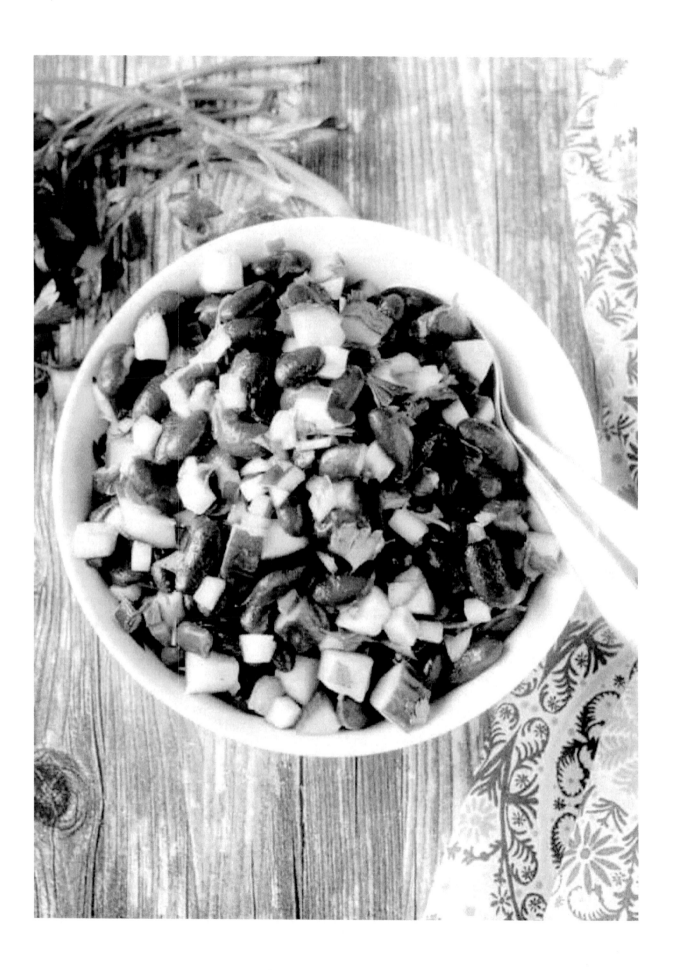

Chapter 12: Salads

Tomato, Cucumber, and Avocado Salad

Prep time: 10 minutes | Cook time: 0 minutes | Serves 4

1 cup cherry tomatoes, halved
1 large cucumber, chopped
1 small red onion, thinly sliced
1 avocado, diced
2 tablespoons
chopped fresh dill
2 tablespoons extra-virgin olive oil
Juice of 1 lemon
¼ teaspoon salt
¼ teaspoon freshly ground black pepper

1. In a large mixing bowl, combine the tomatoes, cucumber, onion, avocado, and dill.
2. In a small bowl, combine the oil, lemon juice, salt, and pepper, and mix well.
3. Drizzle the dressing over the vegetables and toss to combine. Serve.

Per Serving
calories: 152 | fat: 12.1g | protein: 2.1g
carbs: 10.9g | fiber: 4.1g | sugar: 4.0g
sodium: 129mg

Zucchini Salad with Ranch Dip

Prep time: 10 minutes | Cook time: 0 minutes | Serves 4

1 cup cottage cheese
2 tablespoons mayonnaise
Juice of ½ lemon
2 tablespoons chopped fresh chives
2 tablespoons chopped fresh dill
2 scallions, white and green parts, finely chopped
1 garlic clove, minced
½ teaspoon sea salt
2 zucchinis, cut into sticks
8 cherry tomatoes

1. In a small bowl, mix the cottage cheese, mayonnaise, lemon juice, chives, dill, scallions, garlic, and salt.
2. Serve with the zucchini sticks and cherry tomatoes for dipping.

Per Serving
calories: 92 | fat: 4.1g | protein: 7.1g
carbs: 6.9g | fiber: 1.1g | sugar: 5.3g
sodium: 388mg

Cucumber and Kidney Bean Salad

Prep time: 10 minutes | Cook time: 0 minutes | Serves 4

3 cups diced cucumber
1 (15-ounce / 425-g) can low-sodium dark red kidney beans, drained and rinsed
2 avocados, diced
1½ cups diced
tomatoes
1 cup cooked corn
¾ cup sliced red onion
1 tablespoon extra-virgin olive oil
1 tablespoon apple cider vinegar

1. In a large bowl, combine the cucumber, kidney beans, avocados, tomatoes, corn, onion, olive oil, and vinegar.

Per Serving
calories: 320 | fat: 16.1g | protein: 10.1g
carbs: 35.9g | fiber: 14.1g | sugar: 7.0g
sodium: 117mg

Cabbage Slaw

Prep time: 15 minutes | Cook time: 0 minutes | Serves 6

2 cups finely chopped green cabbage
2 cups finely chopped red cabbage
2 cups grated carrots
3 scallions, both white and green parts, sliced
2 tablespoons extra-virgin olive oil
2 tablespoons rice vinegar
1 teaspoon honey
1 garlic clove, minced
¼ teaspoon salt

1. In a large bowl, toss together the green and red cabbage, carrots, and scallions.
2. In a small bowl, whisk together the oil, vinegar, honey, garlic, and salt.
3. Pour the dressing over the veggies and mix to thoroughly combine.
4. Serve immediately, or cover and chill for several hours before serving.

Per Serving
calories: 81 | fat: 5.1g | protein: 1.1g
carbs: 69.9g | fiber: 3.1g | sugar: 6.0g
sodium: 124mg

Triple Bean Salad

Prep time: 10 minutes | Cook time: 0 minutes | Serves 8

1 (15-ounce / 425-g) can low-sodium chickpeas, drained and rinsed
1 (15-ounce / 425-g) can low-sodium kidney beans, drained and rinsed
1 (15-ounce / 425-g) can low-sodium white beans, drained and rinsed
1 red bell pepper, seeded and finely chopped
¼ cup chopped scallions, both white and green parts
¼ cup finely chopped fresh basil
3 garlic cloves, minced
2 tablespoons extra-virgin olive oil
1 tablespoon red wine vinegar
1 teaspoon Dijon mustard
¼ teaspoon freshly ground black pepper

1. In a large mixing bowl, combine the chickpeas, kidney beans, white beans, bell pepper, scallions, basil, and garlic. Toss gently to combine.
2. In a small bowl, combine the olive oil, vinegar, mustard, and pepper. Toss with the salad.
3. Cover and refrigerate for an hour before serving, to allow the flavors to mix.

Per Serving
calories: 194 | fat: 5.1g | protein: 10.1g
carbs: 28.9g | fiber: 8.1g | sugar: 3.0g
sodium: 245mg

Sumptuous Rainbow Salad

Prep time: 15 minutes | Cook time: 0 minutes | Serves 5

1 (15-ounce / 425-g) can low-sodium black beans, drained and rinsed
1 avocado, diced
1 cup cherry
2 tomatoes, halved
1 cup chopped baby spinach
½ cup finely chopped red bell pepper
¼ cup finely chopped jicama
½ cup chopped
scallions, both white and green parts
¼ cup chopped fresh cilantro
2 tablespoons freshly squeezed lime juice
1 tablespoon extra-virgin olive oil
2 garlic cloves, minced
1 teaspoon honey
¼ teaspoon salt
¼ teaspoon freshly ground black pepper

1. In a large bowl, combine the black beans, avocado, tomatoes, spinach, bell pepper, jicama, scallions, and cilantro.
2. In a small bowl, mix the lime juice, oil, garlic, honey, salt, and pepper. Add to the salad and toss.
3. Chill for 1 hour before serving.

Per Serving
calories: 168 | fat: 7.1g | protein: 6.1g
carbs: 21.8g | fiber: 9.1g | sugar: 3.0g
sodium: 236mg

Green Salad with Blackberries Vinaigrette

Prep time: 15 minutes | Cook time: 20 minutes | Serves 4

For the Vinaigrette:
1 pint blackberries
2 tablespoons red wine vinegar
1 tablespoon honey
3 tablespoons extra-
virgin olive oil
¼ teaspoon salt
Freshly ground black pepper

For the Salad:
1 sweet potato, cubed
1 teaspoon extra-virgin olive oil
8 cups salad greens (baby spinach, spicy
greens, romaine)
½ red onion, sliced
¼ cup crumbled goat cheese

To Make the Vinaigrette
1. In a blender jar, combine the blackberries, vinegar, honey, oil, salt, and pepper, and process until smooth. Set aside.

To Make the Salad
1. Preheat the oven to 425ºF (220ºC). Line a baking sheet with parchment paper.
2. In a medium mixing bowl, toss the sweet potato with the olive oil. Transfer to the prepared baking sheet and roast for 20 minutes, stirring once halfway through, until tender. Remove and cool for a few minutes.
3. In a large bowl, toss the greens with the red onion and cooled sweet potato, and drizzle with the vinaigrette. Serve topped with 1 tablespoon of goat cheese **Per Serving**.

Per Serving
calories: 197 | fat: 12.1g | protein: 3.1g
carbs: 20.9g | fiber: 6.1g | sugar: 10.0g
sodium: 185mg

Chickpea Slaw

Prep time: 10 minutes | Cook time: 0 minutes | Serves 6

1 (15-ounce / 425-g) can chickpeas packed in water, rinsed and drained
2 cups shredded kale
1 English cucumber, shredded
1 red bell pepper, seeded and cut into very thin strips
2 tablespoons

balsamic vinegar
1 tablespoon chopped fresh oregano
Sea salt and freshly ground black pepper, to taste
½ cup chopped fresh parsley
½ cup crumbled low-sodium feta cheese

1. In a large bowl, toss together the chickpeas, kale, cucumber, pepper, vinegar, and oregano.
2. Season with salt and pepper.
3. Sprinkle on the parsley and feta, and serve.

Per Serving
calories: 193 | fat: 5.1g | protein: 10.1g
carbs: 30.1g | fiber: 8.1g | sugar: 6.0g
sodium: 169mg

Cobb Salad

Prep time: 10 minutes | Cook time: 30 minutes | Serves 4

For the Salad:
8 (2-ounce / 57-g) chicken tenders
Avocado oil cooking spray
2 slices turkey bacon
2 (9-ounce / 255-
For the Dressing:
3 tablespoons honey mustard
3 tablespoons extra-

g) packages shaved Brussels sprouts
2 hardboiled eggs, chopped
½ cup unsweetened dried cranberries

virgin olive oil
½ tablespoon freshly squeezed lemon juice

To Make the Salad
1. Preheat the oven to 425ºF (220ºC).
2. Lightly coat the chicken tenders with cooking spray, then place them on a baking sheet and bake for 15 to 18 minutes.
3. Meanwhile, heat a large skillet over medium-low heat. When hot, fry the bacon for 5 to 7 minutes until crispy. When the

bacon is done, carefully remove it from the pan, and set it on a plate lined with a paper towel to drain and cool. Crumble when cool enough to handle.
4. Cut the chicken tenders into even pieces. Divide the Brussels sprouts into four equal portions. Top each portion with one-quarter of the chopped eggs, crumbled bacon, dried cranberries, and 2 sliced chicken tenders.
5. Drizzle an equal portion of dressing over each serving.

To Make the Dressing
1. In a small bowl, whisk together the mustard, olive oil, and lemon juice.

Per Serving
calories: 467 | fat: 20.1g | protein: 35.1g
carbs: 36.9g | fiber: 10.1g | sugar: 14.0g
sodium: 243mg

Summer Salad with Honey Dressing

Prep time: 5 minutes | Cook time: 0 minutes | Serves 4

For the Salad:
8 cups mixed greens or preferred lettuce, loosely packed
4 cups arugula, loosely packed
2 peaches, sliced ½
For the Dressing:
4 teaspoons extra-virgin olive oil

cup thinly sliced red onion
½ cup chopped walnuts or pecans
½ cup crumbled feta

4 teaspoons honey

To Make the Salad
1. Combine the mixed greens, arugula, peaches, red onion, walnuts, and feta in a large bowl. Divide the salad into four portions.
2. Drizzle the dressing over each individual serving of salad.

To Make the Dressing
1. In a small bowl, whisk together the olive oil and honey.

Per Serving
calories: 264 | fat: 18.1g | protein: 8.1g
carbs: 21.9g | fiber: 5.1g | sugar: 16.0g
sodium: 223mg

Spinach and Chicken Salad

Prep time: 5 minutes | Cook time: 0 minutes | Serves 4

For the Salad:
8 cups baby spinach
2 cups shredded rotisserie chicken
½ cup sliced strawberries or other

berries
½ cup sliced almonds
1 avocado, sliced
¼ cup crumbled feta (optional)

For the Dressing:
2 tablespoons extra-virgin olive oil
2 teaspoons honey

2 teaspoons balsamic vinegar

To Make the Salad
1. In a large bowl, combine the spinach, chicken, strawberries, and almonds.
2. Pour the dressing over the salad and lightly toss.
3. Divide into four equal portions and top each with sliced avocado and 1 tablespoon of crumbled feta (if using).

To Make the Dressing
In a small bowl, whisk together the olive oil, honey, and balsamic vinegar.

Per Serving
calories: 340 | fat: 22.1g | protein: 25.1g carbs: 12.9g | fiber: 6.1g | sugar: 6.0g sodium: 133mg

Kale, Cantaloupe, and Chicken Salad

Prep time: 10 minutes | Cook time: 0 minutes | Serves 3

For the Salad:
4 cups chopped kale, packed
1½ cups diced cantaloupe

1½ cups shredded rotisserie chicken
½ cup sliced almonds
¼ cup crumbled feta

For the Dressing:
2 teaspoons honey
2 tablespoons extra-virgin olive oil
2 teaspoons apple

cider vinegar or freshly squeezed lemon juice

To Make the Salad
1. Divide the kale into three portions. Layer ⅓ of the cantaloupe, chicken, almonds, and feta on each portion.
2. Drizzle some of the dressing over each portion of salad. Serve immediately.

To Make the Dressing
1. In a small bowl, whisk together the honey, olive oil, and vinegar.

Per Serving
calories: 395 | fat: 22.1g | protein: 27.1g carbs: 23.9g | fiber: 4.1g | sugar: 12.0g sodium: 235mg

Asian Noodle Salad

Prep time: 30 minutes | Cook time: 0 minutes | Serves 4

2 carrots, sliced thin
2 radish, sliced thin
1 English cucumber, sliced thin
1 mango, julienned
1 bell pepper, julienned
1 small serrano pepper, seeded and sliced thin
1 bag tofu Shirataki Fettuccini noodles
¼ cup lime juice
¼ cup fresh basil, chopped

¼ cup fresh cilantro, chopped
2 tablespoons fresh mint, chopped
2 tablespoons rice vinegar
2 tablespoons sweet chili sauce
2 tablespoons roasted peanuts finely chopped
1 tablespoon Splenda
½ teaspoon sesame oil

1. Pickle the vegetables: In a large bowl, place radish, cucumbers, and carrots. Add vinegar, coconut sugar, and lime juice and stir to coat the vegetables. Cover and chill 15 – 20 minutes.
2. Prep the noodles: remove the noodles from the package and rinse under cold water. Cut into smaller pieces. Pat dry with paper towels.
3. To assemble the salad. Remove the vegetables from the marinade, reserving marinade, and place in a large mixing bowl. Add noodles, mango, bell pepper, chili, and herbs.
4. In a small bowl, combine 2 tablespoons marinade with the chili sauce and sesame oil. Pour over salad and toss to coat. Top with peanuts and serve.

Per Serving
calories: 159 | fat: 4.1g | protein: 4.0g carbs: 30.1g | fiber: 6.1g | sugar: 18.9g sodium: 119mg

Kale and Cabbage Salad with Peanuts

Prep time: 15 minutes | Cook time: 0 minutes | Serves 6

2 bunches baby kale, thinly sliced
½ head green savoy cabbage, cored and thinly sliced
Dressing:
¼ cup apple cider

vinegar
Juice of 1 lemon
1 teaspoon ground cumin
¼ teaspoon smoked paprika

1 cup toasted peanuts
1 medium red bell pepper, thinly sliced

1 garlic clove, thinly sliced

1. Toss the kale with cabbage in a large bowl. Set aside.
2. Make the dressing: In a separate bowl, whisk together the vinegar, lemon juice, cumin, and paprika until completely mixed.
3. Pour the dressing into the bowl of greens and using your hands to massage the greens until thickly coated.
4. Add the peanuts, bell peppers, and garlic to the bowl. Gently toss to combine well.
5. Serve chilled or at room temperature.

Per Serving
calories: 200 | fat: 12.3g | protein: 9.8g
carbs: 16.8g | fiber: 4.8g | sugar: 4.2g
sodium: 45mg

Sofrito Steak and Veg Salad

Prep time: 10 minutes | Cook time: 15 minutes | Serves 4

4 ounces (113 g) recaíto cooking base
2 (4-ounce / 113-g) flank steaks
8 cups fresh spinach, loosely packed
½ cup sliced red

onion
2 cups diced tomato
2 avocados, diced
2 cups diced cucumber
$1/_3$ cup crumbled feta

1. Heat a large skillet over medium-low heat. When hot, pour in the recaíto cooking base, add the steaks, and cover. Cook for 8 to 12 minutes.
2. Meanwhile, divide the spinach into four portions. Top each portion with one-quarter of the onion, tomato, avocados, and cucumber.

3. Remove the steak from the skillet, and let it rest for about 2 minutes before slicing. Place one-quarter of the steak and feta on top of each portion.

Per Serving
calories: 346 | fat: 18.1g | protein: 25.1g
carbs: 17.9g | fiber: 8.1g | sugar: 6.0g
sodium: 380mg

Chopped Veggie Salad

Prep time: 15 minutes | Cook time: 0 minutes | Serves 4

1 cucumber, chopped
1 pint cherry tomatoes, cut in half
3 radishes, chopped
1 yellow bell pepper chopped

½ cup fresh parsley, chopped
3 tablespoons lemon juice
1 tablespoon olive oil
Salt, to taste

1. Place all in a large bowl and toss to combine. Serve immediately, or cover and chill until ready to serve.

Per Serving
calories: 71 | fat: 4.1g | protein: 2.0g
carbs: 9.1g | fiber: 2.0g | sugar: 4.9g
sodium: 98mg

Caprese Salad

Prep time: 10 minutes | Cook time: 0 minutes | Serves 4

3 medium tomatoes, cut into 8 slices
2 (1-ounce / 28-g) slices Mozzarella cheese, cut into strips
¼ cup fresh basil,

sliced thin
2 teaspoons extra-virgin olive oil
⅛ teaspoon salt
Pinch black pepper

1. Place tomatoes and cheese on serving plates. Sprinkle with salt and pepper. Drizzle oil over and top with basil. Serve.

Per Serving
calories: 78 | fat: 5.1g | protein: 5.0g
carbs: 4.1g | fiber: 1.0g | sugar: 1.9g
sodium: 84mg

Butternut Squash, Broccoli, and Barley Salad

Prep time: 20 minutes | Cook time: 40 minutes | Serves 8

1 small butternut squash, peeled, deseeded, and diced
3 teaspoons olive oil, divided
2 cups broccoli, cut into florets
1 cup pearl barley
2 cups baby kale
1 cup toasted walnuts, chopped

½ red onion, sliced
Balsamic Vinaigrette:
2 tablespoons balsamic vinegar
2 garlic cloves, minced
½ teaspoon salt
¼ teaspoon freshly ground black pepper
2 tablespoons extra-virgin olive oil

1. Preheat the oven to 400ºF (205ºC).
2. Toss the diced squash with 2 teaspoons of olive oil in a bowl. Put the oiled squash on a baking sheet lined with parchment paper.
3. Roast in the preheated oven for 20 minutes.
4. Meanwhile, toss the broccoli with 1 teaspoon of olive oil in the same bowl.
5. Put the oiled broccoli on the same baking sheet, and turn the squash over. Keep roasting for another 20 minutes or until soft.
6. In the mean time, put the barley in a pot of water. Bring to a boil. Turn down the heat to low. Put the lid on and simmer for 30 minutes until soft. Pat dry with paper towels.
7. Put the cooked squash, broccoli, kale, walnuts, and onion in a large bowl, then add the cooked barley. Toss to combine well.
8. Combine all the ingredients for the balsamic vinaigrette in a separate bowl. Stir to mix well.
9. Pour the balsamic vinaigrette over the salad to dress and stir to serve.

Per Serving
calories: 276 | fat: 14.9g | protein: 6.1g
carbs: 31.8g | fiber: 7.2g | sugar: 3.2g
sodium: 143mg

Shrimp and Avocado Salad

Prep time: 20 minutes | Cook time: 4 minutes | Serves 8

2 tablespoons extra virgin olive oil, divided
1 pound (454 g) large shrimps, peeled and deveined
2 avocados, peeled and cubed
2 ears fresh corn, kernels sliced off
2 cups cherry tomatoes, halved
3 ounces (85 g) reduced-fat feta

cheese, cubed
1 tablespoon balsamic vinegar
¼ teaspoon cumin
¼ teaspoon celery seeds
¼ cup slivered fresh basil
1 tablespoon fresh lemon juice
⅛ teaspoon salt
¼ teaspoon freshly ground black pepper

1. Heat 1 tablespoon of olive oil in a nonstick skillet over medium heat until shimmering.
2. Add the shrimps and grill for 4 minutes or until opaque. Flip the shrimps halfway through the cooking time.
3. Combine the remaining ingredients in a large salad bowl, then add the shrimps and toss to combine well.
4. Serve immediately.

Per Serving
calories: 195 | fat: 10.0g | protein: 17.0g
carbs: 12.0g | fiber: 4.0g | sugar: 3.0g
sodium: 440mg

Pickled Cucumber and Onion Salad

Prep time: 10 minutes | Cook time: 0 minutes | Serves 2

½ cucumber, peeled and sliced
¼ cup red onion, sliced thin

1 tablespoon olive oil
1 tablespoon white vinegar
1 teaspoon dill

1. Place all in a medium bowl and toss to combine. Serve.

Per Serving
calories: 80 | fat: 7.1g | protein: 1.0g
carbs: 4.1g | fiber: 1.0g | sugar: 1.9g
sodium: 2mg

Cantaloupe and Prosciutto Salad

Prep time: 15 minutes | Cook time: 0 minutes | Serves 4

6 Mozzarella balls, quartered
1 medium cantaloupe, peeled and cut into small cubes
4 ounces (113 g) prosciutto, chopped
1 tablespoon fresh lime juice
1 tablespoon fresh mint, chopped
2 tablespoons extra virgin olive oil
1 teaspoon honey

1. In a large bowl, whisk together oil, lime juice, honey, and mint. Season with salt and pepper to taste.
2. Add the cantaloupe and Mozzarella and toss to combine. Arrange the mixture on a serving plate and add prosciutto. Serve.

Per Serving
calories: 241 | fat: 16.1g | protein: 18.0g
carbs: 6.1g | fiber: 0g | sugar: 3.9g
sodium: 701mg

Creamy Crab Slaw

Prep time: 10 minutes | Cook time: 0 minutes | Serves 4

½ pound (227 g) cabbage, shredded
½ pound (227 g) red cabbage, shredded
2 hard-boiled eggs, chopped
Juice of ½ lemon
2 (6-ounce / 170-
g) cans crabmeat, drained
½ cup lite mayonnaise
1 teaspoon celery seeds
Salt and ground black pepper, to taste

1. In a large bowl, combine both kinds of cabbage.
2. In a small bowl, combine mayonnaise, lemon juice, and celery seeds. Add to cabbage and toss to coat.
3. Add crab and eggs and toss to mix, season with salt and pepper. Cover and refrigerate 1 hour before serving.

Per Serving
calories: 381 | fat: 24.1g | protein: 18.0g
carbs: 25.1g | fiber: 8.0g | sugar: 12.9g
sodium: 266mg

Harvest Salad

Prep time: 15 minutes | Cook time: 25 minutes | Serves 6

10 ounces (283 g) kale, deboned and chopped
1½ cup blackberries
½ butternut squash, cubed
¼ cup goat cheese, crumbled
1 cup raw pecans
1/3 cup raw pumpkin seeds
¼ cup dried cranberries
3½ tablespoons olive oil
1½ tablespoons sugar
free maple syrup
⅛ plus ½ teaspoon salt
Pepper, to taste
Nonstick cooking spray
Maple Mustard Salad Dressing:
2 tablespoons balsamic vinegar
2 tablespoons olive oil
1 tablespoon sugar free maple syrup
1 teaspoon Dijon mustard
⅛ teaspoon sea salt

1. Heat oven to 400ºF (205ºC). Spray a baking sheet with cooking spray.
2. Spread squash on the prepared pan, add 1½ tablespoons oil, ⅛ teaspoon salt, and pepper to squash and stir to coat the squash evenly. Bake for 20 to 25 minutes.
3. Place kale in a large bowl. Add 2 tablespoons oil and ½ teaspoon salt and massage it into the kale with your hands for 3 to 4 minutes.
4. Spray a clean baking sheet with cooking spray. In a medium bowl, stir together pecans, pumpkin seeds, and maple syrup until nuts are coated. Pour onto prepared pan and bake for 8 to 10 minutes, these can be baked at the same time as the squash.
5. Meanwhile, combine the ingredients for the dressing in a small bowl.
6. To assemble the salad: place all the ingredients in a large bowl. Pour dressing over and toss to coat. Serve immediately.

Per Serving
calories: 435 | fat: 37.1g | protein: 9.0g
carbs: 24.1g | fiber: 7.0g | sugar: 4.9g
sodium: 161mg

Spinach, Pear, and Walnut Salad

Prep time: 10 minutes | Cook time: 0 minutes | Serves 2

2 tablespoons apple cider vinegar
1 teaspoon peeled and grated fresh ginger
½ teaspoon Dijon mustard
2 tablespoons extra-
virgin olive oil
½ teaspoon sea salt
4 cups baby spinach
½ pear, cored, peeled, and chopped
¼ cup chopped walnuts

1. Combine the vinegar, ginger, mustard, olive oil, and salt in a small bowl. Stir to mix well.
2. Combine the remaining ingredients in a large serving bowl, then toss to combine well.
3. Pour the vinegar dressing in the bowl of salad and toss before serving.

Per Serving
calories: 229 | fat: 20.4g | protein: 3.5g
carbs: 10.7g | fiber: 3.4g | sugar: 4.9g
sodium: 644mg

Asparagus and Bacon Salad

Prep time: 5 minutes | Cook time: 5 minutes | Serves 1

1 hard-boiled egg, peeled and sliced
1²/₃ cups asparagus, chopped
2 slices bacon, cooked crisp and crumbled
1 teaspoon extra
virgin olive oil
1 teaspoon red wine vinegar
½ teaspoon Dijon mustard
Pinch salt and pepper, to taste

1. Bring a pot of water to a boil. Add the asparagus and cook 2 to 3 minutes or until tender-crisp. Drain and add cold water to stop the cooking process.
2. In a small bowl, whisk together, mustard, oil, vinegar, and salt and pepper to taste.
3. Place the asparagus on a plate, top with egg and bacon. Drizzle with vinaigrette and serve.

Per Serving
calories: 357 | fat: 25.1g | protein: 25.0g
carbs: 10.1g | fiber: 5.1g | sugar: 4.9g
sodium: 492mg

Pomegranate and Brussels Sprouts Salad

Prep time: 10 minutes | Cook time: 0 minutes | Serves 6

3 slices bacon, cooked crisp and crumbled
3 cup Brussels sprouts, shredded
3 cup kale, shredded
1½ cup pomegranate seeds
½ cup almonds, toasted and chopped
¼ cup reduced fat Parmesan cheese, grated
Citrus Vinaigrette:
1 orange, zested and juiced
1 lemon, zested and juiced
¼ cup extra virgin olive oil
1 teaspoon Dijon mustard
1 teaspoon honey
1 clove garlic, crushed
Salt and ground black pepper, to taste

1. Combine the ingredient for the citrus vinaigrette in a small bowl.
2. Toss the remaining ingredients with the vinaigrette in a large bowl.
3. Serve garnished with more cheese if desired.

Per Serving
calories: 255 | fat: 18.1g | protein: 9.0g
carbs: 15.1g | fiber: 5.0g | sugar: 4.9g
sodium: 176mg

Asian Style Slaw

Prep time: 5 minutes | Cook time: 0 minutes | Serves 8

1 (1-pound / 454-g) bag coleslaw mix
5 scallions, sliced
1 cup sunflower seeds
1 cup almonds, sliced
3 ounces (85 g)
ramen noodles, broken into small pieces
¾ cup vegetable oil
½ cup Splenda
¹/₃ cup vinegar

1. In a large bowl, combine coleslaw, sunflower seeds, almonds, and scallions.
2. Whisk together the oil, vinegar and Splenda in a large measuring cup. Pour over salad, and stir to combine.
3. Stir in ramen noodles, cover and chill 2 hours.

Per Serving
calories: 355 | fat: 26.1g | protein: 5.0g
carbs: 24.1g | fiber: 3.1g | sugar: 9.9g
sodium: 22mg

Celery Apple Salad

Prep time: 5 minutes | Cook time: 10 minutes | Serves 4

2 green onions, diced
2 Medjool dates, pitted and diced fine
1 honey crisp apple, sliced thin
2 cup celery, sliced
½ cup celery leaves, diced
¼ cup walnuts, chopped
Maple Shallot

Vinaigrette:
1 tablespoon shallot, diced fine
2 tablespoons apple cider vinegar
1 tablespoon spicy brown mustard
1 tablespoon olive oil
2 teaspoon sugar-free maple syrup

1. Heat oven to 375ºF (190ºC). Place walnuts on a cookie sheet and bake 10 minutes, stirring every few minutes, to toast.
2. Meanwhile, combine the ingredients for the vinaigrette in a small bowl. Stir to mix well.
3. When the baking is complete, in a large bowl, combine the baked walnuts with the remaining ingredients and toss to mix.
4. Drizzle vinaigrette over and toss to coat. Serve immediately.

Per Serving
calories: 172 | fat: 8.1g | protein: 3.0g
carbs: 25.1g | fiber: 4.0g | sugar: 14.9g
sodium: 95mg

Baked "Potato" Salad

Prep time: 15 minutes | Cook time: 15 minutes | Serves 8

2 pounds (907 g) cauliflower, separated into small florets
6 to 8 slices bacon, chopped and fried crisp
6 boiled eggs, cooled, peeled, and chopped
1 cup sharp cheddar cheese, grated

½ cup green onion, sliced
1 cup reduced-fat mayonnaise
2 teaspoons yellow mustard
1½ teaspoons onion powder, divided
Salt and fresh-ground black pepper to taste

1. Place cauliflower in a vegetable steamer, or a pot with a steamer insert, and steam 5 to 6 minutes.
2. Drain the cauliflower and set aside.

3. In a small bowl, whisk together mayonnaise, mustard, 1 teaspoon onion powder, salt, and pepper.
4. Pat cauliflower dry with paper towels and place in a large mixing bowl. Add eggs, salt, pepper, remaining ½ teaspoon onion powder, then dressing. Mix gently to combine together.
5. Fold in the bacon, cheese, and green onion. Serve warm or cover and chill before serving.

Per Serving
calories: 248 | fat: 17.1g | protein: 17.0g
carbs: 8.1g | fiber: 3.0g | sugar: 2.9g
sodium: 384mg

Broccoli and Mushroom Salad

Prep time: 10 minutes | Cook time: 0 minutes | Serves 4

4 sun-dried tomatoes, cut in half
3 cup torn leaf lettuce
1½ cup broccoli florets
1 cup mushrooms, sliced
⅓ cup radishes, sliced
2 tablespoons water
1 tablespoon balsamic

vinegar
1 teaspoon vegetable oil
¼ teaspoon chicken bouillon granules
¼ teaspoon parsley
¼ teaspoon dry mustard
⅛ teaspoon cayenne pepper

1. Place tomatoes in a small bowl and pour boiling water over, just enough to cover. Let stand 5 minutes, drain.
2. Chop tomatoes and place in a large bowl. Add lettuce, broccoli, mushrooms, and radishes.
3. In a jar with a tight fitting lid, add remaining and shake well. Pour over salad and toss to coat. Serve.

Per Serving
calories: 55 | fat: 2.1g | protein: 3.0g
carbs: 9.1g | fiber: 2.0g | sugar: 1.9g
sodium: 19mg

Chicken Guacamole Salad

Prep time: 10 minutes | Cook time: 20 minutes | Serves 6

1 pound (454 g) chicken breast, boneless and skinless
2 avocados
1 to 2 jalapeno peppers, seeded and diced
$\frac{1}{3}$ cup onion, diced

3 tablespoons cilantro, diced
2 tablespoons fresh lime juice
2 cloves garlic, diced
1 tablespoon olive oil
Salt and ground black pepper, to taste

1. Heat oven to 400ºF (205ºC). Line a baking sheet with foil.
2. Season chicken with salt and pepper and place on prepared pan. Bake 20 minutes, or until chicken is cooked through. Let cool completely.
3. Once chicken has cooled, shred or dice and add to a large bowl. Add remaining and mix well, mashing the avocado as you mix it in. Taste and season with salt and pepper as desired. Serve immediately.

Per Serving
calories: 325 | fat: 22.1g | protein: 23.0g
carbs: 12.1g | fiber: 7.0g | sugar: 0.9g
sodium: 79mg

Watermelon and Arugula Salad

Prep time: 10 minutes | Cook time: 0 minutes | Serves 6

4 cups watermelon, cut in 1-inch cubes
3 cup arugula
1 lemon, zested
½ cup feta cheese, crumbled
¼ cup fresh mint,

chopped
1 tablespoon fresh lemon juice
3 tablespoons olive oil
Fresh ground black pepper, to taste
Salt, to taste

1. Combine oil, zest, juice and mint in a large bowl. Stir together.
2. Add watermelon and gently toss to coat. Add remaining and toss to combine. Taste and adjust seasoning as desired.
3. Cover and chill at least 1 hour before serving.

Per Serving
calories: 150 | fat: 11.1g | protein: 4.0g
carbs: 10.1g | fiber: 1.0g | sugar: 6.9g
sodium: 145mg

Pecan Pear Salad

Prep time: 15 minutes | Cook time: 0 minutes | Serves 8

10 ounces (283 g) mixed greens
3 pears, chopped
½ cup blue cheese, crumbled
2 cup pecan halves
1 cup dried

cranberries
½ cup olive oil
6 tablespoons champagne vinegar
2 tablespoons Dijon mustard
¼ teaspoon salt

1. In a large bowl combine greens, pears, cranberries and pecans.
2. Whisk remaining , except blue cheese, together in a small bowl Pour over salad and toss to coat. Serve topped with blue cheese crumbles.

Per Serving
calories: 326 | fat: 26.1g | protein: 5.0g
carbs: 20.1g | fiber: 6.0g | sugar: 9.9g
sodium: 294mg

Summer Corn Salad

Prep time: 10 minutes | Cook time: 0 minutes | Serves 8

2 avocados, cut into ½-inch cubes
1 pint cherry tomatoes, cut in half
2 cups fresh corn kernels, cooked
½ cup red onion, diced fine

¼ cup cilantro, chopped
1 tablespoon fresh lime juice
½ teaspoon lime zest
2 tablespoons olive oil
¼ teaspoon salt
¼ teaspoon pepper

1. In a large bowl, combine corn, avocado, tomatoes, and onion.
2. In a small bowl, whisk together remaining until combined. Pour over salad and toss to coat.
3. Cover and chill 2 hours. Serve.

Per Serving
calories: 240 | fat: 18.1g | protein: 4.0g
carbs: 20.1g | fiber: 7.0g | sugar: 3.9g
sodium: 77mg

Festive Holiday Salad

Prep time: 10 minutes | Cook time: 0 minutes | Serves 8

1 head broccoli, separated into florets
1 head cauliflower, separated into florets
1 red onion, sliced thin
2 cup cherry tomatoes, halved
½ cup fat free sour cream
1 cup lite mayonnaise
1 tablespoon Splenda

1. In a large bowl combine vegetables.
2. In a small bowl, whisk together mayonnaise, sour cream and Splenda. Pour over vegetables and toss to mix.
3. Cover and refrigerate at least 1 hour before serving.

Per Serving
calories: 153 | fat: 10.1g | protein: 2.0g
carbs: 12.1g | fiber: 2.0g | sugar: 4.9g
sodium: 264mg

Broccoli and Bacon Salad

Prep time: 10 minutes | Cook time: 0 minutes | Serves 4

2 cups broccoli, separated into florets
4 slices bacon, chopped and cooked crisp
½ cup cheddar cheese, cubed
¼ cup low-fat Greek yogurt
⅛ cup red onion, diced fine
⅛ cup almonds, sliced
¼ cup reduced-fat mayonnaise
1 tablespoon lemon juice
1 tablespoon apple cider vinegar
1 tablespoon granulated sugar substitute
¼ teaspoon salt
¼ teaspoon pepper

1. In a large bowl, combine broccoli, onion, cheese, bacon, and almonds.
2. In a small bowl, whisk remaining together till combined.
3. Pour dressing over broccoli mixture and stir. Cover and chill at least 1 hour before serving.

Per Serving
calories: 220 | fat: 14.1g | protein: 11.0g
carbs: 12.1g | fiber: 2.0g | sugar: 5.9g
sodium: 508mg

Grain, Seafood, and Fruit Salad

Prep time: 30 minutes | Cook time: 20 minutes | Serves 4

1 cup quinoa, rinsed
½ pound (227 g) medium shrimps, peeled and deveined
½ pound (227 g) scallops
1 tablespoon olive oil
½ red bell pepper, chopped
1 roma plum tomatoes, deseeded and chopped
1 jalapeño pepper, stemmed and finely chopped
½ cup cooked black beans
1 mango, chopped
1 avocado, chopped
2 small scallions, chopped
2 tablespoons cilantro leaves, chopped
Citrus Dressing:
2 tablespoons lime juice
2 tablespoons orange juice
1 teaspoon honey
¼ teaspoon cayenne pepper
1 tablespoon extra virgin olive oil
Sea salt, to taste

1. Pour the quinoa in a pot, then pour in enough water to cover. Bring to a boil, then reduce the heat to low and simmer to 10 to 15 minutes or until the liquid has been absorbed. Fluffy with a fork and let stand until ready to use.
2. Meanwhile, combine the ingredients for the citrus dressing in a small bowl. Stir to mix well. Set aside until ready to use.
3. Put the shrimps and scallops in a separate bowl, then drizzle with the olive oil. Toss to coat well.
4. Add the oiled shrimps and scallops in a nonstick skillet and grill over medium-high heat for 4 minutes or until opaque. Flip them halfway through. Remove them from the skillet and allow to cool.
5. Combine the cooked quinoa, shrimp and scallops with bell pepper, tomato, jalapeño, beans, mango, avocado, and scallions in a large salad bowl, then drizzle with the citrus dressing. Toss to combine well.
6. Garnish with cilantro leaves and serve immediately.

Per Serving
calories: 470 | fat: 16.0g | protein: 30.0g
carbs: 56.0g | fiber: 10.0g | sugar: 16.0g
sodium: 320mg

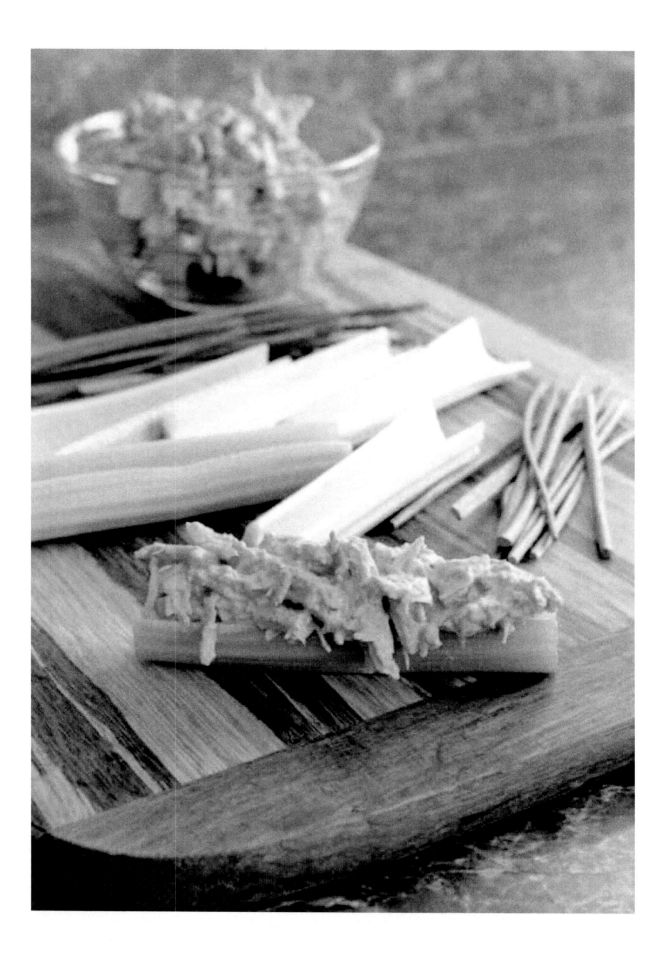

Chapter 13: Snacks and Appetizers

Easy Cauliflower Hush Puppies

Prep time: 15 minutes | Cook time: 10 minutes | Makes 16 hush puppies

1 whole cauliflower, including stalks and florets, roughly chopped
¾ cup buttermilk
¾ cup low-fat milk
1 medium onion, chopped
2 medium eggs
2 cups yellow cornmeal
1½ teaspoons baking powder
½ teaspoon salt

1. In a blender, combine the cauliflower, buttermilk, milk, and onion and purée. Transfer to a large mixing bowl.
2. Crack the eggs into the purée, and gently fold until mixed.
3. In a medium bowl, whisk the cornmeal, baking powder, and salt together.
4. Gently add the dry ingredients to the wet ingredients and mix until just combined, taking care not to overmix.
5. Working in batches, place ⅓-cup portions of the batter into the basket of an air fryer.
6. Set the air fryer to 390ºF (199ºC), close, and cook for 10 minutes. Transfer the hush puppies to a plate. Repeat until no batter remains.
7. Serve warm with greens.

Per Serving
calories: 180 | fat: 8.1g | protein: 4.1g
carbs: 27.9g | fiber: 6.1g | sugar: 11.0g
sodium: 251mg

Cauliflower Mash

Prep time: 7 minutes | Cook time: 20 minutes | Serves 4

1 head cauliflower, cored and cut into large florets
½ teaspoon kosher salt
½ teaspoon garlic pepper
2 tablespoons plain
Greek yogurt
¾ cup freshly grated Parmesan cheese
1 tablespoon unsalted butter or ghee (optional)
Chopped fresh chives

1. Pour 1 cup of water into the electric pressure cooker and insert a steamer basket or wire rack.
2. Place the cauliflower in the basket.
3. Close and lock the lid of the pressure cooker. Set the valve to sealing.
4. Cook on high pressure for 5 minutes.
5. When the cooking is complete, hit Cancel and quick release the pressure.
6. Once the pin drops, unlock and remove the lid.
7. Remove the cauliflower from the pot and pour out the water. Return the cauliflower to the pot and add the salt, garlic pepper, yogurt, and cheese. Use an immersion blender or potato masher to purée or mash the cauliflower in the pot.
8. Spoon into a serving bowl, and garnish with butter (if using) and chives.

Per Serving
calories: 141 | fat: 6.1g | protein: 12.1g
carbs: 11.9g | fiber: 4.1g | sugar: 5.0g
sodium: 591mg

Parmesan Crisps

Prep time: 5 minutes | Cook time: 5 minutes | Serves 2

1 cup grated Parmesan cheese

1. Preheat the oven to 400ºF (205ºC). Line a rimmed baking sheet with parchment paper.
2. Spread the Parmesan on the prepared baking sheet into 4 mounds, spreading each mound out so it is flat but not touching the others.
3. Bake until brown and crisp, 3 to 5 minutes.
4. Cool for 5 minutes. Use a spatula to remove to a plate to continue cooling.

Per Serving
calories: 216 | fat: 14.1g | protein: 19.1g
carbs: 2.0g | fiber: 0g | sugar: 1.5g
sodium: 765mg

Banana and Carrot Flax Muffins

Prep time: 20 minutes | Cook time: 40 minutes | Makes 8 muffins

Dry:

¼ teaspoon cloves	cinnamon
¼ cup tapioca starch	1 teaspoon baking
½ cup stevia	soda
1 teaspoon salt	1 teaspoon baking
1 teaspoon nutmeg	powder
1 tablespoon	1¾ cups almond flour

Wet:

4 tablespoons flax meal	⅓ cup coconut oil
1½ cups water	1 medium banana, mashed
1 teaspoon vanilla extract	1½ cups carrots, shredded

1. Preheat the oven to 350ºF (180ºC). Line an 8-cup muffin tin with paper cups.
2. Soak the flax meal in water in a bowl for 5 minutes to make the flax egg.
3. Combine all the dry ingredients in a large bowl. Stir to mix well.
4. Make a well in the dry mixture, then pour the flax egg, vanilla extract, and coconut oil in the well. Stir to mix well, then mix in the banana and carrots.
5. Divide the mixture among 8 muffins cups, then bake in the preheated oven for 40 minutes or until the top springs back when you press the muffins with your fingers.
6. Remove the muffins from the oven and allow to cool before serving.

Per Serving (1 Muffin)
calories: 135 | fat: 9.5g | protein: 1.5g
carbs: 14.0g | fiber: 1.6g | sugars: 4.2g
sodium: 464mg

Italian Flavor Salmon and Potato Patties

Prep time: 15 minutes | Cook time: 10 minutes | Serves 12 patties

3 medium potatoes, peeled and shredded	cooked flaked salmon
2 eggs	¾ cup dry bread crumbs
1 teaspoon Italian seasoning	¾ cup fresh mushrooms, sliced
Salt and freshly ground pepper, to taste	¾ cup canned banana peppers, chopped
½ pound (227 g)	1 red bell pepper, chopped
2 tablespoons capers, drained	chopped
3 green onions,	¼ cup olive oil, or more as needed

1. Wrap the potatoes in a muslin cloth and squeeze the liquid out as much as possible.
2. Whisk together the eggs, potatoes, Italian seasoning, salt, and pepper in a large bowl to coat the potato well.
3. Combine the remaining ingredients, except for the olive oil, in another large bowl. Stir to mix well.
4. Divide the mixture into 12 equally sized balls, then bash the balls into ¾-inch patties.
5. Heat the olive oil in a nonstick skillet over medium-high heat.
6. Arrange the patties in the skillet and fry for 6 minutes or until lightly browned on both sides. Flip the patties halfway through. You may need to work batches to avoid overcrowding.
7. Place the fried patties on a large plate lined with parchment paper and serve warm.

Per Serving (1 Patty)
calories: 158 | fat: 7.1g | protein: 7.3g
carbs: 16.5g | fiber: 2.3g | sugars: 2.2g
sodium: 200mg

Hot Chicken Stuffed Celery Stalks

Prep time: 10 minutes | Cook time: 0 minutes | Serves 4

1 teaspoon Buffalo hot sauce	chicken meat, shredded
¼ cup chunky blue cheese dressing	8 celery stalks, cut into halves lengthwise
1 cup rotisserie	

1. Combine the hot sauce and blue cheese dressing in a bowl, then dunk the shredded rotisserie chicken in the bowl to coat well.
2. Divide the mixture in the celery stalks and serve.

Per Serving
calories: 148 | fat: 11.9g | protein: 9.1g
carbs: 2.8g | fiber: 1.2g | sugar: 1.6g
sodium: 461mg

Easy Low-Carb Biscuits

Prep time: 10 minutes | Cook time: 15 minutes | Serves 4 biscuits

¼ cup plain Greek yogurt	melted
2 tablespoons unsalted butter,	Pinch salt
	1½ cups finely ground almond flour

1. Preheat the oven to 375ºF (190ºC).
2. Combine the yogurt, butter, and salt in a bowl. Stir to mix well.
3. Fold the almond flour in the mixture. Keep stirring until a dough without lumps forms.
4. Divide the dough into 4 balls, then bash the balls into 1-inch biscuits with your hands.
5. Arrange the biscuits on a baking pan lined with parchment paper. Bake in the preheated oven for 14 minutes or until well browned.
6. Remove the biscuits from the oven and serve warm.

Per Serving
calories: 312 | fat: 27.9g | protein: 10.2g
carbs: 8.9g | fiber: 5.1g | sugar: 2.1g
sodium: 31mg

Zucchini and Banana Bread

Prep time: 15 minutes | Cook time: 45 minutes | Serves 24 slices

Dry:

1½ cups gluten-free all-purpose flour	1 teaspoon salt
½ cup chickpea flour	1 cup almond meal
½ teaspoon ground nutmeg	1 teaspoon baking soda
½ teaspoon ground cinnamon	1 teaspoon baking powder

Wet:

3 medium brown eggs, beaten	oil
2 zucchini, grated, with water squeezed out	2 ripe bananas, mashed
¼ cup sunflower seed	2 teaspoons almond extract

1. Preheat the oven to 350ºF (180ºC).
2. Combine all the dry ingredients in a bowl. Stir to mix well.

3. Whisk together all the wet ingredients in a separate bowl. Stir to mix well.
4. Gently stir the dry ingredients in the wet ingredients until well combined.
5. Pour the mixture in a baking pan lined with parchment paper.
6. Bake in the preheated oven for 40 minutes or until a toothpick inserted in the middle of the bread comes out clean.
7. Remove the bread from the oven and slice it into 24 bread slices, about 2 inch thick, then serve warm.

Per Serving
calories: 205 | fat: 10.9g | protein: 6.2g
carbs: 20.8g | fiber: 4.1g | sugar: 3.8g
sodium: 320mg

Tomato Waffles

Prep time: 15 minutes | Cook time: 40 minutes | Serves 8 waffles

Dry:

½ cup almond flour	chives
½ cup coconut flour	1 cup gluten-free all-purpose flour
½ teaspoon baking soda	2 teaspoons baking powder
½ teaspoon dried	

Wet:

1 tablespoon olive oil	2 medium egg whites
½ cup tomato, crushed	2 cups low-fat buttermilk
1 medium egg	

1. Preheat a waffle iron. Grease the waffle iron with olive oil.
2. Combine all the dry ingredients in a bowl. Stir to mix well.
3. Combine all the remaining wet ingredients in a separate bowl. Stir to mix well.
4. Gently stir the dry ingredients in the wet ingredients until well combined.
5. Pour ¼- to ½-cup of the mixture in the waffle iron and cook for 5 minutes or until the waffle is golden brown. Repeat with remaining mixture.
6. Transfer the waffles onto several serving plates and serve warm.

Per Serving
calories: 142 | fat: 4.1g | protein: 6.9g
carbs: 20.8g | fiber: 5.1g | sugar: 2.8g
sodium: 167mg

Peanut Butter and Chocolate Bites

Prep time: 10 minutes | Cook time: 0 minutes | Serves 16 balls

½ cup sugar-free peanut butter
2 tablespoons unsweetened cocoa powder
2 tablespoons canned coconut milk, or more as needed
¼ cup sugar-free peanut butter powder

1. Combine all the ingredients in a large bowl. Stir to mix well.
2. Divide the mixture into 16 balls with a spoon, then arrange the balls on a baking sheet lined with parchment paper.
3. Place the sheet in the refrigerator to chill the balls for 1 to 2 hours or until the balls are firm
4. Remove the peanut butter balls from the refrigerator and serve chilled.

Per Serving
calories: 65 | fat: 5.1g | protein: 4.1g
carbs: 2.0g | fiber: 0.8g | sugar: 1.2g
sodium: 18mg

Chocolate Almonds

Prep time: 5 minutes | Cook time: 15 minutes | Serves 4

1 cup almonds
2 packets powdered stevia
1 tablespoon cocoa powder

1. Preheat the oven to 350ºF (180ºC).
2. Arrange the almonds in a single layer in a baking pan lined with parchment paper.
3. Bake in the preheated oven for 5 minutes.
4. Meanwhile, combine the stevia and cocoa powder in a small bowl.
5. Dunk the almonds in the bowl of mixture. Toss to coat well.
6. Put the the almonds back to the baking pan, and bake for an additional 5 minutes or until soft.
7. Remove the almonds from the oven and serve warm.

Per Serving
calories: 210 | fat: 18.1g | protein: 8.1g
carbs: 8.9g | fiber: 5.1g | sugar: 3.8g
sodium: 1mg

Aromatic Toasted Pumpkin Seeds

Prep time: 5 minutes | Cook time: 45 minutes | Serves 4

1 cup pumpkin seeds
1 teaspoon cinnamon
2 (0.04-ounce / 1-g) packets stevia
1 tablespoon canola oil
¼ teaspoon sea salt

1. Preheat the oven to 300ºF (150ºC).
2. Combine the pumpkin seeds with cinnamon, stevia, canola oil and salt in a bowl. Stir to mix well.
3. Pour the seeds in the single layer on a baking sheet, then arrange the sheet in the preheated oven.
4. Bake for 45 minutes or until well toasted and fragrant. Shake the sheet twice to bake the seeds evenly.
5. Serve immediately.

Per Serving
calories: 202 | fat: 18.0g | protein: 8.8g
carbs: 5.1g | fiber: 2.3g | sugar: 0.4g
sodium: 151mg

Asian Chicken Wings

Prep time: 5 minutes | Cook time: 30 minutes | Serves 3

24 chicken wings
6 tablespoons soy sauce
6 tablespoons Chinese 5 spice
Salt and ground black pepper, to taste
Nonstick cooking spray

1. Heat oven to 350ºF (180ºC). Spray a baking sheet with cooking spray.
2. Combine the soy sauce, 5 spice, salt, and pepper in a large bowl. Add the wings and toss to coat.
3. Pour the wings onto the prepared pan. Bake for 15 minutes. Turn chicken over and cook another 15 minutes until chicken is cooked through.
4. Serve warm.

Per Serving
calories: 180 | fat: 10.9g | protein: 12.1g
carbs: 8.1g | fiber: 0g | sugar: 1.0g
sodium: 1210mg

Almond Cheesecake Bites

Prep time: 5 minutes | Cook time: 0 minutes | Serves 6

½ cup reduced-fat cream cheese, soft
½ cup almonds,
ground fine
¼ cup almond butter
2 drops liquid stevia

1. In a large bowl, beat cream cheese, almond butter and stevia on high speed until mixture is smooth and creamy. Cover and chill 30 minutes.
2. Use your hands to shape the mixture into 12 balls.
3. Place the ground almonds in a shallow plate. Roll the balls in the nuts completely covering all sides. Store in an airtight container in the refrigerator.

Per Serving
calories: 70 | fat: 4.9g | protein: 5.1g
carbs: 3.1g | fiber: 1g | sugar: 0g
sodium: 73mg

Simple Deviled Eggs

Prep time: 5 minutes | Cook time: 8 minutes | Serves 12

6 large eggs
⅛ teaspoon mustard powder
2 tablespoons plus
1 teaspoon light
mayonnaise
Salt and freshly ground black pepper, to taste

1. Sit the eggs in a saucepan, then pour in enough water to cover the egg. Bring to a boil, then boil the eggs for another 8 minutes. Turn off the heat and cover, then let sit for 15 minutes.
2. Transfer the boiled eggs in a pot of cold water and peel under the water.
3. Transfer the eggs on a large plate, then cut in half. Remove the egg yolks and place them in a bowl, then mash with a fork.
4. Add the mustard powder, mayo, salt, and pepper to the bowl of yolks, then stir to mix well.
5. Spoon the yolk mixture in the egg white on the plate. Serve immediately.

Per Serving
calories: 45 | fat: 3.0g | protein: 3.0g
carbs: 1.0g | fiber: 0g | sugar: 0g
sodium: 70mg

Cinnamon Apple Chips

Prep time: 5 minutes | Cook time: 10 minutes | Serves 2

1 medium apple, sliced thin
¼ teaspoon cinnamon
¼ teaspoon nutmeg
Nonstick cooking spray

1. Heat oven to 375ºF (190ºC). Spray a baking sheet with cooking spray.
2. Place apples in a mixing bowl and add spices. Toss to coat.
3. Arrange apples, in a single layer, on prepared pan. Bake 4 minutes, turn apples over and bake 4 minutes more.
4. Serve immediately or store in airtight container.

Per Serving
calories: 60 | fat: 0g | protein: 0g
carbs: 15.1g | fiber: 3.1g | sugar: 11.2g
sodium: 1mg

Kale Chips

Prep time: 5 minutes | Cook time: 15 minutes | Serves 1

¼ teaspoon garlic powder
Pinch cayenne, to taste
1 tablespoon extra-virgin olive oil
½ teaspoon sea salt, or to taste
1 (8-ounce / 227-g) bunch kale, trimmed and cut into 2-inch pieces, rinsed

1. Preheat the oven to 350ºF (180ºC). Line two baking sheets with parchment paper.
2. Combine the garlic powder, cayenne pepper, olive oil, and salt in a large bowl, then dunk the kale in the bowl. Toss to coat well.
3. Place the kale in the single layer on one of the baking sheet.
4. Arrange the sheet in the preheated oven and bake for 7 minutes. Remove the sheet from the oven and pour the kale in the single layer of the other baking sheet.
5. Move the sheet of kale back to the oven and bake for another 7 minutes or until the kale is crispy.
6. Serve immediately.

Per Serving
calories: 136 | fat: 14.0g | protein: 1.0g
carbs: 3.0g | fiber: 1.1g | sugar: 0.6g
sodium: 1170mg

Bacon-Wrapped Shrimps

Prep time: 10 minutes | Cook time: 6 minutes | Serves 10

20 shrimps, peeled and deveined
7 slices bacon, cut into 3 strips crosswise
4 leaves romaine lettuce

1. Preheat the oven to 400ºF (205ºC).
2. Wrap each shrimp with each bacon strip, then arrange the wrapped shrimps in a single layer on a baking sheet, seam side down.
3. Broil in the preheated oven for 6 minutes or until the bacon is well browned. Flip the shrimps halfway through the cooking time.
4. Remove the shrimps from the oven and serve on lettuce leaves.

Per Serving
calories: 70 | fat: 4.5g | protein: 7.0g
carbs: 0g | fiber: 0g | sugar: 0g
sodium: 150mg

Candied Pecans

Prep time: 5 minutes | Cook time: 10 minutes | Serves 6

1½ teaspoons butter
1½ cup pecan halves
2½ tablespoons Splenda, divided
1 teaspoons cinnamon
¼ teaspoons ginger
⅛ teaspoons cardamom
⅛ teaspoons salt

1. In a small bowl, stir together 1½ teaspoons Splenda, cinnamon, ginger, cardamom and salt. Set aside.
2. Melt butter in a medium skillet over medium-low heat. Add pecans, and two tablespoons Splenda. Reduce heat to low and cook, stirring occasionally, until sweetener melts, about 5 to 8 minutes.
3. Add spice mixture to the skillet and stir to coat pecans. Spread mixture to parchment paper and let cool for 10 to 15 minutes. Store in an airtight container. Serving size is ¼ cup.

Per Serving
calories: 173 | fat: 16.1g | protein: 2.1g
carbs: 8.1g | fiber: 2.1g | sugar: 6.0g
sodium: 52mg

Almond Flour Crackers

Prep time: 5 minutes | Cook time: 15 minutes | Serves 8

½ cup coconut oil, melted
1½ cups almond flour
¼ cup Stevia

1. Heat oven to 350ºF (180ºC). Line a cookie sheet with parchment paper.
2. In a mixing bowl, combine all and mix well.
3. Spread dough onto prepared cookie sheet, ¼-inch thick. Use a paring knife to score into 24 crackers.
4. Bake for 10 to 15 minutes or until golden brown.
5. Separate and store in airtight container.

Per Serving
calories: 282 | fat: 22.9g | protein: 4.1g
carbs: 16.1g | fiber: 2.1g | sugar: 12.9g
sodium: 0mg

Buffalo Bites

Prep time: 5 minutes | Cook time: 10 minutes | Serves 4

1 egg
½ head of cauliflower, separated into florets
1 cup panko bread crumbs
1 cup low-fat ranch dressing
½ cup hot sauce
½ teaspoon salt
½ teaspoon garlic powder
Black pepper, to taste
Nonstick cooking spray

1. Heat oven to 400ºF (205ºC). Spray a baking sheet with cooking spray.
2. Place the egg in a medium bowl and mix in the salt, pepper and garlic. Place the panko crumbs into a small bowl.
3. Dip the florets first in the egg then into the panko crumbs. Place in a single layer on prepared pan.
4. Bake for 8 to 10 minutes, stirring halfway through, until cauliflower is golden brown and crisp on the outside.
5. In a small bowl stir the dressing and hot sauce together. Use for dipping.

Per Serving
calories: 133 | fat: 5.1g | protein: 6.1g
carbs: 15.1g | fiber: 1.1g | sugar: 4.0g
sodium: 1778mg

Cheesy Broccoli Bites

Prep time: 10 minutes | Cook time: 25 minutes | Serves 6

2 tablespoons olive oil
2 heads broccoli, trimmed
1 eggs
1/3 cup reduced-fat shredded Cheddar cheese
1 egg white
½ cup onion, chopped
1/3 cup bread crumbs
¼ teaspoon salt
¼ teaspoon black pepper

1. Preheat the oven to 400ºF (205ºC). Coat a large baking sheet with olive oil.
2. Arrange a colander in a saucepan, then place the broccoli in the colander. Pour the water in the saucepan to cover the bottom. Bring to a boil, then reduce the heat to low. Cover and simmer for 6 minutes or until the broccoli is fork-tender. Allow to cool for 10 minutes.
3. Put the broccoli and remaining ingredients in a food processor. Process to combine until lightly chunky. Let sit for 10 minutes.
4. Make the bites: Drop 1 tablespoon of the mixture on the baking sheet. Repeat with the remaining mixture.
5. Bake in the preheated oven for 25 minutes or until lightly browned. Flip the bites halfway through the cooking time.
6. Serve immediately.

Per Serving
calories: 100 | fat: 3.0g | protein: 7.0g
carbs: 13.0g | fiber: 3.0g | sugar: 3.0g
sodium: 250mg

Almond Coconut Biscotti

Prep time: 5 minutes | Cook time: 50 minutes | Serves 16

1 egg, room temperature
1 egg white, room temperature
½ cup margarine, melted
2½ cup flour
1¹/3 cup unsweetened
coconut, grated
¾ cup almonds, sliced
2/3 cup Splenda
2 teaspoons baking powder
1 teaspoon vanilla
½ teaspoon salt

1. Heat oven to 350ºF (180ºC). Line a baking sheet with parchment paper.
2. In a large bowl, combine dry .

3. In a separate mixing bowl, beat other together. Add to dry and mix until thoroughly combined.
4. Divide dough in half. Shape each half into a loaf measuring 8x2 ¾-inches. Place loaves on pan 3 inches apart.
5. Bake for 25 to 30 minutes or until set and golden brown. Cool on wire rack 10 minutes.
6. With a serrated knife, cut loaf diagonally into ½-inch slices. Place the cookies, cut side down, back on the pan and bake another 20 minutes, or until firm and nicely browned. Store in airtight container. Serving size is 2 cookies.

Per Serving
calories: 235 | fat: 17.9g | protein: 5.1g
carbs: 13.1g | fiber: 3.1g | sugar: 8.9g
sodium: 84mg

Cranberry and Almond Granola Bars

Prep time: 15 minutes | Cook time: 20 minutes | Makes 12 Bars

1 egg
1 egg white
2 cup low-fat granola
¼ cup dried cranberries, sweetened
¼ cup almonds, chopped
2 tablespoons Splenda
1 teaspoon almond extract
½ teaspoon cinnamon

1. Heat oven to 350ºF (180ºC). Line the bottom and sides of a baking dish with parchment paper.
2. In a large bowl, combine dry including the cranberries.
3. In a small bowl, whisk together egg, egg white and extract. Pour over dry and mix until combined.
4. Press mixture into the prepared pan. Bake 20 minutes or until light brown.
5. Cool in the pan for 5 minutes. Then carefully lift the bars from the pan onto a cutting board. Use a sharp knife to cut into 12 bars. Cool completely and store in an airtight container.

Per Serving (1 Bar)
calories: 86 | fat: 3.1g | protein: 3.0g
carbs: 14.1g | fiber: 1.1g | sugar: 4.9g
sodium: 10mg

Apple Pita Pockets

Prep time: 10 minutes | Cook time: 2 minutes | Serves 2

½ apple, cored and chopped
½ teaspoon cinnamon

¼ cup almond butter
1 whole-wheat pita, halved

1. Combine the apple, cinnamon, and almond butter in a bowl. Stir to mix well.
2. Heat the pita in a nonstick skillet over medium heat until lightly browned on both sides.
3. Remove the pita from the skillet. Allow to cool for a few minutes. Spoon the mixture in the halved pita pockets, then serve.

Per Serving
calories: 315 | fat: 20.3g | protein: 8.2g
carbs: 31.3g | fiber: 7.2g | sugar: 20.6g
sodium: 175mg

Cinnamon Apple Popcorn

Prep time: 30 minutes | Cook time: 50 minutes | Serves 11

4 tablespoons margarine, melted
10 cup plain popcorn
2 cup dried apple rings, unsweetened and chopped

½ cup walnuts, chopped
2 tablespoons Splenda brown sugar
1 teaspoon cinnamon
½ teaspoon vanilla

1. Heat oven to 250ºF (121ºC).
2. Place chopped apples in a baking dish and bake 20 minutes. Remove from oven and stir in popcorn and nuts.
3. In a small bowl, whisk together margarine, vanilla, Splenda, and cinnamon. Drizzle evenly over popcorn and toss to coat.
4. Bake 30 minutes, stirring quickly every 10 minutes. If apples start to turn a dark brown, remove immediately.
5. Pout onto waxed paper to cool at least 30 minutes. Store in an airtight container. Serving size is 1 cup.

Per Serving
calories: 135 | fat: 8.1g | protein: 3.0g
carbs: 14.1g | fiber: 3.1g | sugar: 6.9g
sodium: 2mg

Cheese Crisp Crackers

Prep time: 5 minutes | Cook time: 10 minutes | Serves 4

4 slices pepper Jack cheese, quartered
4 slices Colby Jack

cheese, quartered
4 slices cheddar cheese, quartered

1. Heat oven to 400ºF (205ºC). Line a cooking sheet with parchment paper.
2. Place cheese in a single layer on prepared pan and bake 10 minutes, or until cheese gets firm.
3. Transfer to paper towel line surface to absorb excess oil. Let cool, cheese will crisp up more as it cools.
4. Store in airtight container, or Ziploc bag. Serve with your favorite dip or salsa.

Per Serving
calories: 254 | fat: 19.9g | protein: 15.1g
carbs: 1.1g | fiber: 0g | sugar: 0g
sodium: 475mg

Crab and Spinach Dip

Prep time: 10 minutes | Cook time: 2 hours | Serves 10

1 package frozen chopped spinach, thawed and squeezed nearly dry
8 ounces (227 g) reduced-fat cream cheese
6.5 ounces (184 g) can crabmeat, drained and shredded

6 ounces (170 g) jar marinated artichoke hearts, drained and diced fine
¼ teaspoon hot pepper sauce
Melba toast or whole grain crackers (optional)

1. Remove any shells or cartilage from crab.
2. Place all in a small crock pot. Cover and cook on high for 1½ to 2 hours, or until heated through and cream cheese is melted. Stir after 1 hour.
3. Serve with Melba toast or whole grain crackers. Serving size is ¼ cup.

Per Serving
calories: 105 | fat: 8.1g | protein: 5.0g
carbs: 7.1g | fiber: 1.1g | sugar: 2.9g
sodium: 185mg

Cauliflower Hummus

Prep time: 5 minutes | Cook time: 15 minutes | Serves 6

3 cup cauliflower florets
3 tablespoons fresh lemon juice
5 cloves garlic, divided
5 tablespoons olive oil, divided

2 tablespoons water
1½ tablespoons Tahini paste
1¼ teaspoons salt, divided
Smoked paprika and extra olive oil for serving

1. In a microwave safe bowl, combine cauliflower, water, 2 tablespoons oil, ½ teaspoon salt, and 3 whole cloves garlic. Microwave on high 15 minutes, or until cauliflower is soft and darkened.
2. Transfer mixture to a food processor or blender and process until almost smooth. Add tahini paste, lemon juice, remaining garlic cloves, remaining oil, and salt. Blend until almost smooth.
3. Place the hummus in a bowl and drizzle lightly with olive oil and a sprinkle or two of paprika. Serve with your favorite raw vegetables.

Per Serving
calories: 108 | fat: 10.1g | protein: 2.1g
carbs: 5.1g | fiber: 2.1g | sugar: 1.0g
sodium: 506mg

Chewy Granola Bars

Prep time: 10 minutes | Cook time: 35 minutes | Makes 36 Bars

1 egg, beaten
⅔ cup margarine, melted
3½ cup quick oats
1 cup almonds, chopped
½ cup honey
½ cup sunflower kernels
½ cup coconut,

unsweetened
½ cup dried apples
½ cup dried cranberries
½ cup Splenda brown sugar
1 teaspoon vanilla
½ teaspoon cinnamon
Nonstick cooking spray

1. Heat oven to 350ºF (180ºC). Spray a large baking sheet with cooking spray.
2. Spread oats and almonds on prepared pan. Bake for 12 to 15 minutes until toasted, stirring every few minutes.

3. In a large bowl, combine egg, margarine, honey, and vanilla. Stir in remaining .
4. Stir in oat mixture. Press into baking sheet and bake for 13 to 18 minutes, or until edges are light brown.
5. Cool on a wire rack. Cut into bars and store in an airtight container.

Per Serving (1 Bar)
calories: 120 | fat: 5.9g | protein: 2.1g
carbs: 13.1g | fiber: 1.0g | sugar: 7.0g
sodium: 8mg

Fluffy Lemon Bars

Prep time: 15 minutes | Cook time: 0 minutes | Makes 20 Bars

8 ounces (227 g) low fat cream cheese, soft
⅓ cup butter, melted
3 tablespoons fresh lemon juice
12 ounces (340 g) evaporated milk

1 package lemon gelatin, sugar free
1½ cup graham cracker crumbs
1 cup boiling water
¾ cup Splenda
1 teaspoon vanilla

1. Pour milk into a large, metal bowl, place beaters in the bowl, cover and chill 2 hours.
2. In a small bowl, combine cracker crumbs and butter, reserve 1 tablespoon. Press the remaining mixture on the bottom of a baking dish. Cover and chill until set.
3. In a small bowl, dissolve gelatin in boiling water. Stir in lemon juice and let cool.
4. In a large bowl, beat cream cheese, Splenda and vanilla until smooth. Add gelatin and mix well.
5. Beat the chilled milk until soft peaks form. Fold into cream cheese mixture. Pour over chilled crust and sprinkle with reserved crumbs. Cover and chill 2 hours before serving.

Per Serving (1 Bar)
calories: 125 | fat: 5.1g | protein: 3.0g
carbs: 15.1g | fiber: 0g | sugar: 9.9g
sodium: 50mg

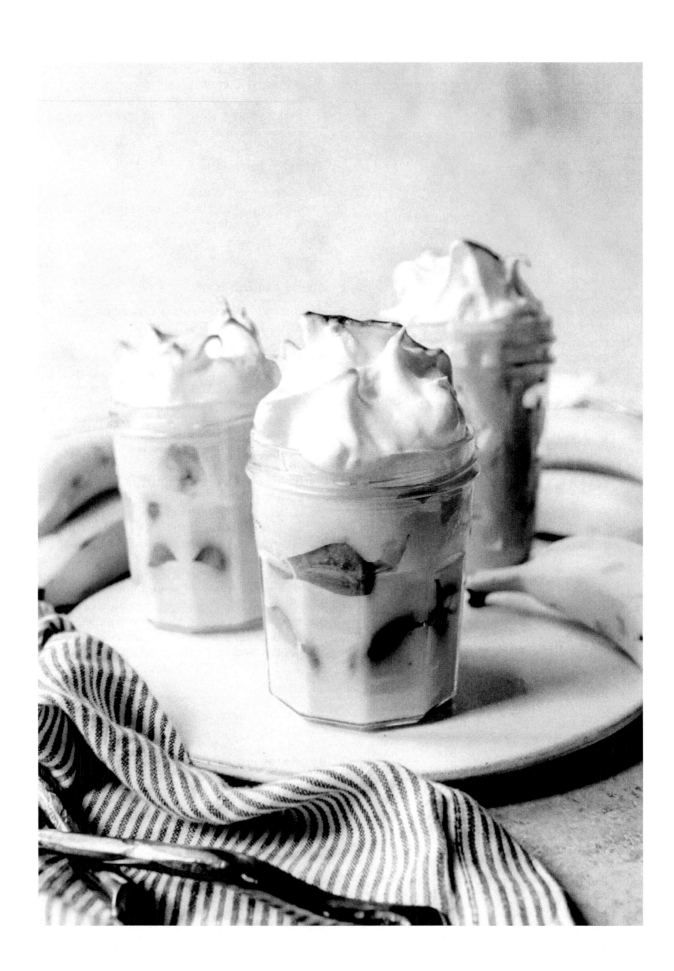

Chapter 14: Desserts

Orange and Peach Ambrosia

Prep time: 10 minutes | Cook time: 0 minutes | Serves 8

3 oranges, peeled, sectioned, and quartered
2 (4-ounce / 113-g) cups diced peaches in water, drained
1 cup shredded, unsweetened coconut
1 (8-ounce / 227-g) container fat-free crème fraîche

1. In a large mixing bowl, combine the oranges, peaches, coconut, and crème fraîche. Gently toss until well mixed. Cover and refrigerate overnight.

Per Serving
calories: 113 | fat: 5.1g | protein: 2.1g
carbs: 12.1g | fiber: 2.9g | sugar: 8.1g
sodium: 8mg

Banana Pudding with Meringue

Prep time: 30 minutes | Cook time: 20 minutes | Serves 10

For the Pudding:
¾ cup erythritol or other sugar replacement
5 teaspoons almond flour
¼ teaspoon salt
2½ cups fat-free milk
6 tablespoons prepared egg
replacement
½ teaspoon vanilla extract
2 (8-ounce / 227-g) containers sugar-free spelt hazelnut biscuits, crushed
5 medium bananas, sliced

For the Meringue:
5 medium egg whites (1 cup)
¼ cup erythritol or other sugar
replacement
½ teaspoon vanilla extract

To Make the Pudding
1. In a saucepan, whisk the erythritol, almond flour, salt, and milk together. Cook over medium heat until the sugar is dissolved.
2. Whisk in the egg replacement and cook for about 10 minutes, or until thickened.
3. Remove from the heat and stir in the vanilla.

4. Spread the thickened pudding onto the bottom of a casserole dish.
5. Arrange a layer of crushed biscuits on top of the pudding.
6. Place a layer of sliced bananas on top of the biscuits.

To Make the Meringue
1. Preheat the oven to 350ºF (180ºC).
2. In a medium bowl, beat the egg whites for about 5 minutes, or until stiff.
3. Add the erythritol and vanilla while continuing to beat for about 3 more minutes.
4. Spread the meringue on top of the banana pudding.
5. Transfer the casserole dish to the oven, and bake for 7 to 10 minutes, or until the top is lightly browned.

Per Serving
calories: 324 | fat: 14.1g | protein: 12.1g
carbs: 42.1g | fiber: 2.9g | sugar: 10.9g
sodium: 149mg

Avocado Mousse with Grilled Watermelon

Prep time: 10 minutes | Cook time: 10 minutes | Serves 8

1 small, seedless watermelon, halved and cut into 1-inch rounds
2 ripe avocados,
pitted and peeled
½ cup fat-free plain yogurt
¼ teaspoon cayenne pepper

1. On a hot grill, grill the watermelon slices for 2 to 3 minutes on each side, or until you can see the grill marks.
2. To make the avocado mousse, in a blender, combine the avocados, yogurt, and cayenne and process until smooth.
3. To serve, cut each watermelon round in half. Top each with a generous dollop of avocado mousse.

Per Serving
calories: 127 | fat: 3.9g | protein: 3.1g
carbs: 24.1g | fiber: 2.9g | sugar: 16.9g
sodium: 15mg

Brown Rice Pudding

Prep time: 5 minutes | Cook time: 35 minutes | Serves 6

2 cups short-grain brown rice
6 cups fat-free milk
1 teaspoon ground nutmeg, plus more for serving
1 teaspoon ground cinnamon, plus more

for serving
¼ teaspoon orange extract
Juice of 2 oranges (about ¾ cup)
½ cup erythritol or other brown sugar replacement

1. In an electric pressure cooker, stir the rice, milk, nutmeg, cinnamon, orange extract, orange juice, and erythritol together.
2. Close and lock the lid, and set the pressure valve to sealing.
3. Select the Manual/Pressure Cook setting, and cook for 35 minutes.
4. Once cooking is complete, quick-release the pressure. Carefully remove the lid.
5. Stir well and spoon into serving dishes. Enjoy with an additional sprinkle of nutmeg and cinnamon.

Per Serving
calories: 321 | fat: 2.1g | protein: 12.9g
carbs: 60.9g | fiber: 2.1g | sugar: 15.1g
sodium: 131mg

Orange Bundt Cake

Prep time: 15 minutes | Cook time: 30 minutes | Serves 24

Unsalted non-hydrogenated plant-based butter, for greasing the pan
1½ cups gluten-free baking flour, plus more for dusting
1½ cups almond flour
½ teaspoon baking soda

½ teaspoon baking powder
9 medium eggs, at room temperature
1 cup coconut sugar
Zest of 3 oranges
Juice of 1 orange
1 cup extra-virgin olive oil

1. Preheat the oven to 325ºF (163ºC).
2. Grease two bundt pans with butter and dust with the baking flour.
3. In a medium bowl, whisk the baking flour, almond flour, baking soda, and baking powder together.
4. In a large bowl, whip the eggs with the coconut sugar until they double in size.

5. Add the orange zest and orange juice.
6. Add the dry ingredients to the wet ingredients, stirring to combine.
7. Add the olive oil, a little at a time, until incorporated.
8. Divide the batter between the two prepared bundt pans.
9. Transfer the bundt pans to the oven, and bake for 30 minutes, or until browned and a toothpick inserted into the center comes out clean.
10. Remove the bundt pans from the oven, and let cool for 15 minutes.
11. Invert the bundt pans onto plates, and gently tap the cakes out of the pan.

Per Serving
calories: 180 | fat: 12.1g | protein: 4.1g
carbs: 14.9g | fiber: 1.1g | sugar: 8.1g
sodium: 51mg

Banana, Peach, and Almond Fritters

Prep time: 15 minutes | Cook time: 15 minutes | Serves 7

4 ripe bananas, peeled
2 cups chopped peaches
1 medium egg

2 medium egg whites
¾ cup almond meal
¼ teaspoon almond extract

1. In a large bowl, mash the bananas and peaches together with a fork or potato masher.
2. Blend in the egg and egg whites.
3. Stir in the almond meal and almond extract.
4. Working in batches, place ¼-cup portions of the batter into the basket of an air fryer.
5. Set the air fryer to 390ºF (199ºC), close, and cook for 12 minutes.
6. Once cooking is complete, transfer the fritters to a plate. Repeat until no batter remains.

Per Serving
calories: 163 | fat: 7.1g | protein: 5.9g
carbs: 21.9g | fiber: 4.1g | sugar: 12.0g
sodium: 24mg

Strawberry and Rhubarb Glazed Ice Cream

Prep time: 10 minutes | Cook time: 15 minutes | Serves 4

1 cup strawberries, sliced
1 cup rhubarb, chopped
1 tablespoon honey
½ teaspoon cinnamon
2 tablespoons water
¼ cup sugar-free vanilla ice cream

1. Combine all the ingredients, except for the ice cream, in a pot.
2. Bring to a boil over medium heat, then turn down the heat to medium-low. Simmer for 15 minutes or until the rhubarb is tender. Stir constantly.
3. Divide the ice cream on four small plates with a spoon, then pour the mixture over the ice cream before serving.

Per Serving
calories: 88 | fat: 2.1g | protein: 3.1g
carbs: 15.8g | fiber: 3.2g | sugar:12.6g
sodium: 35mg

Coconut Yogurt and Pistachio Stuffed Peaches

Prep time: 5 minutes | Cook time: 10 minutes | Serves 4

2 peaches, halved and pitted
1 teaspoon pure vanilla extract
½ cup plain Greek yogurt
2 tablespoons unsalted pistachios, shelled and broken into pieces
¼ cup unsweetened dried coconut flakes

1. Preheat the broiler to high.
2. Place the peach halves on a baking sheet, cut side down, and broil for 7 minutes or until soft and lightly browned.
3. Meanwhile, combine the vanilla and yogurt in a bowl.
4. Divide the mixture among the the pits of peach halves, then scatter the pistachios and coconut flakes on top before serving.

Per Serving
calories: 103 | fat: 4.9g | protein: 5.1g
carbs: 10.8g | fiber: 2.1g | sugars: 7.8g
sodium: 10mg

Peanut Butter and Pineapple Smoothie

Prep time: 10 minutes | Cook time: 0 minutes | Serves 6

1 cup peanut butter
2 cups frozen pineapple
½ cup unsweetened almond milk

1. Put the peanut butter and pineapple in a food processor, then pour the almond milk in the food processor.
2. Pulse until creamy and smooth, then pour the mixture into 6 glasses and serve.

Per Serving
calories: 303 | fat: 21.8g | protein: 14.1g
carbs: 14.8g | fiber: 4.2g | sugars: 7.8g
sodium: 37mg

Easy Banana Mug Cake

Prep time: 10 minutes | Cook time: 1 minutes | Serves 1

½ ripe banana, mashed
3 tablespoons egg white
1 teaspoon oat flour
½ tablespoon vanilla protein powder
1 teaspoon rolled oats
1 teaspoon cocoa powder
½ teaspoon baking powder
2 tablespoons stevia
1 teaspoon olive oil
2 teaspoons chopped walnuts

1. Whisk together the banana and egg whites in a bowl.
2. Add the flour, vanilla protein powder, rolled oats, cocoa powder, baking powder, and stevia to the bowl. Stir to mix well.
3. Grease a microwave-safe mug with olive oil.
4. Pour the mixture in the bowl, then scatter with chopped walnuts.
5. Microwave them for 1 minutes or until puffed.
6. Serve immediately.

Per Serving
calories: 211 | fat: 12.0g | protein: 11.3g
carbs: 46.7g | fiber: 2.8g | sugar: 6.6g
sodium: 97mg

Crispy Apple and Pecan Bake

Prep time: 10 minutes | Cook time: 15 minutes | Serves 4

2 apples, peeled, cored, and chopped
½ teaspoon cinnamon
½ teaspoon ground ginger
2 tablespoons pure maple syrup
¼ cup pecans, chopped

1. Preheat the oven to 350ºF (180ºC).
2. Combine all the ingredients, except for the pecans, in a bowl. Stir to mix well.
3. Pour the mixture in a baking dish, and spread the pecans over the mixture.
4. Bake in the preheated oven for 15 minutes or until the apples are soft.
5. Remove them from the oven and serve warm.

Per Serving

calories: 124 | fat: 5.1g | protein: 1.1g
carbs: 20.8g | fiber: 3.2g| sugar:18.6g
sodium: 1mg

Peach, Banana, and Almond Pancakes

Prep time: 15 minutes | Cook time: 15 minutes | Serves 7

2 cups peaches, chopped
4 ripe bananas, peeled
2 medium egg whites
1 medium egg
¼ teaspoon almond extract
¾ cup almond meal

1. Preheat the oven to 400ºF (205ºC).
2. Put all the ingredients in a food processor, and pulse until mix well and it has a thick consistency.
3. Pour the mixture in a baking dish lined with parchment paper.
4. Bake in the preheated oven for 10 minutes or until a toothpick inserted in the center of the pancakes comes out clean.
5. Remove the pancakes from the oven and slice to serve.

Per Serving

calories: 166 | fat: 6.9g | protein: 6.1g
carbs: 21.8g | fiber: 4.2g | sugars: 11.8g
sodium: 22mg

Apple Cinnamon Chimichanga

Prep time: 15 minutes | Cook time: 15 minutes | Serves 4

2 apple, cored and chopped
3 tablespoons splenda, divided
¼ cup water
½ teaspoon ground
cinnamon
4 (8-inch) whole-wheat flour tortillas
Nonstick cooking spray

Special Equipment:

4 toothpicks, soaked in water for at least 30 minutes

1. Preheat the oven to 400ºF (205ºC). Line a baking sheet with parchment paper and set aside.
2. Make the apple filling: Add the apples, 2 tablespoons of splenda, water, and cinnamon to a medium saucepan over medium heat. Stir to combine and allow the mixture to boil for 5 minutes, or until the apples are fork-tender, but not mushy.
3. Remove the apple filling from the heat and let it cool to room temperature.
4. Make the chimichangas: Place the tortillas on a lightly floured surface.
5. Spoon 2 teaspoons of prepared apple filling onto each tortilla and fold the tortilla over to enclose the filling. Roll each tortilla up and run the toothpicks through to secure. Spritz the tortillas lightly with nonstick cooking spray.
6. Arrange the tortillas on the prepared baking sheet, seam-side down. Scatter the remaining splenda all over the tortillas.
7. Bake in the preheated oven for 10 minutes, flipping the tortillas halfway through, or until they are crispy and golden brown on each side.
8. Remove from the oven to four plates and serve while warm.

Per Serving (1 Chimichanga)

calories: 201 | fat: 6.2g | protein: 3.9g
carbs: 32.8g | fiber: 5.0g | sugar: 7.9g
sodium: 241mg

Crispy Apple Chips

Prep time: 10 minutes | Cook time: 2 hours | Serves 4

2 medium apples, sliced
1 teaspoon ground cinnamon

1. Preheat the oven to 200ºF (93ºC). Line a baking sheet with parchment paper.
2. Arrange the apple slices on the prepared baking sheet, then sprinkle with cinnamon.
3. Bake in the preheated oven for 2 hours or until crispy. Flip the apple chips halfway through the cooking time.
4. Allow to cool for 10 minutes and serve warm.

Per Serving
calories: 50 | fat: 0g | protein: 0g
carbs: 13.0g | fiber: 2.0g | sugar: 9.0g
sodium: 0mg

Date and Almond Balls with Seeds

Prep time: 15 minutes | Cook time: 0 minutes | Serves 36 Balls

1 pound (454 g) pitted dates
½ pound (227 g) blanched almonds
¼ cup water
¼ cup butter, at room temperature
1 teaspoon ground cardamom
1 teaspoon vanilla extract
½ teaspoon ground cinnamon
2 tablespoons ground flaxseed
1 cup toasted sesame seeds

1. In a food processor, add the pitted dates, almonds, water, butter, cardamon, vanilla, and cinnamon, and pulse until the mixture has broken down into a smooth paste.
2. Scoop out the paste and form into 36 equal-sized balls with your hands.
3. Spread out the flaxseed and sesame seeds on a baking sheet. Roll the balls in the seed mixture until they are evenly coated on all sides.
4. Serve immediately or store in an airtight container in the fridge for 2 days.

Per Serving (1 Ball)
calories: 113 | fat: 7.1g | protein: 2.9g
carbs: 12.0g | fiber: 2.0g | sugar: 7.8g
sodium: 10mg

Chia and Raspberry Pudding

Prep time: 1 hours | Cook time: 0 minutes | Serves 4

1 cup unsweetened vanilla almond milk
2 cup plus ½ cup raspberries, divided
¼ cup chia seeds
1½ teaspoons lemon juice
½ teaspoon lemon zest
1 tablespoon honey

1. Stir together the almond milk, 2 cups of raspberries, chia seeds, lemon juice, lemon zest, and honey in a small bowl.
2. Transfer the bowl to the fridge to thicken for at least 1 hour, or until a pudding-like texture is achieved.
3. When the pudding is ready, give it a good stir. Scatter with the remaining ½ cup raspberries and serve immediately.

Per Serving
calories: 122 | fat: 5.2g | protein: 3.1g
carbs: 17.9g | fiber: 9.0g | sugar: 6.8g
sodium: 51mg

Blackberry Crostata

Prep time: 10 minutes | Cook time: 20 minutes | Serves 6

1 (9-inch) pie crust, unbaked
2 cup fresh blackberries
Juice and zest of 1 lemon
2 tablespoons butter, soft
3 tablespoons Splenda, divided
2 tablespoons cornstarch

1. Heat oven to 425ºF (220ºC). Line a large baking sheet with parchment paper and unroll pie crust in pan.
2. In a medium bowl, combine blackberries, 2 tablespoons Splenda, lemon juice and zest, and cornstarch. Spoon onto crust leaving a 2-inch edge. Fold and crimp the edges.
3. Dot the berries with 1 tablespoon butter. Brush the crust edge with remaining butter and sprinkle crust and fruit with remaining Splenda.
4. Bake for 20 to 22 minutes or until golden brown. Cool before cutting and serving.

Per Serving
calories: 207 | fat: 11.1g | protein: 2.0g
carbs: 24.1g | fiber: 3.0g | sugar: 9.1g
sodium: 226mg

Broiled Stone Fruit

Prep time: 5 minutes | Cook time: 5 minutes | Serves 2

1 peach
1 nectarine
2 tablespoons sugar free whipped topping

1 tablespoon Splenda brown sugar
Nonstick cooking spray

1. Heat oven to broil. Line a shallow baking dish with foil and spray with cooking spray.
2. Cut the peach and nectarine in half and remove pits. Place cut side down in prepared dish. Broil 3 minutes.
3. Turn fruit over and sprinkle with Splenda brown sugar. Broil another 2 to 3 minutes.
4. Transfer 1 of each fruit to a dessert bowl and top with 1 tablespoon of whipped topping. Serve.

Per Serving
calories: 100 | fat: 1.0g | protein: 1.0g
carbs: 22.1g | fiber: 2.0g | sugar: 19.1g
sodium: 0mg

Pumpkin and Raspberry Muffins

Prep time: 20 minutes | Cook time: 25 minutes | Serves 12 Muffins

¾ cup blanched almond flour
½ cup coconut flour
3 tablespoons tapioca
1 tablespoon cinnamon
1 tablespoon baking powder
Pinch of nutmeg
½ cup stevia in raw

¼ teaspoon salt
1 cup puréed pumpkin
4 large eggs, whites and yolks separated
1½ teaspoons vanilla extract
½ cup coconut oil
10 drops liquid stevia
1½ cups frozen raspberries

1. Preheat the oven to 350ºF (180ºC). Line a 12-cup muffin pan with paper muffin cups.
2. Combine the flours, tapioca, cinnamon, baking powder, nutmeg, stevia in raw, and salt in a large bowl. Stir to mix well.
3. Mix in the puréed pumpkin, egg yolks, vanilla extract, coconut oil, and liquid stevia until a batter forms. Divide the batter into the muffin cups.
4. Whip the egg whites in a separate large bowl until it forms the stiff peaks.
5. Top the batter with the beaten egg whites and raspberries.

6. Place the muffin pan in the preheated oven and bake for 25 minutes or until a toothpick inserted in the center of the muffins comes out clean.
7. Remove the muffins from the oven and allow to cool for 5 minutes before serving.

Per Serving (1 Muffin)
calories: 223 | fat: 15.6g | protein: 4.4g
carbs: 29.3g | fiber: 2.9g | sugar: 7.7g
sodium: 76mg

Apple Pear and Pecan Dessert Squares

Prep time: 10 minutes | Cook time: 25 minutes | Makes 24 Sqaures

1 Granny Smith apple, sliced, leave peel on
1 Red Delicious apple, sliced, leave peel on
1 ripe pear, sliced, leave peel on
3 eggs
½ cup plain fat-free yogurt
1 tablespoon lemon juice
1 tablespoon

margarine
1 package spice cake mix
1¼ cup water, divided
½ cup pecan pieces
1 tablespoon Splenda
1 teaspoon cinnamon
½ teaspoon vanilla
¼ teaspoon nutmeg
Nonstick cooking spray

1. Heat oven to 350ºF (180ºC). Spray jelly-roll pan with nonstick cooking spray.
2. In a large bowl, beat cake mix, 1 cup water, eggs and yogurt until smooth. Pour into prepared pan and bake 20 minutes or it passes the toothpick test. Cool completely.
3. In a large nonstick skillet, over medium-high heat, toast the pecans, stirring, about 2 minutes or until lightly browned. Remove to a plate.
4. Add the remaining ¼ cup water, sliced fruit, juice and spices to the skillet. Bring to a boil. Reduce heat to medium and cook 3 minutes or until fruit is tender crisp.
5. Remove from heat and stir in Splenda, margarine, vanilla, and pecans. Spoon evenly over cooled cake. Slice into 24 squares and serve.

Per Serving (1 Square)
calories: 131 | fat: 5.1g | protein: 2.0g
carbs: 20.1g | fiber: 1.0g | sugar: 9.9g
sodium: 158mg

Apricot Soufflé

Prep time: 5 minutes | Cook time: 30 minutes | Serves 6

4 egg whites
3 egg yolks, beaten
3 tablespoons margarine
¾ cup sugar free apricot fruit spread
1/3 cup dried apricots,

diced fine
¼ cup warm water
2 tablespoons flour
¼ teaspoon cream of tartar
⅛ teaspoon salt

1. Heat oven to 325ºF (163ºC).
2. In a medium saucepan, over medium heat, melt margarine. Stir in flour and cook, stirring, until bubbly.
3. Stir together the fruit spread and water in a small bowl and add it to the saucepan with the apricots. Cook, stirring, 3 minutes or until mixture thickens.
4. Remove from heat and whisk in egg yolks. Let cool to room temperature, stirring occasionally.
5. In a medium bowl, beat egg whites, salt, and cream of tartar on high speed until stiff peaks form. Gently fold into cooled apricot mixture.
6. Spoon into a 1½–quart soufflé dish. Bake 30 minutes, or until puffed and golden brown. Serve immediately.

Per Serving
calories: 116 | fat: 8.1g | protein: 4.0g
carbs: 7.1g | fiber: 0g | sugar: 1.1g
sodium: 95mg

Autumn Skillet Cake

Prep time: 10 minutes | Cook time: 30 minutes | Serves 10

3 eggs, room temperature
1 cup of fresh cranberries
4 ounces (113 g) cream cheese, soft
3 tablespoons fat free sour cream
2 tablespoons butter, melted
2 cup of almond flour, sifted

¾ cup Splenda
¾ cup pumpkin purée
1½ tablespoons baking powder
2 teaspoons cinnamon
1 teaspoon pumpkin spice
1 teaspoon ginger
¼ teaspoon nutmeg
¼ teaspoon salt
Nonstick cooking spray

1. Heat oven to 350ºF (180ºC). Spray a cast iron skillet or cake pan with cooking spray.
2. In a large bowl, beat Splenda, butter and cream cheese until thoroughly combined. Add eggs, one at a time, beating after each.
3. Add pumpkin and spices and combine. Add the dry and mix well. Stir in the sour cream. Pour into prepared pan.
4. Sprinkle cranberries over the batter and with the back of a spoon, push them halfway into the batter. Bake 30 minutes or the cake passes the toothpick test. Cool completely before serving.

Per Serving
calories: 280 | fat: 17.1g | protein: 7.0g
carbs: 23.1g | fiber: 3.0g | sugar: 16.1g
sodium: 166mg

Baked Maple Custard

Prep time: 5 minutes | Cook time: 1 hour 15 minutes | Serves 6

2½ cup half-and-half
½ cup egg substitute
3 cup boiling water
¼ cup Splenda
2 tablespoons sugar

free maple syrup
2 teaspoons vanilla
Dash nutmeg
Nonstick cooking spray

1. Heat oven to 325ºF (163ºC). Lightly spray 6 custard cups or ramekins with cooking spray.
2. In a large bowl, whisk together half-and-half, egg substitute, Splenda, vanilla, and nutmeg. Pour evenly into prepared custard cups. Place cups in a baking dish.
3. Pour boiling water around, being careful not to splash it into, the cups. Bake 1 hour 15 minutes, centers will not be completely set.
4. Remove cups from pan and cool completely. Cover and chill overnight.
5. Just before serving, drizzle with the maple syrup.

Per Serving
calories: 191 | fat: 12.1g | protein: 5.0g
carbs: 15.1g | fiber: 0g | sugar: 8.1g
sodium: 152mg

Blackberry Soufflés

Prep time: 15 minutes | Cook time: 30 minutes | Serves 4

12 ounces (340 g) blackberries
4 egg whites
⅓ cup Splenda
1 tablespoon water
1 tablespoon Swerve powdered sugar
Nonstick cooking spray

1. Heat oven to 375ºF (190ºC). Spray 4 1-cup ramekins with cooking spray.
2. In a small saucepan, over medium-high heat, combine blackberries and 1 tablespoon water, bring to a boil. Reduce heat and simmer until berries are soft. Add Splenda and stir over medium heat until Splenda dissolves, without boiling.
3. Bring back to boiling, reduce heat and simmer 5 minutes. Remove from heat and cool 5 minutes.
4. Place a fine meshed sieve over a small bowl and push the berry mixture through it using the back of a spoon. Discard the seeds. Cover and chill 15 minutes.
5. In a large bowl, beat egg whites until soft peaks form. Gently fold in berry mixture. Spoon evenly into prepared ramekins and place them on a baking sheet.
6. Bake 12 minutes, or until puffed and light brown. Dust with powdered Swerve and serve immediately.

Per Serving
calories: 142 | fat: 0g | protein: 5.0g
carbs: 26.1g | fiber: 5.0g | sugar: 20.1g
sodium: 56mg

Blueberry Lemon "Cup" Cakes

Prep time: 5 minutes | Cook time: 10 minutes | Serves 5

4 eggs
½ cup coconut milk
½ cup blueberries
2 tablespoons lemon zest
½ cup plus 1 teaspoon coconut flour
¼ cup Splenda
¼ cup coconut oil,
melted
1 teaspoon baking soda
½ teaspoon lemon extract
¼ teaspoon stevia extract
Pinch salt

1. In a small bowl, toss berries in the 1 teaspoon of flour.
2. In a large bowl, stir together remaining flour, Splenda, baking soda, salt, and zest.
3. Add the remaining and mix well. Fold in the blueberries.
4. Divide batter evenly into 5 coffee cups. Microwave, one at a time, for 90 seconds, or until they pass the toothpick test.

Per Serving
calories: 264 | fat: 20.0g | protein: 5.0g
carbs: 14.1g | fiber: 2.0g | sugar: 12.1g
sodium: 87mg

Coconut Cream Pie

Prep time: 5 minutes | Cook time: 10 minutes | Serves 8

2 cup raw coconut, grated and divided
2 cans coconut milk, full fat and refrigerated for 24 hours
½ cup raw coconut,
grated and toasted
2 tablespoons margarine, melted
1 cup Splenda
½ cup macadamia nuts
¼ cup almond flour

1. Heat oven to 350ºF (180ºC).
2. Add the nuts to a food processor and pulse until finely ground. Add flour, ½ cup Splenda, and 1 cup grated coconut. Pulse until are finely ground and resemble cracker crumbs.
3. Add the margarine and pulse until mixture starts to stick together. Press on the bottom and sides of a pie pan. Bake 10 minutes or until golden brown. Cool
4. Turn the canned coconut upside down and open. Pour off the water and scoop the cream into a large bowl. Add remaining ½ cup Splenda and beat on high until stiff peaks form.
5. Fold in remaining 1 cup coconut and pour into crust. Cover and chill at least 2 hours. Sprinkle with toasted coconut, slice, and serve.

Per Serving
calories: 330 | fat: 23.0g | protein: 4.0g
carbs: 15.1g | fiber: 11.0g | sugar: 4.1g
sodium: 24mg

Coconut Milk Shakes

Prep time: 5 minutes | Cook time: 0 minutes | Serves 2

1½ cup vanilla ice cream
½ cup coconut milk, unsweetened
2½ tablespoons coconut flakes
1 teaspoon unsweetened cocoa

1. Heat oven to 350ºF (180ºC).
2. Place coconut on a baking sheet and bake, 2 to 3 minutes, stirring often, until coconut is toasted.
3. Place ice cream, milk, 2 tablespoons coconut, and cocoa in a blender and process until smooth.
4. Pour into glasses and garnish with remaining toasted coconut. Serve immediately.

Per Serving
calories: 324 | fat: 24.0g | protein: 3.0g
carbs: 23.1g | fiber: 4.0g | sugar: 18.1g
sodium: 107mg

Coconutty Pudding Clouds

Prep time: 5 minutes | Cook time: 0 minutes | Serves 4

2 cup heavy whipping cream
½ cup reduced-fat cream cheese, soft
½ cup hazelnuts, ground
4 tablespoons unsweetened coconut
flakes, toasted
2 tablespoons stevia, divided
½ teaspoon of vanilla
½ teaspoon of hazelnut extract
½ teaspoon of cacao powder, unsweetened

1. In a medium bowl, beat cream, vanilla, and 1 tablespoon stevia until soft peaks form.
2. In another mixing bowl, beat cream cheese, cocoa, remaining stevia, and hazelnut extract until smooth.
3. In 4 glasses, place ground nuts on the bottom, add a layer of the cream cheese mixture, then the whip cream, and top with toasted coconut. Serve immediately.

Per Serving
calories: 397 | fat: 35.0g | protein: 6.0g
carbs: 12.1g | fiber: 1.0g | sugar: 9.1g
sodium: 210mg

Peach Custard Tart

Prep time: 5 minutes | Cook time: 40 minutes | Serves 8

12 ounces (340 g) frozen unsweetened peach slices, thaw and drain
2 eggs, separated
1 cup skim milk
4 tablespoons cold margarine, cut into pieces
1 cup flour
3 tablespoons Splenda
2 to 3 tablespoons cold water
1 teaspoon vanilla
¼ teaspoon plus ⅛ teaspoon salt, divided
¼ teaspoon nutmeg

1. Heat oven to 400ºF (205ºC).
2. In a medium bowl, stir together flour and ¼ teaspoon salt. With a pastry blender, cut in margarine until mixture resembles coarse crumbs. Stir in cold water, a tablespoon at a time, just until moistened. Shape into a disc.
3. On a lightly floured surface, roll out dough to an 11-inch circle. Place in bottom of a tart pan with a removable bottom. Turn the edge under and pierce the sides and bottom with a fork.
4. In a small bowl, beat 1 egg white with a fork, discard the other or save for another use. Lightly brush crust with egg. Place the tart pan on a baking sheet and bake 10 minutes. Cool.
5. In a large bowl, whisk together egg yolks, Splenda, vanilla, nutmeg, and ⅛ teaspoon salt until combined.
6. Pour milk in a glass measuring cup and microwave on high for 1 minute. Do not boil. Whisk milk into egg mixture until blended.
7. Arrange peaches on the bottom of the crust and pour egg mixture over the top. Bake for 25 to 30 minutes, or until set. Cool to room temperature. Cover and chill at least 2 hours before serving.

Per Serving
calories: 181 | fat: 7.0g | protein: 5.0g
carbs: 22.1g | fiber: 1.0g | sugar: 9.1g
sodium: 175mg

Carrot Cupcakes

Prep time: 10 minutes | Cook time: 35 minutes | Serves 12

2 cup carrots, grated
1 cup low fat cream cheese, soft
2 eggs
1 to 2 teaspoons skim milk
½ cup coconut oil, melted
¼ cup coconut flour
¼ cup Splenda
¼ cup honey
2 teaspoons vanilla, divided
1 teaspoon baking powder
1 teaspoon cinnamon
Nonstick cooking spray

1. Heat oven to 350ºF (180ºC). Lightly spray a muffin pan with cooking spray, or use paper liners.
2. In a large bowl, stir together the flour, baking powder, and cinnamon.
3. Add the carrots, eggs, oil, Splenda, and vanilla to a food processor. Process until are combined but carrots still have some large chunks remaining. Add to dry and stir to combine.
4. Pour evenly into prepared pan, filling cups ²/₃ full. Bake for 30 to 35 minutes, or until cupcakes pass the toothpick test. Remove from oven and let cool.
5. In a medium bowl, beat cream cheese, honey, and vanilla on high speed until smooth. Add milk, one teaspoon at a time, beating after each addition, until frosting is creamy enough to spread easily.
6. Once cupcakes have cooled, spread each one with about 2 tablespoons of frosting. Chill until ready to serve.

Per Serving
calories: 161 | fat: 10.0g | protein: 4.0g
carbs: 13.1g | fiber: 1.0g | sugar: 11.1g
sodium: 96mg

Cinnamon Bread Pudding

Prep time: 10 minutes | Cook time: 45 minutes | Serves 6

4 cups day-old French or Italian bread, cut into ¾-inch cubes
2 cups skim milk
2 egg whites
1 egg
4 tablespoons
margarine, sliced
5 teaspoons Splenda
1½ teaspoons cinnamon
¼ teaspoon salt
⅛ teaspoon ground cloves

1. Heat oven to 350ºF (180ºC).
2. In a medium sauce pan, heat milk and margarine to simmering. Remove from heat and stir till margarine is completely melted. Let cool 10 minutes.
3. In a large bowl, beat egg and egg whites until foamy. Add Splenda, spices and salt. Beat until combined, then add in cooled milk and bread.
4. Transfer mixture to a 1½ quart baking dish. Place on rack of roasting pan and add 1 inch of hot water to roaster.
5. Bake until pudding is set and knife inserted in center comes out clean, about 40 to 45 minutes.

Per Serving
calories: 363 | fat: 10.0g | protein: 14.0g
carbs: 25.1g | fiber: 2.0g | sugar: 10.1g
sodium: 1090mg

Cream Cheese Pound Cake

Prep time: 10 minutes | Cook time: 35 minutes | Serves 14

4 eggs
3.25 ounces (92 g) cream cheese, soft
4 tablespoons butter, soft
1¼ cup almond flour
¾ cup Splenda
1 teaspoon baking powder
1 teaspoon of vanilla
¼ teaspoon salt
Butter flavored cooking spray

1. Heat oven to 350ºF (180ºC). Spray a loaf pan with cooking spray.
2. In a medium bowl, combine flour, baking powder, and salt.
3. In a large bowl, beat butter and Splenda until light and fluffy. And cream cheese and vanilla and beat well.
4. Add the eggs, one at a time, beating after each one. Stir in the dry until thoroughly combined.
5. Pour into prepared pan and bake for 30 to 40 minutes or cake passes the toothpick test. Let cool 10 minutes in the pan, then invert onto serving plate. Slice and serve.

Per Serving
calories: 203 | fat: 13.0g | protein: 5.0g
carbs: 15.1g | fiber: 1.0g | sugar: 13.1g
sodium: 84mg

Blueberry No Bake Cheesecake

Prep time: 5 minutes | Cook time: 0 minutes | Serves 8

1 pound (454 g) fat free cream cheese, softened
1 cup sugar free frozen whipped topping, thawed
¾ cup blueberries
1 tablespoon

margarine, melted
8 zwieback toasts
1 cup boiling water
⅓ cup Splenda
1 envelope unflavored gelatin
1 teaspoon vanilla

1. Place the toasts and margarine in a food processor. Pulse until mixture resembles coarse crumbs. Press on the bottom of a springform pan.
2. Place gelatin in a medium bowl and add boiling water. Stir until gelatin dissolved completely.
3. In a large bowl, beat cream cheese, Splenda, and vanilla on medium speed until well blended. Beat in whipped topping. Add gelatin, in a steady stream, while beating on low speed. Increase speed to medium and beat 4 minutes or until smooth and creamy.
4. Gently fold in berries and spread over crust. Cover and chill 3 hours or until set.

Per Serving
calories: 315 | fat: 23.0g | protein: 6.0g
carbs: 20.1g | fiber: 0g | sugar: 10.1g
sodium: 417mg

Gingerbread Soufflés

Prep time: 15 minutes | Cook time: 25 minutes | Serves 10

6 eggs, separated
1 cup skim milk
1 cup fat free whipped topping
2 tablespoons butter, soft
½ cup Splenda
⅓ cup molasses
¼ cup flour

2 teaspoons pumpkin pie spice
2 teaspoons vanilla
1 teaspoon ginger
¼ teaspoon salt
⅛ teaspoon cream of tartar
Butter flavored cooking spray

1. Heat oven to 350ºF (180ºC). Spray 10 ramekins with cooking spray and sprinkle with Splenda to coat, shaking out excess. Place on a large baking sheet.

2. In a large saucepan, over medium heat, whisk together milk, Splenda, flour and salt until smooth. Bring to a boil, whisking constantly. Pour into a large bowl and whisk in molasses, butter, vanilla, and spices. Let cool 15 minutes.
3. Once spiced mixture has cooled, whisk in egg yolks.
4. In a large bowl, beat egg whites and cream of tartar on high speed until stiff peaks form. Fold into spiced mixture, a third at a time, until blended completely. Spoon into ramekins.
5. Bake for 25 minutes until puffed and set. Serve immediately with a dollop of whipped topping.

Per Serving
calories: 171 | fat: 5.0g | protein: 4.0g
carbs: 24.1g | fiber: 0g | sugar: 18.1g
sodium: 289mg

Mini Bread Puddings

Prep time: 5 minutes | Cook time: 35 minutes | Serves 12

6 slices cinnamon bread, cut into cubes
1¼ cup skim milk
½ cup egg substitute
1 tablespoon

margarine, melted
⅓ cup Splenda
1 teaspoon vanilla
⅛ teaspoon salt
⅛ teaspoon nutmeg

1. Heat oven to 350ºF (180ºC). Line 12 medium-size muffin cups with paper baking cups.
2. In a large bowl, stir together milk, egg substitute, Splenda, vanilla, salt and nutmeg until combined. Add bread cubes and stir until moistened. Let rest 15 minutes.
3. Spoon evenly into prepared baking cups. Drizzle margarine evenly over the tops. Bake for 30 to 35 minutes or until puffed and golden brown. Remove from oven and let cool completely.

Per Serving
calories: 106 | fat: 2.0g | protein: 4.0g
carbs: 16.1g | fiber: 1.0g | sugar: 9.1g
sodium: 118mg

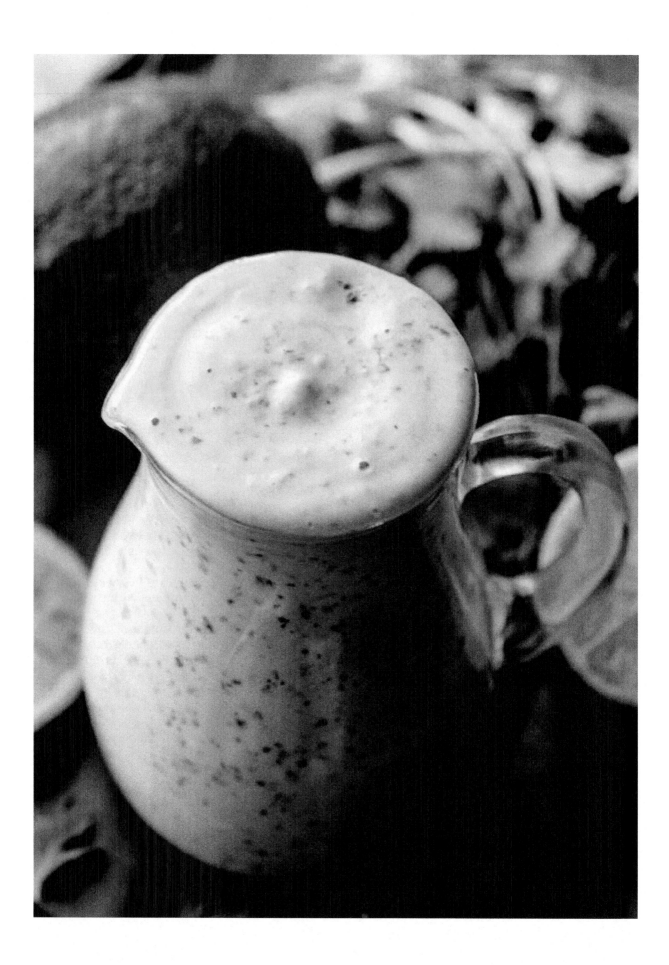

Chapter 15: Sauces, Dips, and Dressing

Creole Seasoning

Prep time: 10 minutes | Cook time: 40 minutes | Makes ¾ cup

2 tablespoons garlic powder
2 tablespoons dried basil
1 tablespoon sweet paprika
1 tablespoon smoked paprika
1 tablespoon freshly ground black pepper

1 tablespoon onion powder
1 tablespoon cayenne pepper
1 tablespoon dried thyme
1 tablespoon dried oregano
1 teaspoon ground red sweet pepper

1. In an airtight container, combine the garlic powder, basil, sweet paprika, smoked paprika, black pepper, onion powder, cayenne, thyme, oregano, and sweet pepper.

Per Serving
calories: 15 | fat: 0g | protein: 1.1g
carbs: 2.9g | fiber: 1.1g | sugar: 1.0g
sodium: 4mg

Avocado Cilantro Dressing

Prep time: 5 minutes | Cook time: 0 minutes | Makes 1 cup

1 large avocado, peeled and pitted
½ cup plain Greek yogurt
¾ cup fresh cilantro
1 tablespoon water

2 teaspoons freshly squeezed lime juice
⅛ teaspoon garlic powder
Pinch salt

1. Process the avocado, yogurt, cilantro, water, lime juice, garlic powder, and salt in a blender until creamy and emulsified.
2. Chill for at least 30 minutes in the refrigerator to let the flavors blend.

Per Serving (¼ Cup)
calories: 92 | fat: 6.8g | protein: 4.1g
carbs: 4.9g | fiber: 2.3g | sugar: 1.0g
sodium: 52mg

Spicy Asian Dipping Sauce

Prep time: 5 minutes | Cook time: 0 minutes | Makes ½ cup

⅓ cup low-fat mayonnaise
1 to 2 teaspoons hot sauce, to your liking

2 teaspoons rice vinegar
1 teaspoon sesame oil

1. Stir together the mayo, hot sauce, rice vinegar, and oil in a small bowl until thoroughly smooth.
2. Chill for at least 30 minutes to blend the flavors.

Per Serving (2 Tablespoons)
calories: 54 | fat: 4.7g | protein: 0g
carbs: 1.7g | fiber: 0g | sugar: 1.0g
sodium: 190mg

BBQ Sauce

Prep time: 5 minutes | Cook time: 15 minutes | Makes 3 cups

1¼ cup tomato purée
1½ cup white vinegar
1 tablespoon yellow mustard
1 teaspoon mustard seeds
1 teaspoon ground turmeric
1 teaspoon sweet paprika

1 teaspoon garlic powder
1 teaspoon celery seeds
½ teaspoon cayenne pepper
½ teaspoon onion powder
½ teaspoon freshly ground black pepper

1. In a medium pot, combine the tomato purée, vinegar, mustard, mustard seeds, turmeric, paprika, garlic powder, celery seeds, cayenne, onion powder, and black pepper. Simmer over low heat for 15 minutes, or until the flavors come together.
2. Remove the sauce from the heat, and let cool for 5 minutes. Transfer to a blender, and purée until smooth.

Per Serving
calories: 10 | fat: 0g | protein: 0.3g
carbs: 1.5g | fiber: 0.3g | sugar: 1.0g
sodium: 14mg

Chicken Gravy

Prep time: 5 minutes | Cook time: 15 minutes | Makes 1½ cup

2 cups low-sodium chicken broth, divided
4 tablespoons whole-wheat flour, divided
1 medium yellow onion, chopped
½ bunch fresh thyme, roughly chopped
2 garlic cloves, minced
1 bay leaf
½ teaspoon celery seeds
Freshly ground black pepper, to taste
1 teaspoon Worcestershire sauce

1. In a shallow stockpot, combine ½ cup of broth and 1 tablespoon of whole-wheat flour and cook over medium-low heat, whisking until the flour is dissolved. Continue to add about ½ cup of broth and the remaining 3 tablespoons of flour in increments for about 2 minutes, or until a thick sauce is formed.
2. Add the onion, thyme, garlic, bay leaf, and ½ cup of broth, stirring well.
3. Add the celery seeds, pepper, Worcestershire sauce, and remaining ½ cup of broth. Stir and cook for 2 to 3 minutes, or until the gravy is thickened. Discard the bay leaf.
4. Serve spooned over Baked Chicken Stuffed with Collard Greens or your protein of choice.

Per Serving
calories: 17 | fat: 0g | protein: 1.1g
carbs: 3.0g | fiber: 0g | sugar: 1.0g
sodium: 17mg

Ranch Dressing

Prep time: 10 minutes | Cook time: 0 minutes | Serves 8 to 10

8 ounces (227 g) fat-free plain Greek yogurt
¼ cup low-fat buttermilk
1 tablespoon garlic powder
1 tablespoon dried dill
1 tablespoon dried chives
1 tablespoon onion powder
1 tablespoon dried parsley
Pinch freshly ground black pepper

1. In a shallow, medium bowl, combine the Greek yogurt and buttermilk.
2. Stir in the garlic powder, dill, chives, onion powder, parsley, and pepper and mix well.
3. Serve with animal protein or vegetable of your choice, or place in an airtight container.

Per Serving
calories: 30 | fat: 0g | protein: 3.0g
carbs: 3.0g | fiber: 0g | sugar: 2.0g
sodium: 24mg

Creamy Lemon Sauce

Prep time: 5 minutes | Cook time: 3 to 5 minutes | Makes 2 cups

1 cup half-and-half
1 tablespoon unsalted butter
2 tablespoons Parmesan cheese, shredded
1 teaspoon freshly squeezed lemon juice
¼ teaspoon garlic powder

1. Add all ingredients to a saucepan and cook over medium-low heat for about 3 to 5 minutes, stirring frequently, or until the sauce is heated through.
2. Remove from the heat to a bowl. Let it cool for a few minutes before serving.

Per Serving
calories: 55 | fat: 5.2g | protein: 3g
carbs: 1g | fiber: 0g | sugar: 0g
sodium: 40mg

Lemony Dill and Yogurt Dressing

Prep time: 5 minutes | Cook time: 0 minutes | Makes ²/₃ cup

2 tablespoons mayonnaise
1 teaspoon freshly squeezed lemon juice
1 teaspoon fresh dill, chopped
½ cup plain Greek yogurt
¼ teaspoon garlic powder
¼ teaspoon salt

1. Combine all the ingredients in a bowl. Stir to mix well.

Per Serving
calories: 36 | fat: 1.0g | protein: 3.2g
carbs: 3.1g | fiber: 0g | sugars: 1.9g
sodium: 176mg

Greek or Italian Vinaigrette

Prep time: 5 minutes | Cook time: 0 minutes | Serves 4

Greek:

¼ cup extra virgin olive oil

3 garlic cloves, minced

1 tablespoon freshly squeezed lemon juice

1 tablespoon red wine vinegar

1 teaspoon dried marjoram

1 teaspoon dried oregano

½ teaspoon lemon zest

¼ teaspoon sea salt

Italian:

¼ cup extra-virgin olive oil

2 tablespoons red wine vinegar

1 teaspoon Dijon mustard

2 teaspoons Italian seasoning

1 garlic clove, finely minced

1 tablespoon minced shallot

¼ teaspoon sea salt

⅛ teaspoon freshly ground black pepper

1. Stir together all ingredients in a medium bowl until completely mixed and emulsified.

Per Serving
calories: 129 | fat: 14.3g | protein: 0g
carbs: 1.1g | fiber: 0.8g | sugar: 0.2g
sodium: 76mg

Quick Peanut Sauce

Prep time: 5 minutes | Cook time: 0 minutes | Serves 4

¼ cup peanut butter

Juice of 1 lime

1 tablespoon honey

1 minced garlic clove

1 tablespoon reduced-

sodium soy sauce

1 tablespoon peeled fresh ginger, grated

Pinch red pepper flakes

1. Put all ingredients in a medium bowl and whisk until well blended.

Per Serving
calories: 120 | fat: 8.3g | protein: 4.2g
carbs: 9.2g | fiber: 1.1g | sugar: 7.3
sodium: 138mg

Fresh Cucumber Dip

Prep time: 10 minutes | Cook time: 0 minutes | Makes 1½ cups

1 medium cucumber, peeled and grated

¼ teaspoon salt

1 cup plain Greek yogurt

2 garlic cloves, minced

1 tablespoon freshly squeezed lemon juice

1 tablespoon extra-virgin olive oil

¼ teaspoon freshly ground black pepper

1. Put the cucumber in a colander, then sprinkle with salt. Set aside.
2. Combine the remaining ingredients in a bowl. Stir to mix well.
3. Wrap the cucumber in a muslin cloth and squeeze the liquid out as much as possible.
4. Put the cucumber in the bowl of mixture, then stir to mix well.
5. Wrap the bowl in plastic and refrigerate to marinate for 2 hours.

Per Serving
calories: 50 | fat: 3.0g | protein: 4.0g
carbs: 3.0g | fiber: 0g | sugars: 2.0g
sodium: 102mg

Lemon Tahini Dressing with Honey

Prep time: 5 minutes | Cook time: 0 minutes | Makes 1 cup

½ cup water

¾ cup unsalted tahini

⅓ cup freshly

squeezed lemon juice

3 tablespoons honey

½ teaspoon salt

1. Mix together the water, tahini, lemon juice, honey, and salt in a medium bowl, and stir vigorously until well incorporated.
2. Store the leftover dressing in an airtight container in the fridge for up to 2 weeks and shake before using.

Per Serving (2 Tablespoons)
calories: 168 | fat: 13.1g | protein: 4.7g
carbs: 10.3g | fiber: 2.8g | sugar: 8.0g
sodium: 148mg

Conclusion

I hope you have enjoyed these recipes as much as I have. Life with diabetes should not be hard. It is not the end—it is the beginning. With healthy dietary management, you can lead a life free from the negative effects of high (or low) blood sugar levels.

With the knowledge I have shared, you now know why you may have become diabetic, you know what this means, and now, you also know how to manage it. You are armed with resources, apps, and recipes to help you along this lifelong journey. Food is not your enemy; it's your friend.

Cook your way to health and vitality with these recipes and tips. Good things are made to share, so please help a friend find out about this way of life. Call them over for a meal, talk about diabetes, and let's help create awareness as we feast on every delectable spoonful of diabetic cooking made easy.

Resources

Centers for Disease Control and Prevention

https://www.cdc.gov/diabetes/basics/type2.html

National Agricultural Library

https://www.nal.usda.gov/fnic/macronutrients

[1] Greger, M., Stone, G. How not to die. (2015) Flatiron Books.

Appendix 1: 21-Day Meal Plan

	Breakfast	Lunch	Dinner	Snack
1	Easy and Creamy Grits	Macaroni and Vegetable Pie	Pita Stuffed with Tabbouleh	Cauliflower Mash
2	Spinach and Cheese Breakfast Tacos	Crab Cakes with Salsa	Linguine with Kale Pesto	Parmesan Crisps
3	Farro with Walnuts and Berries	Triple Bean Chili	Crock Pot Stroganoff	Easy Low-Carb Biscuits
4	Fresh Huevos Rancheros	Lemon Wax Beans	BBQ Pork Tacos	Tomato Waffles
5	Breakfast Grain Porridge	Leek and Cauliflower Soup	Chickpea Tortillas	Asian Chicken Wings
6	Egg Salad Sandwiches	Cilantro Lime Shrimp	Cheesy Chicken Tortilla Soup	Simple Deviled Eggs
7	Portobello and Chicken Sausage Frittata	Grilled Tofu and Veggie Skewers	Blueberry Wild Rice	Peanut Butter and Chocolate Bites
8	Cranberry Grits	Fried Rice with Snap Peas	Turkey Taco	Kale Chips
9	Super Grain Porridge	Citrus Chicken	Baby Spinach Mini Quiches	Candied Pecans
10	Easy Turkey Breakfast Patties	Spicy Beef and Vegetable Soup	Enchilada Black Bean Casserole	Buffalo Bites
11	Ratatouille Egg Bake	Barley Kale and Squash Risotto	Mushroom Rice with Hazelnut	Cheesy Broccoli Bites

12	Scrumptious Orange Muffins	Autumn Pork Chops	Easy Coconut Quinoa	Almond Coconut Biscotti
13	Easy Turkey Breakfast Patties	Quinoa and Lush Vegetable Bowl	Beer Braised Brisket	Cranberry and Almond Granola Bars
14	Breakfast Cheddar Zucchini Casserole	Tempeh Lettuce Wraps	Classic Texas Caviar	Apple Pita Pockets
15	Blueberry and Banana Breakfast Cookies	Zucchini Carbonara	Couscous with Balsamic Dressing	Cinnamon Apple Popcorn
16	Crispy Pita with Canadian Bacon	Crispy Cowboy Black Bean Fritters	Korean Chicken	Cheese Crisp Crackers
17	Farro with Walnuts and Berries	Creamy and Aromatic Chicken	Navy Bean Pico de Gallo	Banana and Carrot Flax Muffins
18	Goat Cheese and Avocado Toast	Tomato and Navy Bean Bake	Shrimp Cocktail	Italian Flavor Salmon and Potato Patties
19	Banana and Zucchini Bread	Red Kidney Beans with Green Beans	Ritzy Jerked Chicken Breasts	Hot Chicken Stuffed Celery Stalks
20	Shrimp with Scallion Grits	Cherry-Glazed Lamb Chops	Farro and Avocado Bowl	Peanut Butter and Chocolate Bites
21	Mushroom Frittata	Black-Eyed Peas Curry	Beef Stroganoff	Aromatic Toasted Pumpkin Seeds

Appendix 2: Measurement Conversion Chart

VOLUME EQUIVALENTS(DRY)

US STANDARD	METRIC (APPROXIMATE)
1/8 teaspoon	0.5 mL
1/4 teaspoon	1 mL
1/2 teaspoon	2 mL
3/4 teaspoon	4 mL
1 teaspoon	5 mL
1 tablespoon	15 mL
1/4 cup	59 mL
1/2 cup	118 mL
3/4 cup	177 mL
1 cup	235 mL
2 cups	475 mL
3 cups	700 mL
4 cups	1 L

VOLUME EQUIVALENTS(LIQUID)

US STANDARD	US STANDARD (OUNCES)	METRIC (APPROXIMATE)
2 tablespoons	1 fl.oz.	30 mL
1/4 cup	2 fl.oz.	60 mL
1/2 cup	4 fl.oz.	120 mL
1 cup	8 fl.oz.	240 mL
1 1/2 cup	12 fl.oz.	355 mL
2 cups or 1 pint	16 fl.oz.	475 mL
4 cups or 1 quart	32 fl.oz.	1 L
1 gallon	128 fl.oz.	4 L

TEMPERATURES EQUIVALENTS

FAHRENHEIT(F)	CELSIUS(C) (APPROXIMATE)
225 °F	107 °C
250 °F	120 °C
275 °F	135 °C
300 °F	150 °C
325 °F	160 °C
350 °F	180 °C
375 °F	190 °C
400 °F	205 °C
425 °F	220 °C
450 °F	235 °C
475 °F	245 °C
500 °F	260 °C

WEIGHT EQUIVALENTS

US STANDARD	METRIC (APPROXIMATE)
1 ounce	28 g
2 ounces	57 g
5 ounces	142 g
10 ounces	284 g
15 ounces	425 g
16 ounces (1 pound)	455 g
1.5 pounds	680 g
2 pounds	907 g

Appendix 3: The Dirty Dozen and Clean Fifteen

The Environmental Working Group (EWG) is a nonprofit, nonpartisan organization dedicated to protecting human health and the environment Its mission is to empower people to live healthier lives in a healthier environment. This organization publishes an annual list of the twelve kinds of produce, in sequence, that have the highest amount of pesticide residue-the Dirty Dozen-as well as a list of the fifteen kinds ofproduce that have the least amount of pesticide residue-the Clean Fifteen.

THE DIRTY DOZEN

- The 2016 Dirty Dozen includes the following produce. These are considered among the year's most important produce to buy organic:

Strawberries	Spinach
Apples	Tomatoes
Nectarines	Bell peppers
Peaches	Cherry tomatoes
Celery	Cucumbers
Grapes	Kale/collard greens
Cherries	Hot peppers

- *The Dirty Dozen list contains two additional itemskale/collard greens and hot peppers-because they tend to contain trace levels of highly hazardous pesticides.*

THE CLEAN FIFTEEN

- The least critical to buy organically are the Clean Fifteen list. The following are on the 2016 list:

Avocados	Papayas
Corn	Kiw
Pineapples	Eggplant
Cabbage	Honeydew
Sweet peas	Grapefruit
Onions	Cantaloupe
Asparagus	Cauliflower
Mangos	

- *Some of the sweet corn sold in the United States are made from genetically engineered (GE) seedstock. Buy organic varieties of these crops to avoid GE produce.*

Appendix 4: Recipe Index

Printed in Great Britain
by Amazon

83681929R10113